Psychosocial perspectives on the management of voice disorders

Psychosocial perspectives on the management of voice disorders

Implications for Patients and Clients
Options and Strategies for Clinicians

Janet Baker, L.A.C.S.T., M.Sc., Ph.D.

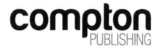
compton
PUBLISHING

This edition first published 2017 © 2017 by Compton Publishing Ltd.

Registered office: Compton Publishing Ltd, 30 St. Giles', Oxford, OX1 3LE, UK

Registered company number: 07831037

Editorial offices: 35 East Street, Braunton, EX33 2EA, UK

Web: www.comptonpublishing.co.uk

ISBN 978-1-909082-04-5

A catalogue record for this book is available from the British Library.

Cover image: **The Green Queen of the Night – Magic Flute, Arthur Boyd (1990)**

Arthur Boyd's work reproduced with kind permission of the Bundanon Trust.

Image from *Arthur Boyd: Art and Life by Janet McKenzie (2000), Thames & Hudson, London*

With further acknowledgement to Margaret and Christopher Burrell

Cover design: David Siddall, http://www.davidsiddall.com

Set in 11pt Adobe Caslon Pro by Regent Typesetting

1   2017

Contents

Part I : Evidence for psychosocial factors contributing to theoretical and causal models for voice disorders

Part II : Addressing psychosocial factors throughout the therapeutic process

Dedication

To Douglas and Jeremy Baker
who have both always been there to hold me

To Professor Arnold Aronson
whose clinical acumen, humanity and academic scholarship have been my inspiration

To Professor David Ben-Tovim
who took me on and gently steered me into believing that clinicians can be scientists too

To Professor Richard Lane
who collaborated so generously with me to take my perspectives on voice and emotion to new levels

To my patients, students and colleagues
with whom it has been such a privilege to work and for whom the door is always open

Acknowledgements

I would like to acknowledge the following people who have all offered me such strong practical, intellectual and emotional nurturing throughout his process.

Johanna Flavell who as read all the chapters as each unfolds and offered diplomatic, helpful, humorous and insightful feedback throughout

Christina Shewell who has read so many of the chapters, offered sensitive feedback that always takes me to another place, and has so generously shared aspects of her work that have been represented in Chapter 12.

Annie Elias, Peter Butcher and Sara Harris for their most stimulating conversations over the years and their unswerving support for this book.

Jenni Oates who has been such a generous mentor to me throughout my career, always asking the searching questions and encouraging me to go further.

Mark Hallett, Jon Stone and Allan Carson whose work and conversations have added immeasurably to my perspectives on functional neurologic disorders including functional voice disorders.

Elaine Butler, David Ben-Tovim, Jane Bickford, Matthew Broadhurst, Peter Butcher, Jean Callaghan, Maria Dietrich, Deborah Hersh, Alison Hodge, Leah Helou, Kate King, Alison Laycock, Linda Matthews, Sharon Moore, Jane Mott, Catherine Sanders, Helen Sjardin and Helen Tiller who have supported me during this process.

Margaret Bowden, Editorial Assistant, who was originally by my side in the preparations of my thesis, and with every other publication since that time including this one. Always so encouraging, meticulous and so much fun.

Trudyanne Brown and Horst Kloss of *BMGART Gallery* in South Australia who have been so extremely generous in contacting artists on my behalf and supporting my book.

Julian Cress, on behalf of the *Fred Cress Estate*, who has kindly given me permission to use the stunning art work of his father Fred Cress who also showed a real interest in my work, especially in relation to the construct of Conflict Over Speaking Out

Håkan Pårup, Editor of Informa Healthcare, publishers for *The International Journal of Speech-Language Pathology (IJSLP)*, who has kindly given me most generous permission to draw upon and re-use parts of articles already published in the IJSLP

To the Department of Speech Pathology and Audiology, and to the staff of the Medical Library at Flinders University and IT Help Desk for their unfailing willingness to assist with finding documents, helping me in practical matters related to Endnote.

To my family and friends – many of whom are mentioned here, but others too, who have waited so patiently – thank you for your understanding.

Noel McPherson who has believed in me from the outset, I thank you.

Foreword

Psychological factors arise in some way and at some time for virtually everyone who experiences a voice disorder, whether as predisposing, causal, exacerbating, or perpetuating influences or as a component of the impact of the voice problem on the individual's activity and participation in everyday life. Those psychological factors may range from slight to far more severe degrees of emotional distress. In order to provide effective care for people with voice disorders, speech-language pathologists and other health professionals who work with such patients therefore require a working knowledge of relevant theory that helps them to explain how and why psychological factors arise. These health professionals also require the knowledge and skills that will assist them to provide effective assessment and management of those psychological factors.

While much has been written and researched about the psychological factors associated with voice disorders from the time of Freud in the early 1900s to the present day, there are very few comprehensive and scholarly expositions devoted to the psychological aspects of voice disorders available to speech-language pathologists and other health professionals. Key figures in the voice literature including Arnold Aronson and Diane Bless, Peter Butcher, Annie Elias and Lesley Cavalli, Linda Rammage, Murray Morrison, and Hamish Nichol, Deborah Rosen and Robert Sataloff have made invaluable contributions through their writing, yet clinicians and scientists remain frustrated at the lack of a contemporary seminal text that provides theoretically driven and evidence-based frameworks for both clinical practice and research. Dr Janet Baker's new book, *Psychosocial Perspectives on the Management of Voice Disorders*, fills this void extremely well and will be a constant source of guidance and inspiration to health professionals and scientists for many years to come.

I had to smile when Janet invited me to write this Foreword. She intimated that she had asked me because I had been an important mentor to her, but the truth is very much the reverse! Having had the privilege of knowing her personally for more than 20 years, reading her many scholarly journal papers, listening to her many conference presentations and workshops, spending enlightening hours with her in in-depth discussion of theoretical and clinical conundrums, and occasionally collaborating with her on research projects, I am not at all surprised that she has produced this extraordinary book. Clinicians and researchers alike should be eternally grateful that she has devoted so much of her life to deep and systematic thought, rigorous research and scholarship, her own professional development and training, and careful documentation of countless clinical cases. *Psychosocial Perspectives on the Management of Voice Disorders* is the culmination of one key aspect of Janet's life work. It will be particularly valuable for qualified and experienced clinicians, academics and researchers in the field of speech-language pathology, but also for those in psychology, psychiatry, laryngology, neurology, social work, family therapy and vocal pedagogy. Student speech-language pathologists and students across these diverse disciplines will also gain from reading Janet's book, albeit with guidance from their teachers to ensure that the more complex theoretical sections are interpreted as intended.

Psychosocial Perspectives on the Management of Voice Disorders provides readers with comprehensive foundation chapters on terminology, a diagnostic classification incorporating functional voice disorders (psychogenic voice disorder and muscle tension voice disorder) and organic voice disorders, and a succinct summary of what is known about the prevalence and demographic/biographic features of people with these disorders. The foundation chapters also introduce the reader to relevant psychosocial and psychobiological models of health and wellbeing, several key theoretical frameworks and associated explanatory propositions for functional voice disorders, and the research evidence underpinning those frameworks and propositions. Models, frameworks and explanatory proposals are explicitly linked and integrated rather than merely listed as a linear catalogue of separate perspectives. Later chapters turn to applications of theory and research evidence to clinical practice, always connected back to underlying theory and aetiological propositions. The more applied chapters address definitions, levels and stages of counselling, the scope of practice of speech-language pathologists in psychosocial interviewing and counselling, and applications of systems theory and family therapy to voice practice. The final chapter guides clinicians working with patients whose voice problems are associated with the most complex emotional and psychosocial issues.

There are many unique aspects to Janet Baker's seminal text, several of which I have already alluded to earlier in this Foreword. This book challenges readers to think for themselves, to critically evaluate theory and research evidence, to continually advance their own knowledge and understanding, and to seek mentoring and supervision from experts. It is certainly not a recipe book, but the guidance and insights it provides are the ingredients required to create the master clinicians, teachers and researchers of the future. It does not emphasise one particular framework, explanatory theory or approach to working with people with voice difficulties, but presents readers with a breadth and depth of relevant material on which to build their clinical practice and research. It draws on evidence, theory and practice knowledge from a range of disciplines and perspectives, more effectively than we see in most texts in the voice field. Although much of the book focusses on functional voice disorders, Janet is careful to discuss the relevance of psychosocial mechanisms and interventions to patients with organic voice disorders; very few books make these important links so convincingly.

Janet's book does not shy away from unresolved theoretical or clinical issues, but takes the reader calmly and logically through several possible approaches to dealing with difficult dilemmas. A holistic and patient-centred approach is taken throughout and rich and highly informative cases examples are discussed. Janet's expertise as an accomplished speech-language pathologist and family therapist shines through the entire book, as does her fundamental regard for her patients, her clinical and research colleagues, and the many prominent researchers whose work she draws upon. Janet shares so much of herself through her writing too; her eloquence, her sense of humour and irony, the occasional foible, her uncanny ability to link the world of art, history and literature to science and practice, and her determination to tackle difficult issues head-on with both scientific rigour and humanity. Dr Baker's achievement in writing this book deserves the admiration and gratitude of all of us who work in the fascinating field of voice.

Jennifer Oates, Ph.D.
Associate Professor, Discipline of Speech Pathology, School of Allied Health,
La Trobe University and Principal, Melbourne Voice Analysis Centre,
Melbourne, Australia

Foreword

During our professional and personal life we may experience a few defining moments that resonate with us and help shape our own journey of discovery. In this book the author, Jan Baker, describes a few such transformational moments. For me, one such enriching experience occurred 30 years ago when I had the good fortune of observing Jan Baker demonstrating her approach to helping a patient with voice loss to find their voice. With expertise, compassion and thoughtful awareness of the complex emotions that may be blocking the voice, Jan worked with great sensitivity to enable the patient to 'peel back the layers' of the block and to gently begin releasing the body, the emotions and the voice. Jan applied no pressure, there was no great ego in the room, she was not seeking a bells and whistles triumphant return of voice, instead she worked with intuition, skill and wisdom. What resonated with me all those years ago was Jan Baker's acknowledgement to the patient that she understood that the voice disturbance was more than a physical manifestation of a disorder of voice, that there were internal pressures and emotions that ran much deeper. Although few words were spoken, the patient felt listened to and responded by lowering their defences and allowed hope and voice to emerge.

At that time the landscape of voice and voice disorders was very different to the picture that we are looking at today. With the development of videostrobolaryngoscopy and specialist voice clinics there was a welcome focus on refining the laryngeal assessment and diagnoses of voice disorders. This led to a more systematic examination and development of the evidence base for physical voice therapy techniques. Less attention however was afforded to considering the psychological and emotional aspects of the voice. With a few exceptions, and most notably the early work of Professor Arnold Aronson, there were few studies that explored the patients with functional voice disorders and examined underlying psychological drivers. Indeed in the United Kingdom in the 1980's one trod tentatively and with some nervousness when suggesting that a voice disorder might have its roots in a psychological basis.

This book defines how much the landscape has changed. Jan Baker sets out an impressive literature base surrounding psychosocial influences on voice disorders including her own robust research and case studies. It is encyclopaedic in the breadth of work and evidence that it covers, including an exploration of the wider psychological research in relation to health. Against this backdrop of evidence that clearly articulates the causal link between psychosocial influences and voice disorders, Jan Baker then takes the reader through an illuminating exploration of the counselling process, systems theory and family therapy and the application of these to the psychosocial interview process and finally the integration of counselling and voice therapy.

This is a serious and scholarly book written with the rare perspective and combined qualities of an expert clinician and scientific researcher. Furthermore Jan Baker is dually qualified as a speech and language pathologist and a family therapist. As an informed scientist Jan Baker presents the evidence with respect for the work of others, with curiosity and with challenges to the reader to think more deeply. Her own versatile thinking and insights and her ability to eloquently translate complex ideas into memorable and accessible information for the reader is enhanced by her humanity, humour, examples from her deep wealth of clinical experience, and the stunning artwork that punctuates the text.

At the heart of this book the author never loses sight of the person with the voice disorder. It is clear that Jan Baker thinks deeply about the patient's dilemmas and struggles, about the therapeutic process and about an evidence based approach to thinking about and treating patients whose voice disorder is inextricably linked to complex psychological factors. In sharing all of this she reveals her talents as an extraordinary therapist and teacher.

This book represents a major contribution to the field of voice. It is special in its devotion to broadening our understanding of psychogenic voice disorders and the psychological skills and approaches required in their therapeutic management. Jan Baker has succeeded in giving us a rich and inspiring text that no student of voice, whether studying, researching or practising voice clinician should be without.

Annie Elias FRCSLT
Consultant Speech and Language Therapist in Voice
Understanding and treating Psychogenic Voice Disorder: A CBT Framework by Peter
Peter Butcher, Annie Elias and Lesley Cavalli

Preface

The earliest foundations of this book are probably deeply rooted in a vibrant family life, where as one of five children there was always such a lot going on. As a middle child I grew up with a fascination for all things medical, psychological and musical, and a school life that fostered an appreciation of literature, public speaking, acting and singing along with the traditional subjects that seemed less memorable. With a G for mathematics, medicine was out of the question, and with a father who didn't want any second daughter of his cleaning toilets in between theatrical or singing engagements, auditioning for the National Institute of Dramatic Art or Conservatorium was a closed door too. This was not meant to be unkind – it was all about getting a proper job. I was far too rebellious to do nursing and play second fiddle to doctors, and speech pathology was the new career on the horizon if one didn't want to do physiotherapy. I envisaged that speech pathology might be a way to foster my interests in medicine and psychology, in voice, language and words, and above all in working closely with people in some capacity or other.

The absolute highlight of every week in our speech therapy training was the Tuesday afternoon sessions devoted to observations through a one-way mirror. Here we watched a master clinician assessing young children and interviewing their parents. In a tantalizing way the therapist would release snippets of assessments from the specialties of medicine, surgery, neurology, otolaryngology, clinical psychology or psychiatry, physiotherapy, and occupational therapy, and invite us to share our observations. We were then required to generate hypotheses and argue for a differential diagnosis, linking the evidence from our observations with our fledgling knowledge. The key was finding a way to integrate what we saw and what we heard, but also to share what we might have sensed more intuitively. We then had to formulate this into some coherent kind of diagnostic explanation that would be useful and helpful to the child and their concerned parents.

Part of the excitement of these sessions was the challenge of 'not knowing'. Another was the permission to consider things from different perspectives, and the knowledge that if our suppositions or final conclusions were wrong there was no shame. Ironically all these years later, approaches just like these have now become the basis of the *problem based learning* approaches that underpin the many of the programs in medicine and speech pathology around the world, including our own programs in the Schools of Medicine and Health Sciences at Flinders University.

In my work with adults, adolescents and children across the full range of voice disorders, those early foundations were a good start. However, as I gained experience, it became increasingly obvious that psychosocial factors contributed to the patterns of onset and clinical presentations of some vocal problems more than others, and that the psychosocial impacts of any voice disorder on a person and their family could be profound.

In order to be more effective in dealing with these complex issues I sought further education and training in counselling, psychotherapy and family therapy. This helped me to think much more respectfully about the individual in the context of his or her family, community, work environment or culture, and to appreciate why some people may be more vulnerable to developing vocal disorders at a particular time in their lives. It has also deepened my interest in the therapeutic processes involved in helping others to change and to understand why some people change, while others find it much more difficult. This advanced training in counselling and psychotherapy also led to serious reflections about the role of the therapeutic relationship and the personal qualities of effective therapists, even those of master clinicians during this whole process. These deliberations also carried into my academic and clinical teaching of students at undergraduate and postgraduate levels, and now into my supervision of experienced colleagues.

The book is structured in two parts. Part 1 incorporates Chapters 1–8. These chapters seek to clarify what is meant by the term *psychosocial,* and how research into the effects of acute and chronic stress in association with a range of other psychosocial factors may affect the physical and mental health of individuals. The empirical evidence for a number of psychosocial factors that have been explored in relation to voice disorders is then discussed. Chapter 8 represents the culmination of Part I by presenting several theoretical models that have been developed to explain how psychosocial factors may interact and operate as risk factors for the development of functional voice disorders, that also comprise the psychogenic voice disorder, and muscle tension voice disorder sub-groups.

Part II includes Chapters 9–12. These chapters are focused on the more practical implications of all that has been discussed in Part I. It addresses issues related to the therapeutic processes that may include different levels of counselling, highlighting a number of principles that underpin family therapy and other models of counselling that can be readily integrated into traditional voice work. Emphasis is given to *incorporating counselling as a way of thinking* that may be helpful throughout the initial consultation and psychosocial interview and then during the action phases of intervention. Reference is made to the importance of the therapeutic relationship, and being alert to restraints to change that indicate the need for seeking a second opinion, inviting collaboration with more experienced therapists, attending supervision or referring on.

The book is intended for all students and particularly for experienced practitioners devoted to the care and management of voice disorders whether they come from speech pathology, otolaryngology, vocal pedagogy, neurology, psychiatry, psychology or family therapy. While the place of counselling across the full range of voice disorders has been discussed, a particular emphasis has been given to more advanced levels of counselling for individuals with psychogenic voice disorders.

Part I

Evidence for psychosocial factors contributing to theoretical and causal models for voice disorders

Terminologies and diagnostic classification of voice disorders

Introduction

In setting out to explore the way in which psychosocial perspectives may influence the management of voice disorders, an important first step is to clarify the meanings of those diagnostic terminologies being used in the current literature, and to highlight the differences in aetiological emphasis of several well-known *diagnostic classification systems*. This has particular significance for the relative weight given to psychosocial factors by speech-language pathologists (SLP) and otolaryngologists, who are the health professionals most commonly involved in the assessment and treatment of individuals with voice disorders. It is also relevant for other doctors, psychologists, family therapists, psychiatrists, neurologists, or medico-legal practitioners who may be involved with their care. Dare we suggest that it might also be of interest and some help to the person with a vocal disorder?

In this chapter, I will briefly outline some of the controversies regarding nomenclature and diagnostic classification, and then discuss the implications of these ongoing dilemmas for overall management. Reference is made to those diagnostic classification systems that highlight possible associations between psychosocial factors, as these may affect the aetiology and patterns of onset for the major groups of voice disorders. The *diagnostic terminologies* for voice disorders to be used in this book are then defined.

Diverse terminologies and different diagnostic classification systems

"What's in a name? That which we call a rose
By any other name would smell as sweet"
Romeo and Juliet Act II, Scene 2, Lines 1–2, William Shakespeare (1597)

When Shakespeare's Romeo made a noble offer to denounce his family name as a mark of his devotion to Juliet, she lovingly reassured him that names are merely superficial conventions. In declaring her love for the man whose family name was «Montague», she reminded him that her allegiance was to Romeo Montague the person, and not to the Montague name and all that would inevitably be associated with his entire family. Such sentiments seemed to be most apt in the setting of this dramatic tragedy, but in the dry and somewhat esoteric context of diagnostic terminology and classification, we too may need to be asking ourselves whether labels given to individual voice disorders and larger families of disorders are merely artificial conventions, or whether they do really matter.

I think that they do matter and would agree with Walsh (2005), who has argued that terminology is more than just a label. In her paper, Walsh challenges the speech pathology profession to recognise and overcome problems of inconsistencies in diagnostic terminologies being perpetuated across all clinical fields. She proposes that terminology refers to the whole problem and includes, even if only by implication, all the current associated nomenclatures, the language used to talk about the problem, the concepts developed about the issue and finally, the diagnostic classification. Walsh urges practitioners to acknowledge that this has significant implications for understanding the essential nature of communication disorders and therefore, how best to intervene.

These notions are directly applicable to the speciality of voice disorders, where experienced clinicians and authors continue to argue for consistency in the use of diagnostic nomenclature, and for classification systems to be founded on reliable empirical evidence, which clearly indicates the primary aetiology of the condition. However, in a recent review of the literature designed to explore the effectiveness and validity of those classification systems most commonly used in the field (Baker *et al.*, 2007) it became evident that there is still a great diversity and confusion amongst terminologies used to refer to voice disorders in general, especially when referring to those classified as 'non-organic' or 'functional' voice disorders. Furthermore, it still remains debatable as to whether the aetiologies within this large heterogeneous group of voice disorders have been reliably established (Baker *et al.*, 2007; Verdolini, Rosen, & Branski, 2006). Some of these diagnostic terms have a strong behavioural emphasis, suggesting that *dysfunctional vocal behaviours* and *laryngeal muscle tension patterns* are causally related. The other terms clearly imply that *disturbed psychological processes* are fundamental to the aetiology (see Table 1.1 and Table 1.2).

Table 1.1 Diagnostic terminologies with a behavioral emphasis

Functional voice and related disorders*
Behavioral emphasis Muscle tension dysphonia Muscle misuse voice disorder Hyperfunctional dysphonia Hypofunctional dysphonia Phonasthenia/Vocal fatigue Ventricular phonation Paradoxical Vocal Fold Dysfunction
Globus pharyngis* Chronic/habitual cough* Hyperventilation syndrome*

*Disorders that might not be construed as disorders of the voice in the strict sense of the word

Table 1.2 Diagnostic terminologies with a psychological emphasis

Functional voice and related disorders*
Psychological emphasis Psychogenic voice disorder Conversion reaction aphonia/dysphonia Hysterical aphonia/dysphonia Medically unexplained voice disorders Mutational falsetto or Puberphonia Phononeurosis/war neurosis of the larynx Iatrogenic
Globus hystericus* Psychogenic cough* Gender dysphoria/transsexualism* Immature speech/childlike voice in adults* Psychogenic and/or Elective Mutism*

*Disorders that might not be construed as disorders of the voice in the strict sense of the word

As we review the range and diversity of terms listed in these tables, some may be more familiar than others, and many may continue to be used indiscriminately, interchangeably and often without clear operational definitions. These choices may be related to professional roles or bias, different clinical settings under which clinicians are operating, or due to cultural traditions. It could also be argued that some of the 'related disorders' in both tables may not seem appropriately placed in the Functional Voice Disorders (FVD) classification because some practitioners may not construe these conditions as disorders of the voice in the strict sense of the term. However, they are included here because they are often listed in well-established diagnostic classification systems within either the 'functional' or 'psychogenic' categories; they often present in association with an aphonia or dysphonia, and serious psychological issues are considered germane to their clinical presentation. These ongoing disparities are tending to perpetuate current controversies over appropriate diagnosis and classification, and to influence the attitudes of clinicians regarding the extent to which attention should be given to emotional and psychological factors in the overall management of voice disorders.

Organic or non-organic voice disorders

One of the ongoing controversies relates to the traditional delineation between 'organic' and 'non-organic' voice disorders often made in speech pathology or otolaryngology textbooks. Here, the terms 'organic' and 'non-organic' are intended to indicate that the neurophysiological state of the larynx or vocal folds is (or is not) the cause of the voice disorder. At first glance, this seems a logical delineation and makes good sense. However, as clinicians from our respective disciplines would acknowledge, organic changes to vocal fold tissue such as vocal nodules, even contact ulcers, polyps or chronic laryngitis can often arise in response to dysfunctional vocal behaviours.

As a consequence, while not denying that the above lesions do constitute organic changes, some practitioners would classify vocal disorders characterised by such organic changes as *behavioural voice disorders* (Mathieson, 2001); some would classify them as *muscle tension disorders* (Rammage, Morrison, & Nichol, 2001), and others would classify them as *psychogenic voice disorders* (Aronson & Bless, 2009). Here, the rationale would be that an individual's motivations to engage in vocally abusive behaviours reflect a degree of psychological vulnerability related to personality traits and coping in the face of life stresses. With all of these possible choices for diagnostic classification, any student of speech pathology or otolaryngology could be forgiven for being uncertain about where to begin.

Controversies over the use of the term 'functional'

Another contentious issue is the use of this term 'functional', which has traditionally been used in medicine, psychiatry and neurology to distinguish between 'organic'- and 'non-organically'-based conditions such as medically unexplained seizures and movement disorders (Hallett *et al.*, 2011), and by otolaryngologists and SLP when differentiating between 'organic' and 'non-organic' voice disorders. The main objection is that the term 'functional' is considered imprecise and ambiguous, and that it fails to denote the essential nature of the problem or its aetiology with sufficient accuracy. It is generally assumed to mean that the problem is due to dysfunction rather than to neurophysiological and structural changes, or that there is a psychological cause. Hallet and his colleagues (2011) also suggest that some clinicians choose to use the term when they consider the problem to be of psychological origin, but would prefer not to confront the patient with such a diagnosis, possibly due to the reaction that this might generate. This is a most valid concern, and one that is particularly relevant for SLP and otolaryngologists.

However, despite several cogent and strong arguments against the use of the term by many highly experienced clinicians and researchers (Aronson & Bless, 2009; Butcher, Elias, & Cavalli, 2007; Mathieson, 2001; Verdolini *et al.*, 2006), it is somewhat surprising to see that the diagnostic term 'functional' has been the most commonly used label referring to 'non-organic' voice disorders throughout our literature during the last 150 years, both across disciplines and countries (Baker, 2002; Baker *et al.*, 2007; Carding, Deary, & Miller, 2013; Roy, 2003). Furthermore, in recent collaborations between neurology and psychiatry, there has been a move to return to the terminology of *'functional movement disorders'* and a range of other *'functional neurologic disorders'* (Carson *et al.*, 2012; Stone, Warlow, & Sharpe, 2010). As Walsh (2005) suggests, 'usefulness' of nomenclature determines whether or not a term persists. Perhaps it is because 'functional' can be interpreted to embrace concepts related to dysregulated vocal behaviours at one end of the spectrum, to disturbed psychological processes at the other end, or even that there may be an interaction between the two, that it remains a reasonable choice, even as a broad first distinction from the *'organic voice disorders'*.

Different emphases in diagnostic classification systems

A number of well-known *diagnostic classification systems* for voice disorders have been developed through the collaborative efforts of many experienced otolaryngologists, SLPs and mental health specialists, with the explicit intention of creating systems based on strong aetiological foundations (Aronson & Bless, 2009; Baker *et al.*, 2007; Butcher *et al.*, 2007; Mathieson, 2001; Morrison & Rammage, 1994; Rammage *et al.*, 2001; Verdolini *et al.*, 2006). Whether or not causality has been confirmed is still questionable, but there does seem to be some consensus over several key issues that need to be taken into account when diagnosing, classifying and planning interventions for all voice disorders. These factors are:

1) The neurophysiological status of the phonatory and respiratory system
2) The vocal behaviours as reflected in laryngeal postures and laryngeal muscle tension patterns observed during laryngoscopic examination
3) The auditory-perceptual and kinaesthetic signs and symptoms that shape the clinical presentation of the particular voice disorder
4) The psychological, emotional and psychosocial issues that are thought to contribute to the pattern of onset and clinical presentation of the voice disorders, those that may serve to aggravate or perpetuate the disorder, or those which may arise as a consequence of the voice problem or in response to intervention.

Although it is reassuring that there is agreement about the relevance of these broad causal factors with all voice disorders, the problem lies in the prominence given to the particular aetiologies, with some being placed in the foreground of the clinical picture and others being placed well into the background. This has inevitable consequences for the way in which clinicians think about the role that psychosocial factors may play, and how this will influence their approaches to both assessment and intervention.

For instance, in the classification system proposed by Aronson and Bless (2009) the term *Psychogenic Voice Disorders* is the preferred term for the 'non-organic' or 'functional' voice disorders. One major sub-group is thought to develop in response to *Emotional Stress with Associated Muscle Tension Patterns*. This group includes disorders without secondary pathology, those characterised by vocal fatigue, and those related to vocal abuse which may also lead to vocal pathologies such as vocal nodules or contact ulcers. The other major sub-group is attributed to *Psychoneurosis* and lists conversion disorder, mutism, aphonia, psychosexual conflict, gender dysphoria, and child-like speech and voice in adults. Interestingly, muscle tension dysphonia is also included under this sub-heading for *Psychoneurosis*. Here, this large *Psychogenic Voice Disorder* classification is strongly influenced by the psychodynamic model, with different degrees of psychopathology considered fundamental to aetiology. The voice disorders are considered to be 'a manifestation of one or more types of psychological disequilibrium, such as anxiety, depression, conversion reaction or personality disorder, that interfere with normal volitional control over phonation' (Aronson & Bless, 2009) (p171). In cases where aberrant muscle tension patterns persist in the form of vocal misuse or abuse, these are thought to reflect psychological instability due to personality disorder or psychiatric disturbance that has led the person to persist in these vocally abusive behaviours.

Another well-known classification system which differentiates the 'non-organic' from the 'organic' voice disorders is that proposed by Rammage and colleagues (2001). These authors prefer the term *Muscle Misuse Voice Disorders*. Here, they argue that the vocal dysfunction resulting in the voice disorder is causally related to the 'misuse of the voluntary muscle systems that are employed for breathing phonation, articulation and resonance' (Rammage *et al.*, 2001) (p.74). Their diagnostic classification is based upon laryngeal postures and visible features at the level of the glottis and supraglottic structures observed during laryngoscopic examination. They emphasise that aberrant muscle tension patterns may be influenced by a range of interacting aetiological factors underpinning all voice disorders, but to a different degree according to the specific circumstances for that individual. These factors are related to the person's technique and vocal skills, to lifestyle situations that may predispose a person to vocal abuses or vocal misuse, to medical issues (particularly the effects of gastroesophageal reflux), and a range of psychological factors including influences from personality traits and emotion. They highlight the fact that a range of factors may contribute to the overall clinical presentation of the voice disorder but stress that muscle misuse patterns are germane to the aetiology of the 'non-organic' voice disorders.

In the comprehensive aetiological classification system by Mathieson (2001), the term *Behavioural Voice Disorders* is used to distinguish between the 'organic' and 'non-organic' voice disorders. One major sub-group is referred to as *Hyperfunctional* and includes the muscle tension dysphonias both with and without pathology, such as nodules, polyps, contact ulcers or chronic laryngitis. The other major sub-group is labelled *Psychogenic* and includes *conversion disorders, puberphonia* and *mutational falsetto, anxiety state* and *transsexual conflict*.

This system proposes a well-balanced conceptual framework with richly detailed clinical profile templates for each disorder within the different sub-groups; these include reference to the pathophysiology, the presumed aetiology, the auditory-perceptual signs and symptoms, laryngoscopic findings, expected vocal profile, acoustic analysis, airflow and volume measures profile, and medicosurgical decisions where relevant. Mathieson emphasises the multifactorial nature of voice disorders, the complexity of the diagnostic process, and the possibility that more than one diagnosis may be relevant where secondary compensatory features may have developed in response to the original voice disorder.

More recently, my colleagues and I developed a modified *Diagnostic Classification System for Voice Disorders (DCSVD)* (Baker *et al.*, 2007). This system draws substantially upon the strengths of the other classification systems mentioned above while also trying to redress some of the problems inherent in each. In our system we use the term *Functional Voice Disorders* (FVD) to refer to the 'non-organic' voice disorders. The choice to revert to this terminology was predicated by the fact that the term has been used so widely across disciplines and countries; it suggests disrupted vocal behaviours that may, over time, lead to poor vocal habits and the subsequent development of organic changes to the vocal folds, and also implies disturbed psychological processes that lead to a loss of volitional control over phonation. We consider that the term *Functional Voice Disorder (FVD)* enables both of these aetiological explanations to stand beside one another as distinct and related entities without the requirement for either entity to necessarily exclude the other, but rather to interact. One major sub-division is referred to as the *Muscle Tension Voice Disorders (MTVD)*. This includes a sub-type where there is no organic pathology, and several other sub-types where the habitual patterns of vocal hyperfunction or misuse lead to minor pathologies such as nodules, polyps, and chronic laryngitis. The other major sub-division is referred to as the *Psychogenic Voice Disorders (PVD)*, with sub-types including *conversion reaction aphonia/dysphonia*, *puberphonia* or *mutational falsetto* and, in rare cases, *psychogenic spasmodic dysphonia*. The DCSVD is a *syndromal diagnostic classification system* that incorporates demographic and psychosocial information from the clinical history reported by the client, the auditory-perceptual and kinaesthetic symptoms, possible phonatory and laryngeal behaviours observed and measured by the SLP and otolaryngologist during laryngoscopy, and detailed operational definitions and guidelines that assist the practitioner in the process of differential diagnosis. These are intended to highlight the primary differences between the major sub-groups and sub-types while allowing for flexibility when the clinical presentation is ambiguous or where multiple factors are operating. The guidelines include:

1. The essential nature of the disorder including the presence or absence of pathophysiology
2. Likely patterns of onset and course of the disorder
3. Symptom congruity in relation to presumed aetiology
4. The possible relationship between muscle tension patterns and co-existing organic conditions
5. Likely responses to techniques used to facilitate improved vocalisation
6. Predictions about possible patterns of resolution
7. The possible role of psychological factors in contributing to onset, aggravation or perpetuation of the condition.

The structure and operational guidelines are intended to reflect our conceptual framework that places a strong emphasis on the interaction between the neurophysiological, behavioural and psychosocial factors rather than on one isolated set of parameters presumed to be aetiologically significant. In this classification system, it is suggested that *psychosocial factors* need to be taken into account across the full range of voice disorders.

Assumptions about psychosocial factors and 'non-organic' voice disorders

As reflected in the various diagnostic classifications for voice disorders discussed above, and following a comprehensive review of the literature (Baker, 2008), it is clear that there are a number of assumptions about the way in which cognitive, psychological or emotional factors may contribute to the patterns of onset and influence the clinical profiles of the large group of 'non-organic' or 'functional' voice disorders. The literature suggests that these same factors, which we might collectively label as *psychosocial factors*, are also likely to affect the patient's ability to cope with changes to their vocal function, their motivation to consolidate vocal changes achieved in the clinic to the wider social or employment setting, or their grief over significant loss of vocal function and identity. They may even precipitate the development of more serious mental illness in response to the voice disorder, such as anxiety state or depression.

Paucity of assumptions about psychosocial factors and 'organic' voice disorders

While there have been many studies devoted to possible causal associations between psychosocial factors and 'functional' voice disorders (to be discussed in more detail in later chapters), it is interesting to note that there have been relatively few studies in which the organic voice disorder groups have been the primary focus. It could be argued that this is logical because causality with organic conditions is generally more straightforward, especially where acute infections, mass lesions, endocrine changes, structural anomalies or neurologic disorders can be readily identified, but considering the breadth and depth of research into possible associations between psychosocial factors and other medical disorders, such as cardiovascular disease, diabetes, cancer, endocrine disorders and skin complaints (Nyklicek, Temoshok, & Vingerhoets, 2004; Vingerhoets, Nyklicek, & Denollet, 2008), this could well be a fruitful area for deeper consideration. For instance, it would be very helpful to understand how psychosocial factors might contribute to medical or mental health conditions that may render an individual vulnerable to the development of organically-based voice disorders, such as acute viral laryngitis, thyroid disease leading to surgical intervention with implications for recurrent laryngeal nerve function, or cancer leading to total laryngectomy. It is also possible that patients with organic voice disorders, by virtue of their medical aetiologies and the extent to which these conditions alter their vocal function, may indeed face very different challenges in dealing with their voice problems from those with functional voice disorders.

Implications for clinical practice and research studies

Clearly, finding terminologies in common and developing clinically reliable diagnostic classification systems is a complex task. As expressed so cogently by Mathieson (2001), while the process is intended to help us to be 'conveniently tidy', the clinical reality is more difficult. The discussion above is intended to emphasise that these ongoing dilemmas over terminology and diagnostic classification may contribute to practitioners remaining conceptually muddled about what constitutes a symptom and what may be the true aetiology. Most significantly of all it can lead to feelings of nervousness about making a confident diagnosis (Butcher *et al.*, 2007). This inevitably leads to confusion when communicating diagnostic findings and decisions to other voice practitioners and health professionals, to the client's employers or associated medico-legal advisors. Most significantly of all, it directly affects the way in which practitioners give information and explanations to their clients and families about the essential nature of their voice disorder, how they intend to approach the initial case history interview and decide which causal factors seem to be the most relevant and deserving of attention, what the focus of the assessment procedures will be and finally, their rationale for treatment strategies selected to facilitate the best outcomes.

Terminologies and definitions to be used

For the purposes of this book, I have chosen to apply the terminologies which I developed with my colleagues for the *Diagnostic Classification System of Voice Disorders (DCSVD)* (Baker *et al.*, 2007) as shown in Box 1.1.

Box 1.1 Diagnostic Terminologies Baker et al. (2007)

Organic Voice Disorder (OVD) refers to an aphonia/dysphonia due to mass lesions, structural changes to the vocal folds or cartilaginous structures, or interruption to neurological innervations of the laryngeal mechanism. Psychosocial factors often arise in response to, or may aggravate the situation.

Functional Voice Disorder (FVD) refers broadly to an aphonia/dysphonia where there is no organic pathology, or if there is, it is either insufficient to account for the nature and severity of the voice disorder or is considered secondary to the functional problem. There are two main sub-divisions within the FVD classification:

Muscle Tension Voice Disorder (MTVD) refers to a dysphonia that develops as a result of psychological processes that lead to patterns of dysregulated vocal behaviours that over time may result in secondary organic changes such as vocal nodules, polyps or contact ulcers, and which are generally amenable to resolution through behavioural change. While psychosocial factors play a role in the onset or aggravation of the dysphonia, they may appear to be secondary to the vocal trauma produced by dysregulated vocal behaviors.

Psychogenic Voice Disorder (PVD) refers to an aphonia/dysphonia that occurs as a result of disturbed psychological processes leading to sudden or intermittent loss of volitional control over the initiation and maintenance of phonation, in the absence of structural or neurological pathology sufficient to account for the dysphonia. Symptom incongruity and reversibility are demonstrable, and psychosocial factors are often linked to onset. Whilst muscle tension patterns may be observed, such patterns are secondary to the psychological processes operating.

From The Diagnostic Classification System of Voice Disorders, Baker et.al (2007)

References

Aronson, A. E., & Bless, D. M. (2009). *Clinical voice disorders* (4th ed.). New York: Thieme.

Baker, J. (2002). Psychogenic voice disorders-heroes or hysterics? A brief overview with questions and discussion. *Logopedics Phoniatrics Vocology, 27*, 84–91.

Baker, J. (2008). The role of psychogenic and psychosocial factors in the development of functional voice disorders. *International Journal of Speech-Language Pathology, 10*(4), 210–230.

Baker, J., Ben-Tovim, D. I., Butcher, A., Esterman, A., & McLaughlin, K. (2007). Development of a modified diagnostic classification system for voice disorders with inter-rater reliability study. *Logopedics Phoniatrics Vocology, 32*, 99–112.

Butcher, P., Elias, A., & Cavalli, L. (2007). *Understanding and treating psychogenic voice disorder: A CBT framework.* Chichester: Wiley.

Carding, P., Deary, V., & Miller, T. (2013). Cognitive behavioural therapy in the treatment of functional dysphonia in the United Kingdom. In E. M.-L. Yiu (Ed.), *International perspectives on voice disorders* (pp. 133–148). UK: Multilingual Matters/ Channel View Publications.

Carson, A. J., Brown, R., David, A. S., *et al.* (2012). Functional (conversion) neurological sysmptoms: Research since the millennium. *Journal of Neurology, Neurosurgery and Psychiatry, 83*, 842–850.

Hallett, M., Lang, A., Jankovic, J., Fahn, S., Halligan, P. W., Voon, V., & Cloninger, C. R. (Eds.). (2011). *Psychogenic movement disorders and other conversion disorders.* Cambridge: Cambridge University Press.

Mathieson, L. (2001). *Greene and Mathieson's: The voice and its disorders.* (6th ed.). London: Whurr.

Morrison, M. D., & Rammage, L. (1994). *The management of voice disorders.* San Diego: Singular Publishing Group.

Nyklicek, I., Temoshok, L., & Vingerhoets, A. (Eds.). (2004). *Emotional expression and health.* Hove: Brunner-Routledge.

Rammage, L., Morrison, M., & Nichol, H. (2001). *Management of the voice and its disorders.* San Diego: Singular Publishing Group.

Roy, N. (2003). Functional dysphonia. *Current Opinion in Otolaryngology and Head and Neck Surgery, 11*(3), 144–148.

Stone, J., Warlow, C., & Sharpe, M. (2010). The symptom of functional weakness: A controlled study of 107 patients. *Brain, 133*, 1537–1551.

Verdolini, K., Rosen, C. A., & Branski, R. C. (Eds.). (2006). *Classification Manual for Voice Disorders – I.* Mahwah: Laurence Erlbaum Associates.

Vingerhoets, A., Nyklicek, I., & Denollet, J. (Eds.). (2008). *Emotion regulation: Conceptual and clinical issues.* New York: Springer.

Walsh, R. (2005). A response to eight views on terminology: Is it possible to tame the wild beast of inconsistency? *Advances in Speech-Language Pathology, 7*(2), 105–111.

2

Psychosocial factors in context

Introduction

There is a substantial body of research devoted to the exploration of possible associations between psychosocial factors and a range of physical and mental health conditions. Three fundamental propositions have driven much of this psychosocial research:

1) Heightened levels of emotion in response to external and internal influences may impact upon an individual's thoughts, feelings, behaviours and neuro-biological functioning
2) Biopsychosocial systems of human beings reflect the complexity typical of all living systems, where any one part of that system operates in a dynamic relationship with the whole
3) The health concerns of people need to be considered within the context of their wider social network.

In this chapter, I discuss the different ways in which the term *'psychosocial'* has been used throughout the literature, and relate current definitions to the wider contexts of the *Social Determinants of Health (SDH)*, the *International Classification of Functioning, Disability and Health (ICF)*, and how these conceptual frameworks reflect the broad principles of *Systems Theory and Cybernetics*. It is suggested that psychosocial perspectives may inform our thinking about the management of voice disorders without detracting from traditional and established neurophysiological knowledge, or from direct approaches to voice therapy shown to be reasonably effective.

Approaching the same phenomena from different perspectives

'Everything that one thinks one understands has to be understood over and over again, in its different aspects, each time with the same new shock of discovery' (Psychoanalyst, Marion Milner (2011) (p. 47) (as quoted by Australian author Helen Garner, Inaugural Stella Prize Ceremony, April 16, 2013).

There are probably several experiences in our student and professional lives that we recall as pivotal and transformational. One of these inspiring experiences occurred when I attended a speech pathology conference as a student, where the highly revered otolaryngologist, Dr Paul Moore, presented his remarkable video-filmed images of the vocal folds during phonation. The first images were taken using the flexible nasendoscope with plain light giving an excellent functional view of the vocal folds during phonation (Fig. 2.1). The second images were filmed using the rigid Stortz laryngoscope with a stroboscopic light source, providing an image of the mucosal wave on the surface of the vocal fold, and a level of detail surpassing anything the naked eye could normally see or the mind could imagine (Fig. 2.2).

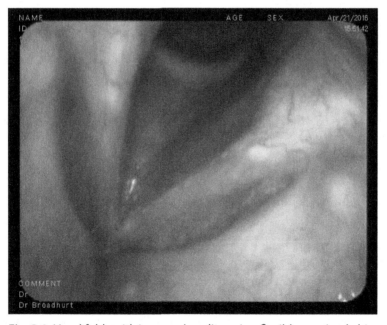

Fig. 2.1 Vocal folds with 'average' quality using flexible proximal chip endoscope (under plain light)

Image courtesy of Dr. Matthew Broadhurst, Laryngeal surgeon

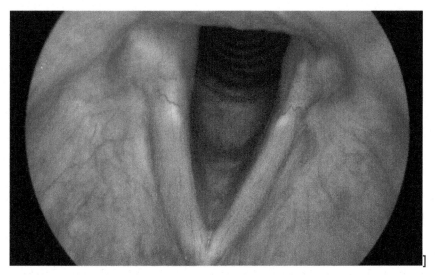

Fig. 2.2 Vocal folds using high definition magnified view of the rigid telescope (under stroboscopic light)

Image courtesy of Dr. Matthew Broadhurst, Laryngeal surgeon

Dr Moore's films highlighted how another lens or light source could produce new perspectives on what was essentially the same set of structures and series of vocal fold behaviours. These different ways of conducting laryngoscopic examination led the field in a new understanding of the normal and abnormal structure and function of the vocal folds, and established the foundations for the 'gold standard' of diagnostic assessment in voice analysis clinics around the world. For most otolaryngologists and speech pathologists there has been no going back, but even if there are situations where this, and even more sophisticated instrumentation such as *videokymography* is not readily accessible, or where there is a clinical choice not to seek these different perspectives, we know that the means to obtain these rich levels of detail do exist.

Another transformational experience occurred many years later when I attended a keynote address by the Welsh family therapist, Brian Cade, which was entitled "Stuckness, Unpredictability and Change" (1985). His main message was that in order for clinicians to be therapeutic and effective, it is crucial that they do not constrain themselves with the reification of one theoretical position or set of beliefs which predetermines their approaches to intervention. In quoting one of his own texts he said *"It is vital that we never believe what we believe, that way lies The Inquisition"*. He also suggested the scientific principles underpinning the phenomena involved in holography might be an apt metaphor for therapists to consider.

Holograms were new to me at the time, but I now understand that the process of creating these three dimensional images requires the projection of *holographic images* onto a plate with a selected frequency and intensity of refracted light from a stipulated direction. An interesting property of holograms is that if the same frequency and intensity of light is projected, and from the same direction, the primary object and its figure–ground associations will always be perceived in the same way. However, if the light source is projected from a new angle, with a different frequency or intensity, the original target image can still be recognized but new aspects will predominate while others will become more indistinct. Another fascinating feature of holograms is that every part of any hologram contains the image of the whole object, so that even if one piece of the hologram is removed and scrutinised more closely, the gestalt of the entire image is retained.

In applying this metaphor to family or therapeutic systems that may be stuck, Cade suggested that one of the key *restraints to change* often lies in the clinician's very firm set of beliefs about a problem. This will then predetermine the therapist's focus for intervention while other issues become relegated to the background. He proposed that for change to occur, some unpredictability would need to be introduced into the system, with the therapist viewing issues through an entirely different lens and considering approaches from an alternative direction. With a new way of thinking about the problem, different aspects of the family system could be brought to light, and those usually given primacy, although still being taken into account, would no longer be the main target of attention.

These two pivotal experiences, although very different, highlighted for me how a willingness to view clinical issues from an alternative viewpoint can bring a depth of insight and a new kind of clarity to the situation. They have also continued to remind me that it is possible to focus on one particular aspect, or at another time to attend to the whole, without the eye or the mind necessarily losing an appreciation of the other.

What do we mean by the terms 'psychosocial' and 'psychosocial factors'?

While considering how best to introduce the notion that psychosocial perspectives may improve our understanding and management of voice disorders, it has been interesting to note how widely the term *psychosocial* is used in research studies exploring possible social and psychological pathways underlying health and illness. In a challenging editorial discussion about the extensive epidemiological research in this area, Martikainen, Bartley and Lahelma (2002) refer to the rather loose use of the term *psychosocial* across studies with very different research questions, and warn that it may become an 'umbrella label' that 'refers to everything and nothing in particular' (p.1091). Their extensive Medline search on this topic revealed numerous phrases referring to three main areas of psychosocial research into health related areas (Table 2.1).

Table 2.1 Diverse uses of the term 'Psychosocial' following Medline search

Causes and risk factors	Mediating factors and contexts	Outcomes
Psychosocial causation	Psychosocial mechanisms	Psychosocial distress
Psychosocial influences	Psychosocial environment	Psychosocial well-being
Psychosocial risk factors	Psychosocial context	Psychosocial health
	Psychosocial resources	

Adapted from Editorial material collated by Martikainen et al. (2002) p1091.

As defined by *The Oxford English Dictionary*, the word *psychosocial* refers to 'the influence of social factors on an individual's mind or behavior, and to the interrelationship between behavioural and social factors' (http://dictionary.oed.com.). Martikainen *et al.* (2002) propose that it is the metaphorical space representing the interactions between these external societal and internal personal factors that provide the operational domain for psychosocial factors. These authors argue that while a person may experience a stressful life event, it is only when that external social experience causes psychological changes for that individual, such as the negative emotions of anxiety or loss of self esteem which then affects the person's neurophysiological system, behavior or health, that it can be said that *psychosocial processes* are operating. Only then can this type of event be legitimately referred to as a *psychosocial risk factor* for that condition, mediated by the individual *psychosocial context* of that person with the potential to precipitate *psychosocial outcomes* such as altered sense of well-being, behaviours or health.

Psychosocial factors in the context of the Social Determinants of Health

'Conceptualising our mental life as some sort of enclosed world residing inside the skull does not do justice to the lived reality of human experience. It systematically neglects the importance of social context' (Bracken & Thomas, 2002) (p.1433).

The complex processes mentioned above are clearly reflected in the way psychosocial factors have been located within the context of the most recently formulated *Conceptual Framework on Social Determinants of Health (SDH)* (Solar & Irwin, 2010) (Fig. 2.3) This rich schematic model pulls together the major external structural and societal influences that interact with intermediary factors such as living arrangements, biological and behavioural issues, and those psychosocial factors which include personality traits, coping strategies, social supports and interpersonal relationships. The inclusion of the health system as an intermediary factor is, in my opinion, a highly significant addition and one that can operate as a powerful psychosocial force in the management of voice disorders. This is particularly so when involving worker's compensation or medico-legal issues. The model illustrates that it is the interrelationship between the external and internal factors, rather than one or the other, that determines the social and psychological pathways underlying changes to the sense of well-being or health.

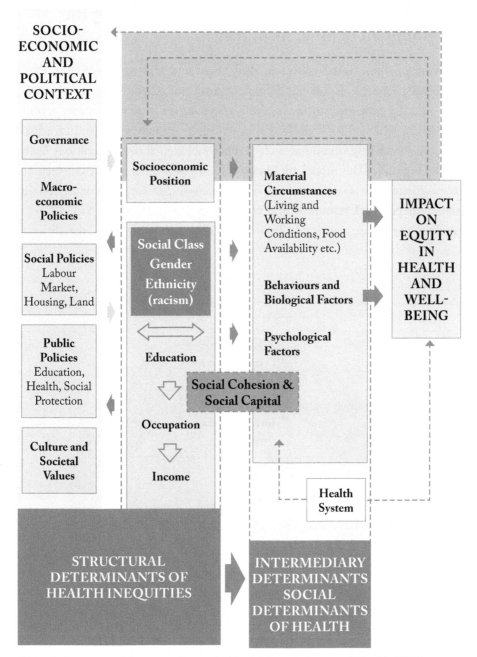

Fig. 2.3 Conceptual frameworks on the Social Determinants of Health (SDH)

Reproduced with kind permission: World Health Organization/Solar & Irwin (2010)

Psychosocial factors in the context of mediating the development of inner resources

Drawing on these same concepts, Paul Ward and colleagues (Muller, Ward, Winefield, Tsouros, & Lawn, 2009; Tsourtos *et al.*, 2011; Ward *et al.*, 2011) have recently proposed an *interactive psychosocial model of resilience* to account for ways in which this particular coping mechanism may affect an individual's responses to adverse situations, such as those included above, and various health issues (Fig. 2.4). The model highlights the ongoing interactions between the *external social determinants* and *internal psychological factors*, such as personality traits and personal resources, and shows how this capacity to face adversity develops over time, inevitably influenced by transitions within the different

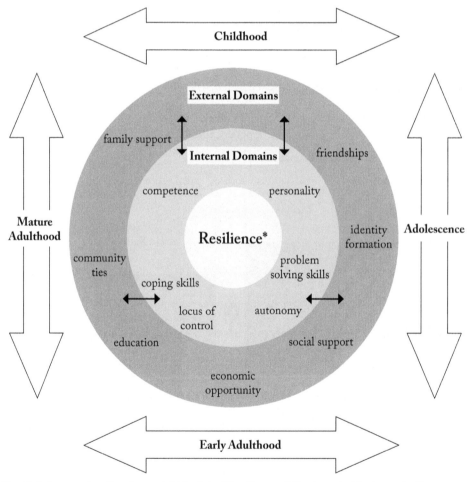

Fig. 2.4 Interactive Psychosocial Model of Resilience (Ward et al., 2011, p. 1142)

Reproduced by kind permission Ward et al., and Elsevier

stages of the family life cycle. This *interactive psychosocial model* lends further support for any operational definition of the term *psychosocial* encompassing the interrelationship between external social and internal psychological factors, and provides a useful platform for thinking about how other psychosocial resources may develop in relation to a range of physical and mental health conditions, including voice disorders.

Psychosocial factors in the context of the International Classification of Functioning, Disability and Health (ICF)

This dynamic interplay between external and internal factors is also inherent in the philosophical foundations of the *International Classification of Functioning, Disability and Health* (ICF) (World Health Organization, 2001), which is a comprehensive classification system that aims to account for the relative status of an individual's health in holistic and functional terms. At one end of the spectrum, the ICF has been designed to assist leaders on global health matters and at the other end of the continuum, it is now being used to guide the thinking of individuals and their medical and health practitioners on clinical matters with respect to assessment, intervention, outcomes and research.

The original edition of the framework, the *International Classification of Impairments, Disabilities and Handicaps* (ICIDH) (World Health Organization, 1980), focused primarily on consequences of disorders in terms of impairment, leading to disability and finally, to handicap. The main criticisms of this original edition were that the model suggested a linear and causal relationship between the different levels of disablement. Further, *Environmental Factors* were depicted as largely negative barriers to be overcome by the individual concerned, and *Personal Factors*, those that could be identified as being unrelated to the current health condition, were not included in the framework at all (Ma, Threats, & Worrall, 2008).

The modified and current conceptual framework for the ICF now shows how the health status of an individual can be construed from a number of different perspectives in which the emphasis may be on the alterations to bodily structures and their functions (*impairments*) which in turn, may or may not lead to changes in activity levels (*limitations*) and which may or may not alter the capacity of the person to participate in those activities previously part of his or her lifestyle (*restrictions*) (Fig. 2.5).

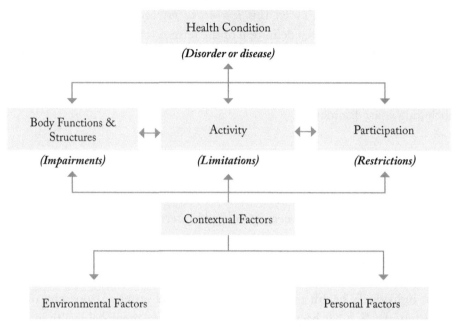

Fig. 2.5 Graphical representation of the International Classification of Functioning, Disability and Health (ICF) WHO [2001]

Reproduced with kind permission WHO

In this current model, the philosophical emphasis is on the different components being construed as complex and interactive rather than linear, and that across all of these domains, *Contextual Factors* need to be taken into account. These include the external influences of *Environmental Factors* and the internal influences of *Personal factors*. Aronson (1990) has led the field in highlighting this, so cogently, in relation to disorders of the voice, and it is these factors 'that represent the complete background of an individual's life and living' (WHO, 2001, p.16).

Environmental Factors are defined within the ICF as 'the physical, social and attitudinal environment in which people live and conduct their lives' (WHO, 2001, p.10). In this model, they may be positive if they operate as facilitators, or they may be negative if they form barriers; and in some cases they may be relatively neutral, having no effect on the system at all. In the light of this emphasis on *Environmental Factors* within the ICF model, it has been pleasing to note that the *scope of practice* for SLPs in the USA (American Speech-Language-Hearing Association, 2001) and Australia (Speech Pathology Australia, 2002) now encourages a focus on *Environmental Factors*, as these may impact on a person's functioning in relation to their communication disorders and in therapists' approaches to planning for clinical intervention. It is difficult to believe that this ever needed formal ratification.

Personal Factors within the ICF framework refer to those features pertinent to an individual that are *not* part of the health condition as such but are likely to have a direct impact on how individuals respond to the limitations arising from any health condition, such as a voice disorder. These may include 'age, gender, race, coping styles, fitness, lifestyle, habits, upbringing, social background, education, profession, past and current experience (past life events, and concurrent events), overall behavior patterns and character style, individual psychological assets and other characteristics' (WHO, 2001, p 17). These *Personal Factors*, although part of the framework, have not been coded in a detailed manner in the ICF, and it has been strongly argued that they should not be separated, either conceptually or visually, but embedded within all components of the model, especially in relation to Activities and Participation (Threats, 2008).

The structural framework and philosophical foundations of the ICF with respect to their relevance to the speech-language pathology profession are discussed in two recent special issue journals. In the *International Journal of Speech-Language Pathology* (2008), several excellent papers provide an overview of the nature and functions of the different components of the ICF model (Ma *et al.*, 2008; Threats, 2008); followed by papers highlighting ways in which the particular elements of the conceptual framework may be applied to domains of speech pathology, including clinical practice, research, education and training of clinicians. In a special issue of *Seminars in Speech and Language* (2007), also devoted to the ICF framework and speech-language pathology practice, there are two papers devoted to voice-related matters: one focuses on the application of the ICF to laryngectomy (Eadie, 2007) and the other in relation to the management of voice disorders (Ma, Yiu, & Verdolini Abbott, 2007). These two publications are very timely and strongly support the discussion above which proposes that psychosocial factors in association with physical or mental health conditions need to be viewed against the larger backdrop of the social context of each individual.

Ma *et al.* (2007), clearly outline ways in which the ICF can be adapted to describe a voice disorder and its consequences, consequences that have been shown to impact on individuals as markedly as more life-threatening illnesses such as cancer (Smith *et al.*, 1996). The authors then outline ways in which the ICF may guide a clinician's approaches to assessment and treatment. Reference is made to key domains of Body Functions, Body Structures, Activities and Participation, with an excellent section on those Contextual Factors (Environmental and Personal Factors) that need to be considered across all elements. Helpful examples of Environmental Factors relevant to individuals with voice disorders are described. For example, with respect to teaching, these may include access to adequate amplification technology, suitability of the teaching environment, appropriate support from employers if leave for voice rest is required; community attitudes to the teacher's vocal disorder; and sufficient educational programmes to promote healthy use and care of the voice. Emphasis is placed on those Personal Factors that may influence how an individual responds to the various limitations caused by dysphonia whether due to age, personality traits or introversion, or profession. In conclusion, these authors strongly believe that the application of the ICF to the management of voice disorders 'is essential to achieve the ultimate goal of enhancing the quality of life of the individual' (Ma *et al.*, 2007) (p.349).

Psychosocial factors in relation to systems theory, cybernetics and family therapy

The three conceptual frameworks described above exemplify the complexity of living systems; they also provide a timely space to introduce several of the key principles of systems theory and cybernetics and their application to human beings. This application may be at a cellular level with respect to bodily functions such as respiratory-phonatory systems, to relationships between individuals and their close family, friendships or the wider social context.

As summarised most effectively by Wallis and Rhodes (2011), one of the basic tenets of *systems theory* is that changes to any one part of a system will influence other parts, and this will affect the larger system to which these components belong. Furthermore, while living systems are always seeking to evolve through growth and development, they also use energy to maintain homeostasis and stability in the face of external or internal influences (Bateson, 1972). When these systemic principles are applied to families, for example where external pressures may come from loss of employment or when internal demands may arise during the *family life cycle* such as loss of a parent through acrimonious divorce, these 'nodal points' and external situations will both require adjustments in order to maintain the status quo (Vetere & Dallos, 2003). According to systems theory, the maintenance of this *dynamic steady state* is achieved via complex *feedback loops* involving ongoing communication between individuals with one another, or between individuals and their wider social context (von Bertalanffy, 1968).

The other pivotal theoretical influences underpinning family therapy are drawn from *cybernetics* and *information theories*. These relate to the study of communication in the context of mechanical systems, where communication between one part and another within a system then leads 'automatically' to actions or adjustments in another part of the system (Weiner, 1961). Wallis and Rhodes (2011) suggest that this 'recursive' interplay between 'influencing and being influenced' reflects a *circular* rather than a *linear* causation, which is certainly a more realistic way of thinking about communication and interactions between family members, or between individuals and their social networks.

These *principles of systems theory* support the conceptual framework for the Social Determinants of Health (SDH) which seeks to account for the social and psychological pathways underpinning the course and onset of various physical and mental health conditions. They can be recognised in the recursive communication loops that evolve between individuals facing adverse situations and as they develop personal resources, such as resilience, to deal with these challenges over time. They are also clearly reflected in the ICF framework which may guide our thoughts regarding the health status of an individual in functional and contextual terms (Titze & Verdolini Abbott, 2012). The dynamic interrelationships that emerge between the principles of living systems and those psychosocial factors embedded within these different models challenge traditional mind-body dualities and biomedical models based upon *linear causal assumptions*. However, this need not diminish established knowledge but rather, provide an appreciation of the complexity of those neurophysiological processes involved in physical and mental health, and in relation to normal and abnormal vocal function. Furthermore, I have found that the integration of *psychosocial perspectives* into clinical voice work serves to complement the more direct approaches to voice therapy without detracting from them in any way.

As previously mentioned it is possible to view the management of voice disorders through different lenses, real and metaphorical. At times, the focus may be either on individual parts or, as these components may interact with one another, with a holistic approach that embraces *biopsychosocial perspectives*. It is acknowledged by a number of authors that focusing on psychosocial factors may not be encouraged or prioritised in some clinical settings, and that this is most unfortunate (Aronson & Bless, 2009; Baker, Ben-Tovim, Butcher, Esterman, & McLaughlin, 2013; de Jong *et al.*, 2003; Dietrich & Verdolini Abbott, 2012; Nichol, Morrison, & Rammage, 1993). However, as with the flexible nasendoscope under plain light or the rigid storz under a stroboscopic light source, the detail and its surrounding context are there: they do exist, regardless of whether or not a practitioner chooses to access this rich and relevant material.

References

American Speech-Language-Hearing Association. (2001). *Scope of practice in speech-language pathology*. Rockville: ASHA.

Aronson, A. E. (1990). Psychogenic voice disorders. *Clinical voice disorders: An interdisciplinary approach*. (3rd ed., pp. 116–159). New York: Thieme.

Aronson, A. E., & Bless, D. M. (2009). *Clinical voice disorders* (4th ed.). New York: Thieme.

Baker, J., Ben-Tovim, D. I., Butcher, A., Esterman, A., & McLaughlin, K. (2013). Psychosocial risk factors which may differentiate between women with functional voice disorder, organic voice disorder, and control group. *International Journal of Speech-Language Pathology, 15*(6), 547–563.

Bateson, G. (1972). *Steps to an ecology of mind: Collected essays in anthropology, psychiatry, evolution, and epistemology*. New York: Ballantine Books.

Bracken, P., & Thomas, P. (2002). Time to move beyond the mind-body split. *British Medical Journal, 325*(7378), 1433.

Cade, B. (1985). Stuckness, unpredictability and change. *Australian and New Zealand Journal of Family Therapy, 6*(1), 9–15.

de Jong, F. I. C. R. S., Cornelius, B. E., Wuyts, F. L., Kooijman, P. G. C., Schutte, H. K., Oudes, M. J., & Graamans, K. (2003). A psychological cascade model for persisting voice problems in teachers. *Folia Phoniatrica et Logopaedia, 55*(2).

Dietrich, M., & Verdolini Abbott, K. (2012). Vocal function in introverts and extraverts during a psychological stress reactivity protocol. *Journal of Speech, Language and Hearing Research, 55*, 973–987.

Eadie, T. L. (2007). Application of the ICF in communication after total laryngectomy. *Seminars in Speech and Language, 28*, 291–300.

Ma, E. P.-M., Threats, T. T., & Worrall, L. E. (2008). An introduction to the International Classification of Functioning, Disability and Health (ICF) for speech-language pathology: Its past, present and future. *International Journal of Speech-Language Pathology, 10*(1–2), 2–8.

Ma, E. P.-M., Yiu, E. M.-L., & Verdolini Abbott, K. (2007). Application of the ICF in voice disorders. *Seminars in Speech and Language, 28*, 343–350.

Martikainen, P., Bartley, M., & Lahelma, E. (2002). Psychosocial determinants of health in social epidemiology. *International Journal of Epidemiology, 31*, 1091–1093.

Milner, M. (2011). *An experiment in leisure* (Revised edition). London: Taylor & Francis Ltd.

Muller, R., Ward, P. R., Winefield, T., Tsouros, G., & Lawn, S. (2009). The importance of resilience to primary care practitioners: an interactive psycho-social model. *Australasian Medical Journal, 1*(1), 1–15.

Nichol, H., Morrison, M. D., & Rammage, L. (1993). Interdisciplinary approach to functional voice disorders: The psychiatrist's role. *Otolaryngology-Head and Neck Surgery, 108*(6), 643–647.

Smith, E., Verdolini, K., Gray, S. D., Nichols, S., Lemke, J., Barkmeier, J., Dove, H., & Hoffman, H. (1996). Effect of voice disorders on quality of life. *Journal of Medical Speech-Language Pathology, 4*(4), 223–244.

Solar, O., & Irwin, A. (2010). A conceptual framework for action on the social determinants of health. Social Determinants of Health Discussion. Paper 2 (Policy and Practice) *Commission on Social Determinants of Health*. Geneva: World Health Organization.

Speech Pathology Australia. (2002). *Scope of practice in speech pathology*. Melbourne: Speech Pathology Australia.

Threats, T. T. (2008). Use of the ICF for clinical practice in speech-language pathology. *International Journal of Speech-Language Pathology, 10*(1–2), 50–60.

Titze, I. R., & Verdolini Abbott, K. (2012). *Vocology. The science and practice of voice habilitation*. Salt Lake City: National Center for Voice and Speech.

Tsourtos, G., Ward, P. R., Muller, R., Lawn, S., Winefield, A. H., Hersh, D., & Coveney, J. (2011). The importance of resilience and stress to maintaining smoking abstinence and cessation: A qualitative study in Australia. *Health and Social Care in the Community, 19*(3), 299–306.

Vetere, A., & Dallos, R. (2003). *Working systematically with families: Formulation, intervention and evaluation*. London: Karnac Books.

von Bertalanffy, L. (1968). *General systems theory: Foundation, development, application*. New York: Braziller.

Wallis, A., & Rhodes, P. (2011). Structured guidelines for the first session of post-Milan systemic therapy. In P. Rhodes & A. Wallis (Eds.), *A practical guide to family therapy*. Melbourne: IP Communications, Pty.Ltd.

Ward, P. R., Muller, R., Tsouros, G., Hersh, D., Lawn, S., Winefield, A. H., & Coveney, J. (2011). Additive and subtractive resilience strategies as enablers of biographical reinvention: A qualitative study of ex-smokers and never-smokers. *Social Science and Medicine, 72*, 1140–1148.

Weiner, N. (1961). *Cybernetics*. Cambridge: MIT Press.

World Health Organization. (1980). *ICIDH: International Classification of Impairments, Disabilities and Handicaps*. Geneva: World Health Organization.

World Health Organization. (2001). *International Classification of Functioning, Disability, and Health (ICF)*. Geneva: World Health Organization.

3

Trends in the psychosocial research in relation to physical and mental health

Introduction

There are several different approaches to *psychosocial research* in relation to physical and mental health conditions. These include clinical studies, large population studies within epidemiological programmes, and neurophysiological studies exploring possible *psychobiological pathways*. Underlying many of the research efforts across these different perspectives are the hypotheses that *positive* and *negative emotions* and their related cognitions are going to affect the mind and the body, and that negative emotions and cognitions in response to *different types of stressors* are likely to be deleterious to our health.

In order to appreciate how these propositions may help to explain possible associations between psychosocial factors and voice disorders, the role of negative emotions in the *neurobiology of acute and chronic stress* responses is briefly described, with recent evidence highlighting those features of *chronic stress* shown to create greater risk for health. It is suggested that the findings that have emerged from this psychosocial research have provided a strong framework for similar studies in relation to voice disorders. It is also proposed that the trends in recent evidence, including some of the controversies arising in relation to physical and mental health research, may continue to influence the clinical questions that need to be pursued in the different areas of *vocology*.

Trends in psychosocial research associated with physical and mental health

'Health commissioners, budgetary systems, health care professionals, and the public all act as if there is some clear, inescapable separation between physical and mental health problems, ignoring evidence that a person's emotional state always affects their function and presentation of physical symptoms' (Wade & Halligan, 2004) (p.1399).

It is not within the scope of this book to provide an adequate overview of the vast field of psychosocial research in relation to physical and mental health conditions. It is, however, relevant to highlight where the focus of this research has been placed, and how a number of these same research questions have influenced the directions of recent studies with respect to voice disorders. Broadly speaking, research efforts over the last 30 years have focused upon possible associations between psychosocial factors and health as these may contribute to causal pathways when accounting for the aggravation or perpetuation of conditions which may influence *quality of life* and outcomes. While the focus for many studies has been on particular external variables such as *stressful life events*, or internal variables such as *personality traits* and *coping styles*, other studies have sought to show how these external and internal factors may interact, culminating in the development of *theoretical models* to explain the underlying psychological and neurophysiological processes operating.

Inevitably, there has been more funding for research into possible psychosocial contributions across the widespread chronic or life-threatening illnesses such cardiovascular disease, stroke, diabetes, asthma, infectious diseases, and cancer (E. M. A. Bleiker, Van der Ploeg, Hendriks, & Adèr, 1996; Marmot & Wilkinson, 2006; Nyklicek, Temoshok, & Vingerhoets, 2004). However, more recently, attention has been given to *musculoskeletal disorders*, which represent some of the most frequently reported occupational health issues (Menzel, 2007), to *progressive neurological diseases* such as Motor Neuron Disease (McLeod & Clarke, 2007), and to dementia, representing an urgent response to our expanding elderly populations (Karp, 2005; Matsuoka & Yamaguchi, 2011).

The mental health conditions traditionally attracting attention have been the *mood disorders* related to *anxiety* and *depression* (Brown, Bifulco, & Harris, 1987; Fisher & Baum, 2010), with recent concerns over the increased suicide rates in young men in response to unemployment and job insecurity throughout the world (Page, Milner, Morrell, & Taylor, 2013). There is now a burgeoning literature with respect to *post-traumatic stress disorder (PTSD)*, whether triggered by what appears to be relatively innocuous work-place bullying (McFarlane & Bryant, 2007), or following more obviously catastrophic events related to combat in war, political persecution and migration, floods, and fire (McFarlane, 2010; van der Kolk, McFarlane, & Weisarth, 1996). Other conditions receiving attention have been the less well understood but just as disabling '*medically unexplained*', 'functional', or 'psychogenic' disorders which are estimated to account for 15–30% of medical consultations (Kirmayer, Groleau, Looper, & Dao, 2004). These include the *somatization disorders, fibromyalgia, irritable bowel disorder*, and *chronic fatigue syndromes*, and the 'functional' or *psychogenic neurologic disorders* (Akagi & House, 2001; Carson *et al.*, 2012; Hallett *et al.*, 2006; Hallett *et al.*, 2011; Halligan, 2011; Stone, 2016; Stone, Warlow, & Sharpe, 2011).

Clinical studies

Clinical studies have focused on individual or small group differences across a range of psychosocial factors and their possible associations with many physical and *mental health conditions*. These have included: prevalence and demographic profiles; the nature of stressful situations preceding onset; personality and psychological correlates that may predispose individuals to certain illnesses or ways of coping; interpersonal issues related to seeking social supports and responsiveness to intervention; and the ways in which these may be reflected in compliance and other aspects of the practitioner–patient relationship.

Epidemiological and public health programmes

Large population studies have been devoted to tracking interactions between different external social determinants and internal personal factors, as these may have led to various physical and mental health disorders either within populations or across populations on a global scale. For instance, *low socioeconomic status (SES)* is a major social determinant that is known to be a reliable correlate with poor physical health. In an extensive review of the status of the research in this area, Matthews and Gallo (2011) have critiqued the available evidence, highlighted the ambiguities or controversies, and proposed a most helpful conceptual model which seeks to explain how *psychosocial pathways* may interact with low SES and poor health, as shown in Fig.3.1.

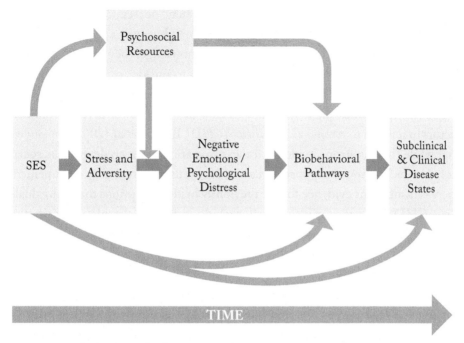

Fig. 3.1 Psychobiological influences on the socioeconomic status-health gradient (Matthews & Gallo, 2011)

Reproduced with kind permission Matthews & Gallo and Courtesy Annual Reviews®.

The model shows how low SES may trigger *stress* and the associated *psychological distress* responses, which then interact with the psychological and social resources available to that person as a possible protection against the adverse situations and the negative emotional responses elicited. These pathways are then thought to precipitate adverse biological processes and negative health behaviours that may facilitate sub-clinical illness and eventually, frank disease.

One of the most positive outcomes of these large population studies has been the co-operation between countries under the auspices of the *World Health Organization (WHO)*, with the pooling of data on prevalence and possible causal pathways, and the establishment of public policy guidelines in relation to prevention, early intervention, and management. There is now a comprehensive literature base of systematic reviews and government-funded reports led by panels of international experts whose primary objectives have been: to distil and present the strongest evidence in a clear and unequivocal manner; to highlight limitations from ambiguous data and gaps in current evidence; to raise new burning questions (Bunker *et al.*, 2003; Marmot, Allen, Bell, Bloomer, & Goldblatt, 2012).

While some of these big picture reports may be seen to diminish the significance of findings from some relatively small but well-conducted studies, even to challenge what has become accepted knowledge, they do enable health practitioners and national health authorities to reconsider earlier assumptions, and to be better informed about new trends in the scientific evidence.

For example, following a systematic review of evidence for psychosocial risk factors in relation to *coronary heart disease (CHD)*, Bunker *et al.* (2003) concluded that while there is strong evidence for an association between depression, social isolation, lack of social support, and acute life events, as previously documented, there is insufficient evidence for the previously held assumptions that individuals with CHD are necessarily exposed to high levels of chronic stress in the workplace, or that these individuals necessarily demonstrate a *Type A Personality* (typically described as being hostile, impatient, intolerant, competitive, and ambitious).

Similarly, following many years of studies implicating the *suppression* or *repression of negative emotion* and its possible association with development of breast cancer in women, Bleiker *et al.* (2008) have now clearly shown, in several large prospective population studies, that there is insufficient evidence to suggest that women who develop breast cancer are likely to reveal personality traits which reflect a reticence to express negative emotions. The findings from these two examples above are significant not only for the health practitioners involved in the care of patients with CHD or breast cancer but also, for the individuals themselves. Dealing with the diagnosis and treatments of these conditions is demanding enough, let *alone* having to cope with the additional guilt or shame of knowing that aspects of their personalities may have actively contributed to the development of their life-threatening illnesses.

Neurophysiological research investigating psychobiological pathways

Many studies using *structural* and *functional neuro-imaging* have been undertaken in animals and human beings to explain how psychosocial factors may influence the neurological and biochemical interactions between the brain and major systems of the body (Goleman & Gurin, 1995). These processes can be visualised as 'the pathways through which psychosocial factors stimulate biological systems via central nervous system activation of the autonomic, neuroendocrine and immunological responses' (Steptoe & Marmot, 2002) (p.13). This is represented in the schematic diagram below that draws upon the original source material from Marmot and Wilkinson (1999) with respect to the social determinants of health, and then on data presented by Fran Baum (2009) in a keynote address entitled '*Participation and the Social Determinants of Health: Citizen Action for Health Equity*'. The diagram highlights the complex interactions between adverse situations and personal vulnerabilities, and then on the *psychobiological stress responses* that may affect the different systems in the body, leading eventually to serious illness (see Fig. 3.2).

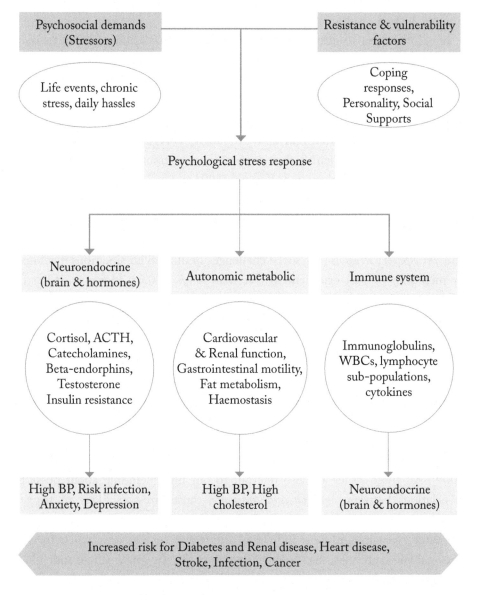

Fig. 3.2 Psychobiological Pathways-Image compiled by Baum from multiple sources, Baum (2009) and Marmot & Wilkinson (1999)

Negative emotions and cognitions and stress

There appear to be two fundamental propositions inherent in the different models and research paradigms outlined in this chapter. The first is that positive and negative emotions, and associated cognitions, are likely to affect the mind and the body. The second is that negative emotions and cognitions in response to stressors sustained over time are likely to be deleterious to our health, including mental illnesses and both organic and functional health conditions (Fava & Sonino, 2000; Kessler, 1997; Selye & Fortier, 1950).

It is interesting to note, however, that with all that is known about stress, research efforts are still being made to distinguish between the *neural correlates of emotions* as distinct from feelings, cognitions, and stress (Damasio, 2000; Dedovic, D'Aguiar, & Pruessner, 2009; Lane, 2000). Many studies have focused on ways in which the experience of negative emotions and responses to stress may manifest in the brain and body (Dedovic, D'Aguiar, *et al.*, 2009), while others have sought to identify the nature of those stressors most likely to trigger a cortisol response (Dickerson & Kemeny, 2004).

It is now acknowledged that there are different ways of distinguishing between types of stressors, such as those posing *physical* versus *psychological* threat, *reactive stressors* (e.g. bodily injury, pain, or challenge to the immune system), and *anticipatory stressors* (e.g. social challenges or unfamiliar situations mediated by memories of past experiences) (Herman *et al.*, 2003). However, it is still not entirely clear which of these stressors are most likely to influence physical health, those likely to affect mental health, and, more importantly, those that may be implicated in both. Furthermore, research efforts are still being directed towards the understanding of how responses to these different types of stressors may be influenced by individual differences as determined by *stress reactivity*, and how *personality traits*, *coping styles*, *emotional expressiveness*, *social support*, and *interpersonal relationships* may influence ways in which people react to such incidents (Dedovic, Duchesne, Andrews, Engert, & Pruessner, 2009; Nyklicek *et al.*, 2004; Vingerhoets, Nyklicek, & Denollet, 2008; Wilkinson & Pickett, 2009). All these issues are also relevant to our understanding about possible associations between *emotion and the voice*, those stressors likely to trigger negative emotions and responses in the body that impact on the respiratory and phonatory systems, and those individual differences, such as stress reactivity and personal vulnerabilities, that are likely to affect the way in which an individual copes with these external and internal challenges.

Biology of acute and chronic stress

There are numerous texts explaining the neurobiology of stress but for the purposes of this book, several key issues are highlighted for discussion. These ideas have contributed to current knowledge about the ways in which stress and negative emotions can lead to the development of physical or mental health conditions, including voice disorders.

Original stress theory as, proposed by Lazarus and Folkman (1984), suggested that animals and human beings perceive a situation as being stressful when the demands of a particular event are experienced as exceeding available resources and capacity to adapt, followed then by the feeling of stress. Broadly speaking, *stress* refers to a psychological experience that has emotional, cognitive, physiological, and behavioural consequences.

When an individual perceives the environment as being stressful, a number of responses are mediated in the brain via the limbic system and its interaction with the hypothalamic-pituitary-adrenal (HPA) axis, the autonomic nervous system, and the whole body. These effects have been referred to as allostatic load, which refers to the wear and tear on the body in response to repeated cycles of stress, and manifests in stress responses. These include physiological, cognitive, psychological, emotional, and behavioural changes, culminating in a freezing response or readiness for action with an acute fight or flight response as shown in Box 3.1. Although such an acute stress reaction may be perceived as a negative experience, it may also have relatively positive consequences, leading to adaptive healthy learning (Fisher & Baum, 2010).

On the other hand, chronic stress is reflected in a higher allostatic load and produces stabilised, dysregulated forms of chronic hyper- or hypo-activity of the stress system (Chrousos, 2009). This is thought to represent the final common pathway to disease that can be manifest in various ways (McFarlane, 2010). In the shorter term, this may begin with increased muscle tension throughout the body, headaches, insomnia, and impaired memory or concentration (Rosen & Sataloff, 1997). When repeated and prolonged over longer periods of time, the heightened stress reactivity of the HPA axis has been shown to be associated with a range of physical and mental health conditions (Chrousos, 2009; Chrousos & Gold, 1992; Marmot & Wilkinson, 2003) (Box 3.2).

Box 3.1 Acute Stress Responses

- Physiological changes which include: dilated pupils, cold sweaty palms, dry mouth, increased secretion of stomach acid; increased heart rate and blood pressure, with more blood directed to the muscles and less to organs such as the kidneys and liver; lowered perception of pain
- Endocrine changes leading to the release of hormones that mobilise energy supplies, increased insulin, adrenalin, and the core stress marker cortisol which targets both peripheral systems and central processes
- Reproductive organs temporarily suppressed
- Cognitive changes which may include heightened vigilance and attention
- Behavioural changes motivated by the perceived threat

Box 3.2 Chronic Stress Responses

- Physiological changes which include generalised muscle tension, headaches, insomnia, with longer term risks for obesity, hypertension and cardiovascular disease, stroke; altered insulin levels, diabetes and renal disease; chronic fatigue syndrome and fibromyalgia; susceptibility to infections; cancer
- Endocrine changes which trigger hyperactivity of the HPA axis; higher resting levels of stress markers such as cortisol; slower recovery from stress; lowering of the immune system functions and susceptibility to infections; slower wound healing; and autoimmune dysfunction etc.
- Reproductive changes with higher risk of infertility and miscarriage
- Cognitive changes which include: impaired sleep; poor memory; reduced concentration; lowered motivation and application to tasks of daily living
- Behavioural changes such as increased use of alcohol, tobacco, illegal drugs
- Greater risks for mental health disorders related to anxiety, depression, post-traumatic stress disorder

In a compelling discussion paper reviewing the neural correlates of *cortisol regulation in response to stress*, Dedovic *et al.* (2009) comment upon substantial evidence which indicates that stress sensitivity and responsivity of the HPA-axis (as reflected in cortisol levels) are influenced by many factors. These include genetic predisposition, personality traits, coping mechanisms, and life events in general. They also include *early adverse life experiences* during critical developmental periods, such as childhood abuse and perceptions of poor quality of early maternal care and *attachment* (Fries, Shirtcliff, & Pollak, 2008). Significantly, stress and the associated mental health disorders of anxiety and depression are reported more often by women than men, to the extent that some writers construe stress as a women's health issue (Dietrich, Verdolini Abbott, Gartner-Schmidt, & Rosen, 2008).

In seeking to identify the particular kinds of stressors that may operate as more powerful risk factors for mental illness, Fisher and Baum (2010) recently suggested that it is important to distinguish between those social determinants known to trigger reasonable levels of *acute stress conditions* which, in the short term, are not usually deleterious to health, and those conditions of stress that tip the system into a *chronic stress reaction phase* with higher risks for either physical or mental illness. In reviewing the evidence for those social determinants that may contribute to chronic stress and mental health disorders, Fisher and Baum (2010) have drawn on a series of animal studies. These have shown that where chronic stress is associated with unpredictable and inconsistent *hierarchical control* (Sapolsky, 1993) with no apparent avenue to avoid this behaviourally, coupled with chronic inescapable exposure to the sight or smell of the dominant animal, this *anxious anticipation* produces a stronger and more chronic HPA-axis activation with elevated basal levels of cortisol secretion than in controllable stressors (de Kloet, Joëls, & Holsboer, 2005; Joëls, Karst, Krugers, & Lucassen, 2007).

Fisher and Baum propose that these findings from animal studies support some of the major public health research programmes seeking to determine risk factors for serious physical and mental health disorders. They refer to the well-known Whitehall II studies conducted by Michael Marmot (2004) over a period of 15 years with 10,000 British public servants. These studies repeatedly revealed a *social gradient in health*, with those individuals at the lower end of the social scale being more likely to suffer changes to their physical and mental health. Among the salient features experienced by those lower down the social scale were the lack of control, fewer choices for work variety, and less opportunity for the use and development of skills and initiative (Bosma *et al.*, 1997).

These features associated with chronic stress have also been reflected in the conclusions drawn by Dickerson and Kemeny (2004). These authors recently conducted a comprehensive meta-analysis of over 200 laboratory studies using cortisol levels as an indicator of *psychological stress* in healthy human subjects. The accumulated evidence showed that where individuals were exposed to situations demanding high achievement coupled with social evaluation and serious consequences pending, or where there was a lack of control and anticipation of ongoing conflicting or inconsistent demands from supervisors, these chronic conditions lead to higher levels of cortisol. Both separately and together these conditions were shown to act as significant risk factors for deterioration in health.

In drawing the findings from these studies together, Fisher and Baum (2010) suggest that the shift from acute to more chronic states of arousal may occur 'when current stimulus conditions predict the possibility of a future aversive or emotionally unpleasant event, based upon prior learning, and when this is combined with a lack of perceived behavioural opportunities to decisively avoid or resolve the predicted event' (p. 1061). Consequently, chronic stress is as much about the repetitive or extended anticipation of possible unpleasant events as it is about direct exposure to such events, along with a lack of behavioural options to resolve such difficulties.

For instance, in the work place setting this may occur in the form of anticipating undermining or subtly manipulative behaviour from those with influence, with implicit threats of isolation or loss of social position. As pointed out by Fisher and Baum, an ongoing situation such as this, coupled with a person's perception that he/she has little or nothing to offer for avoiding or resolving the situation, is the other major feature of chronic stress. This may be due to a lack of cognitive or behavioural resources because of limited education or employment opportunities. Alternatively, it may be based upon past experiences, knowing that the consequences of doing something are likely to be as damaging as the consequences of doing nothing. It has been suggested that these factors support *social self-preservation theory*, which proposes that humans have a strong need to preserve their social selves (social values, esteem, and status), and that chronic stress responses are perpetuated when individuals remain alert to threats that may jeopardise this identity (Gruenewald *et al.*, 2004).

All of these factors are directly pertinent to our understanding of predisposing, precipitating or perpetuating factors in relation to voice disorders. The implications of these issues for the clinical management of voice disorders will be discussed in later chapters. A summary of features associated with chronic stress as these may affect physical and mental health, as extrapolated from the publications cited above, are shown in Box 3.3.

Box 3.3 Features of Chronic Stress Situations Affecting Physical and Mental Health

- Long-term and repeated exposure to stressful situations
- Hierarchical or social structures which promote sense of powerlessness
- Ongoing sense of little control over one's own environment and destiny
- Frequent exposure to social evaluative conditions with serious consequences
- Inconsistent but likely presence of threatening authority figures with powers of evaluative judgment
- Conscious or sub-conscious anticipatory anxiety of these threats
- Lack of personal resources to respond cognitively or behaviourally
- Previous experiences where responding was as likely to have poor consequences, as not responding at all
- Underlying vulnerability associated with memories of early adverse life situations such as abuse or poor quality of 'maternal' care (insecure attachment)
- Consistent threats to one's social values, sense of self and identity
- Serious challenge to one's self preservation

(Extrapolated from Dickerson & Kemeny, 2004; Fisher & Baum, 2010; Gruenewald, Kemeny, Aziz, & Fahey, 2004; Marmot, 2004)

Stress in relation to life events and difficulties

These recent findings delineating possible features of chronic stress serve to highlight the extensive research efforts by Brown and Harris. These began over 36 years ago with their studies using the *Life Events and Difficulties Schedule (LEDS)* to explore the Social Origins of Depression (1978). Their research programme has since been expanded, beyond the original focus on depression in women, to explore possible interactions between external socio-demographic variables and internal factors as these may then contribute to the onset of various medical conditions, both functional and organic. For instance, the LEDS has been used to explore the role of threatening life experiences with physical health conditions such as amenorrhea and breast cancer in women (Chen *et al.*, 1995; T. O. Harris, 1989; Protheroe *et al.*, 1999). It has also been used in several studies exploring functional health conditions such as digestive problems (Craig, 1989), pain in association with appendectomy (Creed, Craig, & Farmer, 1988), globus pharyngis (M. B. Harris, Deary, & Wilson, 1996), and chronic fatigue syndrome (Hatcher & House, 2003).

The vast body of Brown and Harris's work, and that of many other following studies using the LEDS, has shown that while there may be many universally recognised stressful situations that could operate as risk factors, or personality traits that could render a person more vulnerable in their ways of responding, it is the interaction between the external and internal factors that generates different degrees of negative emotion and psychological distress. Together, these interacting factors may be experienced as a direct threat or as a contribution to a sense of loss for that individual. In her book *'Where Inner and Outer Worlds Meet: Psychosocial Research in the Tradition of George W. Brown'*, Tirril Harris (2000) poignantly emphasises that it is 'through understanding the meaning' of these interactions and mediating psychological mechanisms that health professionals have now come to appreciate the ways in which people's physical and mental health is affected by their social frameworks.

Introduction to the trends in psychosocial research into voice disorders

This rich field of research into such a wide range of physical and mental health conditions serves as an excellent foundation for similar explorations into psychosocial factors that may be associated with disorders of the voice. As I have mentioned in a previous publication reviewing the evidence for the role of psychogenic and psychosocial factors in the development of functional voice disorders (FVD) (Baker, 2008), many of our earlier findings derived from single case reports and small descriptive studies. However, as discussed in this review article, the trends have changed during the last 10–15 years, with efforts to conduct more carefully designed case-control studies, larger cohort studies, and randomised control trials to assess different treatment approaches and outcomes. These more recent studies have drawn upon both qualitative and quantitative methodologies, with the use of standardised measures and more appropriate statistical analyses. It is interesting to note that much of the psychosocial research has been predominantly directed towards the FVD groups, but the climate is changing and more recently, there have been a number of studies which include organic voice disorder (OVD) groups, even if only for comparison with experimental FVD groups. The psychosocial research into other domains of physical and mental health would suggest that the additional focus on OVD would be an important direction to follow.

In the following chapters, the evidence from the different domains of psychosocial research in relation to voice disorders is presented with implications for patients and the ways in which these findings might provide options and strategies for clinicians. The findings are then discussed in relation to the development of several theoretical models that seek to explain the neural correlates of emotion, and stress and how these factors influence vocal function. Each model highlights the interactions between particular external and internal psychosocial factors that may operate as significant risk factors for the development, perpetuation, or outcomes of voice disorders. The areas of psychosocial research undertaken by a number of writers to date in relation to a number of physical and mental health conditions, including voice disorders, form a framework to guide the discussion in the following chapters. These domains are shown in Box 3.4.

Box 3.4 Psychosocial Research in relation Functional and Organic Voice Disorders (Baker, 2008)

- Prevalence and demographics of individuals with voice disorders
- Physical and mental health profiles
- Daily hassles, stressful life events, longer-term difficulties
- Personality traits and other psychological correlates
- Psychiatric co-morbidity
- Emotional expressiveness, suppression or repression of negative emotion
- Coping styles
- Interpersonal factors, social support, and attachment style
- Quality of life
- Intervention and outcome studies
- Doctor-patient relationship and therapeutic processes
- Theoretical and causal models including neural correlates of negative emotion and stress

References

Akagi, H., & House, A. (2001). Epidemiology of conversion hysteria. In P. W. Halligan, C. Bass & J. Marshall (Eds.), *Contemporary approaches to the study of hysteria.* Oxford: Oxford University Press.

Baker, J. (2008). The role of psychogenic and psychosocial factors in the development of functional voice disorders. *International Journal of Speech-Language Pathology, 10*(4), 210–230.

Baum, F. (2009). *Participation and the social determinants of health: Citizen action for health equity.* Faculty of Health Sciences. Southgate Institute for Health, Society & Equity. Available at http://healthissuescentre.org.au/images/uploads/resources/Participation-and-the-social-determinants-of-health.pdf [Accessed October 2016]

Bleiker, E. M., Hendriks, J. H., Otten, J. D., Verbeek, A. L., & van der Ploeg, H. M. (2008). Personality factors and breast cancer risk. *Journal of the National Cancer Institute, 100*(3), 213–218.

Bleiker, E. M. A., Van der Ploeg, H. M., Hendriks, J. H. C., & Adèr, H. J. (1996). Personality factors and breast cancer development: A prospective longitudinal study. *Journal of the National Cancer Institute, 88,* 1478–1482.

Bosma, B., Marmot, M. G., Hemingway, H., Nicholson, A. C., Brunner, E., & Stansfeld, S. A. (1997). Low job control and risk of coronary heart disease in Whitehall II (prospective cohort) study. *British Medical Journal, 1997,* 314–558.

Brown, G. W., Bifulco, A., & Harris, T. O. (1987). Life events, vulnerability and onset of depression: Some refinements. *British Journal of Psychiatry, 150,* 30–42.

Brown, G. W., & Harris, T. O. (1978). *Social origins of depression.* London: Tavistock Publications.

Bunker, S. J., Colquhoun, D. M., Esler, M. D., *et al.* (2003). "Stress" and coronary heart disease: Psychosocial risk factors. *Medical Journal of Australia, 178,* 272–276.

Carson, A. J., Brown, R., David, A. S., *et al.* (2012). Functional (conversion) neurological sysmptoms: Research since the millennium. *Journal of Neurology, Neurosurgery and Psychiatry, 83,* 842–850.

Chen, C. C., David, A. S., Nunnerly, H., *et al.* (1995). Adverse life events and breast cancer: Case-control study. *British Medical Journal, 311,* 1527–1530.

Chrousos, G. P. (2009). Stress and disorders of the stress system. *National Review of Endocrinology, 5,* 374–381.

Chrousos, G. P., & Gold, P. W. (1992). The concepts of stress and stress system disorders: Overview of physical and behavioural homeostasis. *Journal of the American Medical Association, 267*(9), 1244–1252.

Craig, T. K. J. (1989). Abdominal pain. In G. W. Brown & T. O. Harris (Eds.), *Life events and illness.* New York: Guilford Press.

Creed, F., Craig, T., & Farmer, R. (1988). Functional abdominal pain, psychiatric illness, and life events. *Gut, 1988*(29), 235–242.

Damasio, A. R. (2000). A second chance for emotion. In R. D. Lane & L. Nadel (Eds.), *Cognitive neuroscience of emotion* (pp. 12–23). New York: Oxford University Press.

de Kloet, E. R., Joëls, M., & Holsboer, F. (2005). Stress and the brain: From adaptation to disease. *Nature Reviews. Neuroscience, 6*, 463–475.

Dedovic, K., D'Aguiar, A., & Pruessner, J. C. (2009). What stress does to your brain: A review of neuroimaging studies. *Canadian Journal of Psychiatry, 54*, 6–14.

Dedovic, K., Duchesne, A., Andrews, J., Engert, V., & Pruessner, J. C. (2009). The brain and the stress axis: The neural correlates of cortisol regulation in response to stress. *NeuroImage, 47*, 864–871.

Dickerson, S. S., & Kemeny, M. E. (2004). Acute stressors and cortisol responses: A theoretical integration and synthesis of laboratory research. *Psychological Bulletin, 2004*(130), 355–391.

Dietrich, M., Verdolini Abbott, K., Gartner-Schmidt, J., & Rosen, C. L. (2008). The frequency of perceived stress, anxiety, and depression in patients with common pathologies affecting voice. *Journal of Voice, 22*(4), 472–487.

Fava, G. A., & Sonino, N. (2000). Psychosomatic medicine: Emerging trends and perspectives. *Psychotherapy and Psychosomatics, 69*(4), 184.

Fisher, M., & Baum, F. (2010). The social determinants of mental health: Implications for research and health promotion. *Australian and New Zealand Journal of Psychiatry, 44*, 1057–1063.

Fries, A. B., Shirtcliff, E. A., & Pollak, S. D. (2008). Neuroendocrine dysregulation following early social deprivation in children. *Developmental Psychobiology, 50*, 588–599.

Goleman, D., & Gurin, J. (Eds.). (1995). *Mind body medicine. How to use your mind for better health*. Marrickville: Choice Books.

Gruenewald, T. L., Kemeny, M. E., Aziz, N., & Fahey, J. L. (2004). Acute threat to the social self: Shame, social self-esteem, and cortisol activity. *Psychosomatic Medicine, 66*(6), 915–924.

Hallett, M., Fahn, S., Jankovic, J., Lang, A. E., Cloninger, C. R., & Yudofsky, S. C. (Eds.). (2006). *Psychogenic movement disorders: Neurology and neuropsychiatry*. Philadelphia: Lippincott Williams & Wilkins.

Hallett, M., Lang, A., Jankovic, J., Fahn, S., Halligan, P. W., Voon, V., & Cloninger, C. R. (Eds.). (2011). *Psychogenic movement disorders and other conversion disorders*. Cambridge: Cambridge University Press.

Halligan, P. W. (2011). Psychogenic movement disorders: Illness in search of disease? In M. Hallet, A. E. Lang, J. Jankovic, S. Fahn, P. W. Halligan, V. Voon & C. R. Cloninger (Eds.), *Psychogenic movement disorders and other conversion disorders* (pp. 120–133). Cambridge: Cambridge University Press.

Harris, M. B., Deary, I. J., & Wilson, J. A. (1996). Life events and difficulties in relation to the onset of globus pharyngis. *Journal of Psychosomatic Research, 40*, 603–615.

Harris, T. (Ed.). (2000). *Where inner and outer worlds meet. Psychosocial research in the tradition of George Brown*. London: Routledge.

Harris, T. O. (1989). Disorders of menstruation. In G. W. Brown & T. O. Harris (Eds.), *Life events and illness*. London: The Guilford Press.

Hatcher, S., & House, A. (2003). Life events, difficulties and dilemmas in the onset of chronic fatigue syndrome: A case–control study. *Psychological Medicine, 33*, 1185–1192.

Herman, J. P., Figueiredo, H., Mueller, N. K., Ulrich-Lai, Y., Ostrander, M. M., Choi, D. C., & Cullinan, W. E. (2003). Central mechanisms of stress integration: Hierarchical circuitry controlling hypothalamic-pituitary-adrenocortical responsiveness. *Frontiers in Endocrinology, 24*, 151–180.

Joëls, M., Karst, H., Krugers, J. J., & Lucassen, P. J. (2007). Chronic stress: Implicatons for neuronal morphology, function and neurogenesis. *Frontiers in Neuroendocrinology, 28*(2–3):72–96.

Karp, A. (2005). *Psychosocial factors in relation to development of dementia in late-life: A life course approach within the Kungsholmen Project.* (Ph.D. thesis), Karolinska Institutet, Stockholm.

Kessler, R. C. (1997). The effects of stressful life events on depression. *Annual Review of Psychology, 48*, 191–214.

Kirmayer, L. J., Groleau, D., Looper, K. L., & Dao, M. D. (2004). Explaining medically unexplained symptoms. *Canadian Journal of Psychiatry, 49*(10), 663–671.

Lane, R. D. (2000). Neural correlates of conscious emotional experience. In R. D. Lane & L. Nadel (Eds.), *Cognitive neuroscience of emotion.* (pp. 345–370). Oxford: Oxford University Press.

Lazarus, R. L., & Folkman, S. (1984). *Stress appraisal and coping.* New York: Springer.

Marmot, M. (2004). *Status syndrome: How your social standing directly affects your health and life expectancy.* London: Bloomsbury.

Marmot, M., Allen, J., Bell, R., Bloomer, E., & Goldblatt, P. (2012). WHO European review of social determinants of health and the health divide. *Lancet, 380*(9846), 1011–1029.

Marmot, M., & Wilkinson, R. (2006). *Social determinants of health* (2nd ed.). Oxford: Oxford University Press.

Marmot, M., & Wilkinson, R. (Eds.). (1999). *Social determinants of health.* Oxford: Oxford Universtiy Press.

Marmot, M., & Wilkinson, R. (Eds.). (2003). *Social determinants of health: The solid facts.* Geneva: World Health Organization.

Matsuoka, H., & Yamaguchi, H. (2011). Path dependence in social and psychological risk factors for dementia. *Dementia Psychologia, 5*(1), 2–7.

Matthews, K. A., & Gallo, L. C. (2011). Psychological perspectives on pathways linking socioeconomic status and physical health. *Annual Review of Psychology, 62*, 501–530.

McFarlane, A. (2010). The long-term costs of traumatic stress: intertwined physical and psychological consequences. *World Psychiatry, 9*, 3–10.

McFarlane, A., & Bryant, R. A. (2007). Post-traumatic stress disorder in occupational settings: Anticipating and managing the risk. *Occupational Medicine, 57*(6), 404–410.

McLeod, J. E., & Clarke, D. M. (2007). A review of psychosocial aspects of motor neurone disease. *Journal of Neurological Sciences, 258*, 4–10.

Menzel, N. N. (2007). Psychosocial factors in musculoskeltal disorders. *Critical Care Nursing Clinics North America, 19*(2), 145–153.

Nyklicek, I., Temoshok, L., & Vingerhoets, A. (Eds.). (2004). *Emotional expression and health.* Hove: Brunner-Routledge.

Page, A., Milner, A., Morrell, S., & Taylor, R. (2013). The role of under-employment and unemployment in recent birth cohort effects in Australian suicide. *Social Science and Medicine, 93*, 155–162.

Protheroe, D., Turvey, K., Horgan, K., Benson, E., Bowers, D., & House, A. (1999). Stressful life events and difficulties and onset of breast cancer: Case-control study. *British Medical Journal, 319*.

Rosen, D. C., & Sataloff, R. T. (1997). *Psychology of voice disorders.* San Diego: Singular Publishing Group.

Sapolsky, R. M. (1993). Endocrinology alfresco: Psychoendocrine studies of wild baboons. *Recent Progress in Hormone Research, 48*, 437–468.

Selye, H., & Fortier, C. (1950). Adaptive reaction to stress. *Psychosomatic Medicine, 12*(3), 149–157.

Steptoe, A., & Marmot, M. (2002). The role of psychobiological pathways in socio-economic inequalities in cardiovascular disease and risk. *European Heart Journal, 23*, 13–25.

Stone, J. (2016). Functional neurological disorders: The neurological assessment as treatment. *Practical Neurology, 16*, 7–17. doi: 10.1136/practneurol-2015-001241

Stone, J., Warlow, C., & Sharpe, M. (2011). Functional weakness: Clues to mechanism from the nature of onset. *Journal of Neurology, Neurosurgery and Psychiatry*. doi: 10.1136/jnnp-2011-300125

van der Kolk, B., McFarlane, A., & Weisarth, L. (1996). *Traumatic stress.* New York: The Guilford Press.

Vingerhoets, A., Nyklicek, I., & Denollet, J. (Eds.). (2008). *Emotion regulation: Conceptual and clinical issues.* New York: Springer.

Wade, D. T., & Halligan, P. W. (2004). Do biomedical models of illness make for good healthcare systems? *British Medical Journal, 329*(11), 1398–1401.

Wilkinson, R., & Pickett, K. (2009). *The spirit level: Why more equal societies almost always do better.* London: Penguin.

4

Prevalence, demographics and biographical details of individuals with voice disorders

Introduction

'The patient's essential being is very relevant in the higher reaches of neurology and psychology; for here the patient's personhood is essentially involved, and the study of disease and identity cannot be disjoined' (Sacks, 1985) (Preface, p. x).

As we begin to consider many of the psychosocial factors associated with disorders of the voice, perhaps the first question we need to ask is 'Who are our patients?' An awareness of the prevalence of voice disorders in the general population and within specific sub-groups is an important first step. Secondly, an appreciation of the demographics and biographical details of individuals with voice disorders is essential because without having a sense of who these people are, I would suggest we risk becoming merely technicians.

In this chapter I refer to estimates for the *prevalence of voice disorders* in relation to: 1) the general population, 2) specific occupational groups where more reliable estimates have been made, and 3) clinical sub-groups where such data are available. I then discuss the paucity of biographical details often gathered in relation to people with voice disorders, highlighting trends in the demographic data where these have been obtained. It is suggested that we need to be more rigorous in recording *biographical details* about our patients and research participants. This knowledge will enhance the voice practitioner's understanding of the different kinds of voice disorders, and may also influence ways of helping patients and their families to resolve these problems more effectively.

Who are our patients?

'Of the many meanings of voice in our lives, perhaps the most important is that it lies at the heart of our personal identity, as indelibly implanted in our consciousness as our faces' Arnold E. Aronson (2009) (Preface to the Fourth Edition, p. x).

In thinking about the patients that we seek to help, I am reminded of two other significant experiences that have shaped my practice and affirmed my research into psychosocial factors in relation to voice disorders. Throughout my entire career I have been inspired by the writings of Dr Arnold Aronson and many years ago, I had the privilege of spending five days with him at the Mayo Clinic in Minnesota. I was permitted to sit in on assessment sessions with his patients, all of whom had been referred to the Mayo Clinic with very complex voice disorders. Here, I was able to observe Dr Aronson obtain extensive biographical details, carry out a formal assessment of the vocal problem, explore sensitive psychosocial issues and then offer his opinion and recommendations. While already convinced from my reading and limited experience that attention to psychosocial perspectives should be an integral part of all of our work as *speech-language pathologists (SLP)*, it was both inspirational and extremely humbling to see a *master clinician* at work. I have continued to believe that there is no substitute in our clinical education and later, during our clinical practice, for observing a master clinician at work.

Dr Aronson recorded his notes in meticulous printed handwriting on tiny cards held discretely in the palm of his hand. At the end of the session, he drew together all the medical, neurophysiological, and psychological issues, with explanations about how these different factors might be interacting to account for the clinical presentation of that person's voice problem. This was communicated to his patient in a manner that exemplified his *holistic approach* to understanding voice disorders, with a genuine appreciation of the person, his or her family, and his or her wider *social context*.

Several aspects of this experience seemed particularly remarkable to me. First, at no time did any patient behave as though the biographical and personal questions relating to psychosocial issues were unduly intrusive or inappropriate. Secondly, all the patients responded as though they appreciated Dr Aronson taking the time to enquire about their concerns, and to understand a little more about their lives and the impact that the voice problem was having on them and their close ties. Thirdly, after each session I had a sense of having met a person, and his or her family whether they were present or not. I came away with the strong conviction that if we are to help patients to understand the meaning of their voice problem in a way that resonates with who they are we must begin by obtaining rich biographical details and when the time is right, explore their psychosocial issues further.

The other transformational experience occurred more recently when I went to Washington DC to attend the *Psychogenic Movement Disorder Conference* and managed to obtain a ticket to a jazz concert. I have often found that in seeking to understand how best to help our patients it is often in stepping outside one's traditional milieu that alternative ways of thinking become possible. A concert with a jazz band and trumpeter was a bit off the beaten track from my usual classical music orientation and naturally, too, my mind was buzzing with all things psychological as befits a diligent delegate attending a conference about psychogenic or medically unexplained movement and pain disorders. The concert was held at the John F. Kennedy Center and to my delight was to be led by the world famous trumpeter Wynton Marsalis, who was also going to deliver the Nancy Hanks Lecture on Arts and Public Policy. All of this was somewhat unexpected and seemingly far away from any philosophical musings about psychogenic movement and related voice disorders.

Marsalis delivered a most erudite and scholarly oration. He spoke about the journey travelled by black Americans from slavery to the present time with new hope for people across the world engendered by the election of the President, Barak Obama. He reminded the almost exclusively white audience, all dressed in their elegant black suits and evening dress, of America's cultural heritage, with so much of it founded on 'black music', and how music and arts unites people across generations. He then slipped into the nitty-gritty, protesting against government cuts to funding for the performing arts across all sectors of the community, and especially in schools (see Fig. 4.1).

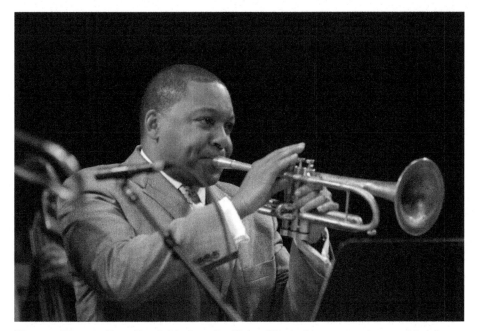

Fig. 4.1 Wynton Marsalis, delivering the Nancy Hanks Lecture on Arts and Public Policy (2009)

Photo Jim Saah, reproduced with kind permission.

Wynton Marsalis and his band punctuated his passionate speech with musical excerpts that had the audience laughing and crying and tapping their feet and, as so often happens when situations are experienced with such heightened emotion, it was both thrilling and unforgettable. He said many things that were serious, moving and inspiring, but for the purposes of this discussion I would like to highlight one of the points that I found particularly relevant. He said:

> *'Great art forms come out of people's experience with their own environments, with their way of life and their need to express their attitude about their very existence... if an artist sings deep enough he takes you to the frontiers of your soul... and while the American Constitution told us **what we are**, artists speak about the undeniable truth about where we belong and who we are, and **it is who we are that matters**'. Wynton Marsalis* (Personal communication, March 30, 2009).

Although many years apart, these two transformational experiences have served to highlight another of my basic tenets: that if we are to be effective in helping our patients to find their 'lost voice', both real and metaphorical, we need to have a sense of who they are, where they have come from, and the meaning of this loss of voice both to the person seeking help and to those around them.

Prevalence and broad psychosocial implications of voice disorders

Understanding the prevalence of voice disorders is a good place to start as this enables us to appreciate those populations most at risk. We can then consider possible causal pathways and make recommendations for prevention and the most appropriate forms of intervention. Voice problems are common and we know from personal and clinical experience that loss of voice has debilitating effects on communication in close relationships and the wider social context.

Voice disorders in children have been associated with developmental and behavioural problems, with implications for participation in the classroom, peer relationships, and communication with teachers (Ramig & Verdolini, 1998). Disorders of the voice in *children* often increase feelings of sadness, anxiety, and self-consciousness (Connor *et al.*, 2008), and when persisting into *adolescence*, they may lead to embarrassment and low self-esteem, with subtle behavioural strategies reflected in withdrawal or isolation from peers and school activities (Baker, 2002a). At the other extreme, in *elderly adults* recent preliminary findings suggest that voice disorders affect quality of life due to the 'increased effort and discomfort, combined with increased anxiety and frustration' with requests to repeat utterances (Roy, Stemple, Merrill, & Thomas, 2007).

In adults, voice problems often affect relationships with immediate and extended family members, work colleagues, and community relationships. For some people, a voice disorder may lead them to withdraw from their normal social activities and for others, it can compromise their capacity to carry out their work. For those adults, such as teachers, who rely on their voices as their primary tools of trade, or for those who depend on the excellence of their voices for artistic performance, such as singers, a voice disorder can be emotionally traumatic with serious implications for health, employment, and financial security. In more extreme cases it may mean the end of their chosen career (Rosen & Sataloff, 1997). Perhaps most alarmingly of all, the effects on many individuals with voice disorders have been shown to be similar to those experienced by individuals with more life-threatening illnesses (Smith *et al.*, 1996; Yiu, 2002). While these broad psychosocial and economic ramifications have been recognised for some time, they are of sufficient magnitude to confirm that disorders of the voice are now a significant public health issue (Baker, 1991; Roy, Merrill, Gray, & Smith, 2005; Russell, Oates, & Greenwood, 2005; Vilkman, 2000).

General population

The true prevalence of voice disorders in the general population still remains uncertain, and there are marked discrepancies in estimates both for the general population and for specific voice disorder groups. This is due to the different ways in which 'voice disorder' or 'voice problem' has been defined, the different methodologies in sampling procedures including target populations and sample sizes, and importantly, whether the judgment has been made on the basis of self-report of voice problems or professional diagnosis of a voice disorder (Roy et al., 2005). Perhaps the best we can do is to extrapolate from trends in the data from a number of prevalence studies across the world in the following areas: 1) the general population, 2) occupational groups known to be at risk of voice disorders, and 3) within specific voice disorder sub-groups where such data are available.

A broad overview of prevalence studies from Australia and a number of other Western countries shows that prevalence of voice disorders in the general population ranges between 3 and 17%, taking into account that some of these studies included adults and children, and allowing for differences in terms of reference and methodologies as outlined above (Aronson & Bless, 2009; Mathieson, 2001; Ramig & Verdolini, 1998; Roy et al., 2004a; Russell et al., 2005). Recent statistics compiled by ASHA (2008) indicate that if an average is taken from studies across the world, including estimates for life-time, year and point prevalence, then the prevalence of voice disorders in the general population is approximately 10%, making disorders of the voice the most commonly occurring communication disorder across the lifespan (Titze & Verdolini Abbott, 2012). When we consider the relatively low weighting given to topics related to voice disorders in the curricula for SLP courses as reported by many academics and practitioners in the edited volume *International Perspectives on Voice Disorders* (Yiu, 2013), and as we note the markedly diminishing priority given to provision of services for the treatment for voice disorders in many of our teaching hospitals and community based-health centres, this is a most troubling anomaly.

Prevalence of voice disorders in occupational groups at risk

It is readily acknowledged that for many occupational groups such as teachers, performers, ministers, aerobics teachers, auctioneers, and politicians etc., the voice is the primary tool of trade. For others, such as doctors, therapists, sport coaches, and sales personnel, the use of the voice is required for major components of the job. Recent figures from the Bureau of Labor Statistics in the US indicate that approximately 25% of the working population (30 million people) rely on their voices for some essential aspects of their work (Titze, Lemke, & Montequin, 1997; U.S. Department of Labor, 2008). With these factors in mind, it has been suggested 'that loss or serious impairment of voice constitutes an occupational limitation similar to limb loss in the industrial age' (Titze & Verdolini Abbott, 2012, p.15).

Teaching is reported to be one of the most common occupations in many Western countries, and in view of the heavy vocal load undertaken by teachers on a daily and yearly basis, teachers have been identified as a high-risk group for voice disorders. Consequently, the *prevalence of voice problems in teachers* has been the focus of numerous studies from around the world (Angelillo, Di Maio, Costa, Angelillo, & Barillari, 2009; de Jong *et al.*, 2006; Roy *et al.*, 2004a; Russell, Oates, & Greenwood, 1998; Smith, Kirchner, Taylor, Hoffman, & Lemke, 1998a; Vilkman, 2000). Extrapolating reliable estimates of the prevalence of voice disorders for teachers is somewhat fraught because of the diversity in terms of reference and methodologies used, and the various distinctions between life, career, year, and point prevalence. However, in reviewing several key trends in the various prevalence studies cited above, and with recent financial data justifying a major prevention programme conducted in Australia, it is now possible to appreciate the magnitude of this problem and understand a little more about who these people are (Pemberton, 2010; Pemberton, McCormack, & Comensoli, 2009). Some trends in the estimates extrapolated from the references cited above are summarised in Box 4.1.

Box 4.1 General trends in the prevalence of voice problems in teachers

- Teachers represent a significant component of the employed workforce
- Teachers are significantly more at risk for self-reported voice problems and diagnosed voice disorders than general population (3 to 5 times more likely)
- Teachers are 32 times more likely to seek referral to voice centres relative to their representation in the workforce, and in comparison to non-teachers
- Teachers have higher point, year, career, and lifetime prevalence than non-teachers, with 20% of teachers experiencing voice problems each year
- Female teachers outnumber male teachers throughout the world
- Female teachers are two times more likely to report voice problems than male teachers (*a similar pattern in the general population*)
- Teachers between 40 and 60 years of age are more prone to experiencing voice problems (*a similar pattern in non-teachers*)
- Teachers are more prone to voice problems in the first 5 years and after 15 years of teaching
- Teachers of the performing arts, physical education, languages, and those teaching at pre-school and primary schools most commonly report voice problems
- Annual cost of vocal injury to teachers based upon sick leave is approximately AS$55,000,000 (Australia)
- Workers' compensation estimates are AS$44,000 per claim (NSW, Australia)
- Voice problems in teachers are generally related to vocal load and phono-trauma and would *generally* be classified as FVD (MTVD sub-group)

(Extrapolated from data collated by Pemberton (2010)).

Prevalence of particular voice disorders in clinical populations

It is difficult to draw definitive conclusions about the prevalence of organic voice disorders (OVD) as distinct from the broad heterogeneous group of functional voice disorders (FVD), and from the estimates for the general population. Furthermore, as different clinics attract particular patient groups it is unlikely that the true prevalence of specific voice disorder sub-groups throughout the world is known. However, there are trends emerging in the treatment-seeking populations, both from anecdotal reports of individual clinicians and from estimates for different geographical catchment areas. These relate primarily to the relative proportions of patients with OVD versus FVD, and to some extent between the FVD sub-groups of muscle tension voice disorder (MTVD) and psychogenic voice disorder (PVD). Some detailed estimates of prevalence, incidence, likely ages of onset, and gender ratios for specific voice disorders are documented in a number of excellent seminal texts and diagnostic classification systems where such information is currently available (Aronson & Bless, 2009; Mathieson, 2001; Verdolini, Rosen, & Branski, 2006). It is perhaps significant to note how often this basic information is not systematically determined.

However, if we consider the broad picture there does seem to be some consensus. For instance, estimates from The Glasgow Infirmary in Scotland suggest a 'substantial proportion' suffer from FVD (Wilson, Deary, & MacKenzie, 1995). In the US it is suggested that at least 10–40% of any caseload are likely to be diagnosed with FVD, acknowledging that these figures include a diversity of terminologies to classify the FVD patients (Roy, 2003). Data from the UK give estimates for 50,000 new cases of dysphonia per year with FVD diagnosed 'most commonly' (Carding, 2003), and according to Oates (2000), the majority of patients seeking help for a voice disorder across many countries are troubled by 'non-organic' or FVD. Following an audit of patients diagnosed according to the Diagnostic Classification System of Voice disorders (DCSVD) (Baker, Ben-Tovim, Butcher, Esterman, & McLaughlin, 2007) at one teaching hospital in South Australia between 2003 and 2006, 60% (n = 232/396) had a FVD and 40% (n = 164/396) had an OVD. Within the total FVD group of 232 patients, 91% (n = 211/232) were diagnosed with MTVD and 9% (n = 21/232) with PVD. Therefore, while there are no widely accepted figures for the prevalence of either FVD or OVD, it appears there are substantially more individuals likely to experience a FVD in the general population, and particularly within occupational groups where use of the voice is fundamental to the work required.

Prevalence of voice disorders in relation to gender and age

If we then view these broad trends in the data from a psychosocial perspective, one or two significant demographic features emerge. The first is the *preponderance of women* reporting vocal problems. Across the larger prevalence studies for the general population, and within occupational groups such as teachers or clinical treatment-seeking populations, females are approximately twice as likely to report and seek help for voice problems than males (Mathieson, 2001; Roy *et al.*, 2005; Russell *et al.*, 2005; Russell *et al.*, 1998). Amongst clinical populations, Morton and Watson (1998) suggest that women comprise approximately 76% of voice referrals to voice specialists. Furthermore, in a comprehensive review of literature dating from 1870 to 2005 focusing on psychogenic and psychosocial aetiological factors that may contribute to the onset of FVD (Baker, 2008), within the broad group of FVD, females were shown to present more often than males in ratios ranging from 2:1 to 19:1 (Gerritsma, 1991; White, Deary, & Wilson, 1997), and within the PVD sub-group, at a ratio of at least 8:1, females to males (Aronson, Peterson, & Litin, 1964; Baker, 2002b; Wilson *et al.*, 1995).

It needs to be acknowledged here that there are exceptions to this pattern. Boys are more likely to present with FVD characterised by hyperfunctional vocal problems and vocal nodules than girls. Significantly too, with respect to some OVDs where structural pathologies such as malignant vocal fold lesions, keratosis, and recurrent papillomatosis are found, these conditions present more commonly in males than in women (Verdolini *et al.*, 2006). In developed countries, men are seven times more likely to be diagnosed with laryngeal cancer than women, with risk factors such as heavy tobacco smoking, alcohol consumption, and lower SES, educational achievement, and aging have been shown to operate (Bickford, Coveney, Baker, & Hersh, 2012). This in itself should raise searching questions about those factors that may contribute to this different psychosocial profile for men and the development of this life-threatening condition.

The second noteworthy trend relates to the higher prevalence of women with voice problems between the ages of 40 and 60 both within the general population and occupational groups such as teachers (Pemberton *et al.*, 2009; Roy *et al.*, 2004a; Roy *et al.*, 2004b; Russell *et al.*, 1998). Furthermore, in that same review of the literature cited above (Baker, 2008), women's ages ranged from 13 to 81 years (mean age 40 years) across all studies and in males, from 21 to 71 years (mean age 47 years).

This profile reflecting a higher prevalence of voice problems in women, peaking at a particular time of their lives (40 to 60 years of age), raises some interesting issues. Recent explanations for the increased prevalence amongst females in general often refer to structural differences in laryngeal physiology. These differences contribute to the higher frequency of vocal fold vibration used by women, coupled with typically lower levels of *hyaluronic acid*, which normally assists with shock absorption in tissues. They may thus render females more prone to *vocal injury*, *reduced wound healing* and *increased scarring* after phonotrauma (Butler, Hammond, & Gray, 2001; Hunter, Smith, & Tanner, 2011; Titze, Hunter, & Svec, 2007).

These explanations are entirely relevant, especially when considering how early on in many careers with high vocal load, vocal skills and fitness need to be developed to manage these high demands. This might be one possible explanation for the higher prevalence of voice problems in teachers in the first 5 years of their careers, as noted by Pemberton (2010). Furthermore, if we consider possible reasons for the second increase in prevalence noted after 15 or more years in vocally-demanding careers, this is a time when vocal stamina needs to be maintained along with the inevitable 'wear and tear' that would accompany repetitive physical activity of any kind over so many years.

However, it may also be relevant to consider another hypothesis. I would suggest that in addition to the physiological factors, there are a number of psychosocial issues likely to be confronting many women at that point in their career when they have been teaching or doing other forms of vocally and psychologically demanding work for 15 years or more. Ironically too, this stage of women's careers would also place them generally in that 40 to 60 year-old age bracket where prevalence rates for voice problems in women, both in the general population and teaching professions, have been shown to be high (Roy *et al.*, 2004a; Russell *et al.*, 1998). These psychosocial factors might relate to confidence over security of employment, promotion and leadership, changes in workplace expectations, shifts in processes and leadership structures, and being in or out of control with anxieties about one's destiny in the large ever-changing workplace environment. These scenarios are not unlike those depicted in the previous chapters, with work situations known to contribute to *anticipatory chronic stress* and a threat to self preservation.

Also, during this pivotal stage in an individual's and family's life cycle, we might anticipate that women would be coping with many psychosocial factors in relation to their own physical and mental health (such as hormonal changes), and also in relation to others for whom they have considerable responsibilities of one kind or another. These people may include partners, children, parents, extended family members, confidantes, and significant community members. It is for these very reasons that obtaining comprehensive *demographic information* and *biographical details* about our patients or research participants is so crucial. I would suggest, that without this information we have little sense of who our patients are, the meaning that their voice problem has for them, and the implications of this, both for themselves and others.

Limited biographical details about individuals with FVD and their social context

'You can know the number of houses and trees in every street, but you need to know what it's like to live there – the nature of the street – you have to understand the person, not the issue' (Mark Textor, Political Analyst, One Plus One, Australian Broadcasting Commission – personal communication, September 29, 2013).

The recent review of the literature cited above (Baker, 2008) included references to 42 single case reports, 19 case series, and 18 comparative group studies published between 1870 and 2005. While not exhaustive it was reasonably comprehensive in referring to the key purpose of each study, the patient groups involved, and an estimate of the *Levels of Evidence* emerging from the key findings. The emphases of these studies reflected *psychosocial theories of causality* with respect to FVD that included: negative emotions following stressful life events; predisposing personality traits and ways of coping; ambivalence over expressing negative emotions; and the development of tensional symptoms resulting in poorly regulated laryngeal muscle tension patterns. The most startling discovery was the absolute dearth of systematically reported demographic and biographical data about this clinical population. Furthermore, any available information was documented somewhat haphazardly and could only be determined by extrapolation. In the majority of single case reports, descriptive case series, or case control studies, only two biographical features were regularly documented. These were *age* and gender. It should be noted that the review cited above did not include the substantial literature with regard to prevalence and risk factors for *occupational voice disorders*, such as teachers who commonly present with FVD. In some of the more recent studies related to specific occupational groups at risk, it is evident that more detailed demographic information *has* been sought with respect to employment, educational background, and socioeconomic status (Roy *et al.*, 2004a; Verdolini & Ramig, 2001).

Occupation

With respect to *occupation*, amongst the 42 single case reports in the review cited above (Baker, 2008) employment of patients was only mentioned in 60% of the cases, with a weak trend towards the 'helping' or 'educational' professions in female patients, and insufficient numbers of males to comment upon any trend. Across 19 of the descriptive case series, only two studies provided specific and complete occupation data, and in two others related to 'war neuroses of the larynx', it was reasonable to extrapolate that the men were soldiers on active military service (Andersson & Schalen, 1998; Schalen & Andersson, 1992; Smurthwaite, 1919; Sokolowsky & Junkermann, 1944). Several of the comparative studies mentioned percentages of their samples being employed in occupations of 'high vocal demand' (House & Andrews, 1987), or as being represented in 'a range of occupations', without being specific as to the numbers and percentages in each (McHugh-Munier, Scherer, Lehmann, & Scherer, 1997). In the majority of the studies, data for the occupations of participants were not reported at all. This omission of occupation in the demographic and biographical data does seem very strange, especially when we consider how much of a person's time is spent at work where interpersonal issues and psychosocial factors are fundamental to day-to-day experiences.

Educational and socioeconomic status

In a similar vein, this literature review also exposed the dearth of information with respect to the *educational levels* and *socioeconomic status (SES)* of patients with FVD. In commenting upon the occupations of 74 of his male and female patients with FVD, Brodnitz (1969) alluded to the fact that a number of them were teachers, doctors, and secretaries and that at the time of his reporting, 'no clinic catering to patients on a lower social level has reported any significant number of cases' (p. 1246). In my opinion, Brodnitz has been one of the most thorough clinicians in seeking and reporting explicit biographical information about his patients, and while the language used in his observation above may bring a gentle smile to the mind, it can also be concluded that in his experience, which is vast, patients with FVD were generally middle class!

A similar conclusion can also be extrapolated from the recent studies cited earlier in this chapter in relation to voice problems in specific occupational groups such as teachers or *professional voice users*. Here, the majority of individuals would probably be diagnosed with a FVD – either MTVD or PVD – (Oates, 2000, 2005), and from this we might conclude that many voice patients participating in the occupational health studies came from a middle SES with education to tertiary levels.

There was a somewhat paradoxical picture with regard to PVD and in particular, where patients had been diagnosed with *conversion reaction* or *hysterical aphonia*. As pointed out by Akagi and House (2001) in their systematic critique of the literature on the epidemiology of hysterical conversion, Freud's patients with hysterical conversion were essentially from a middle class background, and 'hysteria' had been assumed to be an 'illness of affluence' (p. 80). However, other epidemiological studies have shown the condition to be more common in those of a lower SES (Folks, Ford, & Regan, 1984) and in a subsequent study exploring the social demographic and clinical details of 25 patients with hysterical aphonia in India (Bhatia & Vaid, 2000), the majority of cases had only been educated to primary or high school level. In another study exploring sociodemographic characteristics of 164 patients diagnosed with hysterical conditions, including patients with hysterical aphonia, although the illness occurred in all educational groups 'the illiterate predominated over all others' (Jain, Verma, Solanki, & Sidana, 2000), (p. 396).

Therefore, on the basis of those studies reviewed up until 2005 that were specifically devoted to exploring psychosocial factors contributing to FVD, it was only possible to suggest that most individuals with FVD in Western society were educated to high school levels, but that in specific occupational groups such as teachers the majority would be educated to tertiary levels. There was no clear indication of SES or educational levels of individuals with PVD that included those diagnosed with conversion reaction aphonia.

Relationship status and current family constellation

In this same review of the literature, there were virtually no data regularly sought or reported for individuals with FVD with respect to their *relationship status*, the numbers, ages and sex of children in their care, or their *current family constellation*. These details were sometimes deeply embedded in a number of the single case reports, but virtually no such data were systematically reported in the majority of group studies. Drawing on estimates and extrapolations from the limited information above, it was only possible to suggest that approximately 54–76% of individuals with FVD were in a 'formal' conjugal relationship of some kind, 12–18% were divorced or separated at the time of assessment, and 10–25% were single or living alone. These figures are comparable with those taken from the *Australian Bureau of Statistics (ABS)* in South Australia (Trewin, 2001).

This paucity of data with regard to relationship status of individuals with FVD, and the absence of any information with respect to children in their care, was a staggering finding, particularly when we consider how the developmental stages of children and the life cycle of the parental relationship and family as a whole can make such different demands on individuals at various times. It was all the more curious in the light of the numerous anecdotal comments by clinicians regarding those women that develop FVD in relation to stressful events characterised by conflicts over discipline of adolescent children and conflicts with family members (Butcher & Cavalli, 1998; Seifert & Kollbrunner, 2005), or problems with communication of negative emotions with partners and others close to them (Andersson & Schalen, 1998; Aronson, 1990; Baker, 1998, 2003; Butcher, Elias, & Raven, 1993; House & Andrews, 1988).

Family-of-origin including ethnic and cultural background

Similarly, very few systematically recorded demographic data in relation to *family-of-origin* were obtained for individuals with FVD in terms of: parents' physical and mental health status, whether they were alive or deceased, and time of death; numbers, ages, and health of siblings in the patient's family, and their order in the family. Significantly, there were no data regarding history of *sexual abuse*, exposure to *violence* or *traumatic stress experience*, other than in several isolated case reports (Aronson, 1990; Baker, 2003; Butcher *et al.*, 1993) and in those studies outlining the unusual cases of FVD experienced by men during times of war (Barker, 1991; Smurthwaite, 1919; Sokolowsky & Junkermann, 1944). While it was possible to extrapolate from the authors of the respective studies in the literature review country of origin and probable language spoken at home, only two of the studies specifically differentiated between patients being designated as 'black' or 'white'. In general, there was no information about family-of-origin or the ethnic and cultural background of research participants with FVD.[1]

This dearth of demographic data in relation to family and the wider social context for individuals with voice disorders seems most alarming, especially when we note that almost every study exploring psychosocial factors related to individuals presenting with FVD begins with the premise that stressful life circumstances, psychological correlates, personality traits or psychiatric co-

---

1 In more recent studies conducted since this literature review details regarding race and ethnicity have sometimes been included (Dietrich, Verdolini Abbott, Gartner-Schmidt, & Rosen, 2008).

morbidity may contribute in some way to onset and course of the disorder. These same factors are also thought likely to contribute to the aggravation, perpetuation, or longer-term outcomes for all individuals with voice disorders, both functional and organic. The omission of so much basic personal data seems all the more ironic because we know from so many other areas of physical and mental health research that the current family constellation and extended family members influence interpersonal relationships both at work and at home, with the inevitable potential to impact upon physical and mental health. So, too, do issues related to family-of-origin and wider sociocultural systems which might include details about prior traumatic experiences, ethnicity, religious faith, and cultural factors.[2]

With so little biographical and demographic information available in much of our published literature there is a sense that people with voice disorders are viewed as individuals of a certain age and gender, possibly in a particular occupation, living in a somewhat disembodied, social, and contextual vacuum. I would suggest that if we are to be truly effective as clinicians, sensitivity to such issues is not only desirable, it is essential.

Demographic profiles of women with functional and organic voice disorders

As a way of supporting this suggestion, the form that we developed for collecting a range of biographic and demographic details in a recent study (Baker *et al.*, 2013) is shown in Fig. 4.2.

Here, we investigated a range of *psychosocial risk factors* that may contribute to onset, and differentiated between a group of women with FVD (*n* = 73) and OVD (*n* = 55) and a control group of women with no voice disorders (*n* = 66). The form included information about the patient, her current family situation, a little about her family-of-origin, and some sensitive information in relation to any experience of sexual abuse or violence, including strangulation, in her lifetime.[3] For the purposes of this discussion, a number of the key features from

---

2   This is particularly relevant throughout the world at the present when literally hundreds of thousands of people are choosing to migrate or are seeking asylum in countries other than their own, either following catastrophes related to earthquake, fire, drought or flood, or due to politically oppressive regimes and civil wars in their countries of origin.

3   The full details of this biographical information, both in relation to those with FVD and OVD and controls, and then in relation to the FVD sub-groups, MTVD (*n* = 36) and PVD (*n* = 37, are to be found in the reference as cited above.

Name _____ Age: _____
DOB_____
Country of Birth_____
Year person arrived in Australia_____
Language spoken at home now_____
Language spoken during childhood_____

Education
☐ Secondary
☐ Tafe/Trade School
☐ College of Advanced Education
☐ University

Occupation_____ Employment status ☐ Yes ☐ No
How long in present job? _____ (months)   In present occupation?_____ (years)
☐ FT ____ Hours/wk.   ☐ PT ____Hours/wk.

If retired, previous occupation_____
☐ Worker's Compensation   ☐ Medico-legal   ☐ Health Insurance Cover

Occupation of spouse/partner_____
Employment status   ☐ Yes   ☐ No
☐ FT ___ Hours/Week   ☐ PT__Hours/Week

S/E Status [Postcode]_____

Marital status
  ☐ Married
  ☐ Divorced
  ☐ Separated
  ☐ De-facto
  ☐ Single
  ☐ Widowed

Children   ☐ Yes   ☐ No
Ages and genders of Children_____

Family of Origin:
Mother ☐ Alive   ☐ Deceased   Age of subject when mother died_____
Father ☐ Alive   ☐ Deceased   Age of subject when father died_____
Siblings_____ Position in the family in relation to siblings_____

Any experience in your lifetime of:
Sexual abuse   ☐ Yes   ☐ No
Violence   ☐ Yes   ☐ No
Strangulation   ☐ Yes   ☐ No

Total number of close confidantes or social supports_____

Fig. 4.2 Demographic and biographical data form (Baker et al., 2013)

the data have been drawn together in order to map out the possible *demographic profiles* of those women who participated in this study, and to show how these data support or differ from the trends in the prevalence studies and literature (Table 4.1).

Table 4.1 Selected demographics of women with FVD and OVD
(Baker et al., 2013)

Age	23–73yrs (Mean age 47.2 yrs)		22–77yrs (Mean age 48.4 yrs)	
	FVD (n=73)	Percentage	OVD (n=55)	Percentage
Employed	63	86%	33	60%
Full-time	38	60%	21	64%
Occupations				
Managerial, professional, supervisory	50	69%	24	42%
Education/teaching	23	32%	10	18%
Educational level				
Secondary	22	30%	29	53%
TAFE/Trade	11	15%	4	7%
Tertiary	40	55%	22	40%
Married	50	68%	38	69%
Divorce separated	13	18%	8	15%
Single, living alone	10	14%	9	16%
1–3 children	48	66%	34	62%
Family of origin *Born Australia*	52	71%	44	80%
Siblings (1–3)	71	97%	55	100%
Middle child	35	48%	27	49%
Any sexual abuse, violence or strangulation	36	49%	18	33%
Sexual abuse	23	32%	10	18%
Violence	30	41%	16	29%
Strangulation	10	14%	4	7%

Age, education, occupation, and socioeconomic status

As can be seen in Table 4.1, women with FVD (n = 73) had a mean age of 47.2 years (range 23–73) and those with OVD (n = 55) had a mean age of 48.4 years (range 22–77). This reflected similar findings in the prevalence studies cited above. Most of the women were employed, with the majority working full time. Women with FVD were more likely to be middle class and educated to tertiary levels. While teaching was the predominant profession for this voice disorder group, many of the other women were employed in jobs with professional, managerial, or supervisory responsibilities. This was an interesting finding. Significantly, women with OVD were more likely to live in areas with a postcode reflecting a lower level of SES than the FVD group women, they were less likely to have undertaken tertiary studies, and they were more likely to be unemployed, retired, or engaged in home duties.

Current family constellation and family-of-origin data

There were few differences between the FVD and OVD groups with respect to relationship status and numbers of children in current family. The majority of women were in a conjugal relationship of some kind, with one or more children. Family-of-origin data showed that most women came from families with one or more siblings and interestingly, with respect to order in the family, they were most likely to be the middle child.[4] With regard to women who had *at least one experience in their lifetime* of sexual abuse, violence or strangulation the data revealed, somewhat astonishingly, that 36/73 (49%) of the FVD group had reported such an incident, and that for either *sexual abuse*, or *violence*, or *strangulation*, more women with FVD reported such experiences than those in the OVD group. For some, these experiences had occurred during their formative years but for others, the incidents had happened during the 12 months prior to onset of the voice disorder.

---

4   Otolaryngologist, Dr Tom Harris, has often commented upon this same phenomenon amongst patients seen in both his private and public clinics in the UK.

While not unexpected, given the mean ages of women in this cohort, many had experienced the death of either one or both of their parents. One of the more poignant features concerning this was that when the father died, the median ages of FVD and OVD group women were 37 and 42 years, respectively, and when the mother died, the median age of FVD and OVD group women was 50 and 45 years, respectively.

Drawing on these same dimensions, we then compared the demographic profiles of women within the FVD sub-groups of PVD (n = 37) and MTVD (n = 36). Overall, the comparisons showed similarities for most of the variables, but there were several statistically significant differences. These are of interest in relation to the trends in the literature discussed above, and as we consider how biographical details may influence the way in which we consider the best approaches to management. (See Box 4.2).

While drawing attention to the different demographic profiles from this particular study no causal associations are being implied. It is suggested, however, that as the mean age of the women falls well within the *40 to 60 year age band* (identified as a period of increased risk for voice disorders in women), and taking into account that the majority of the women were working full time while simultaneously supporting partners and young families, and coping with ageing, ailing, and for some, the death of their parents, we now have a stronger sense of who these people are. I propose that armed with information like this, researchers and clinicians will be in a better position to understand how differences in the demographic and psychosocial profiles may impact on individuals with voice disorders, and how this may influence approaches to management.

Box 4.2 Significant differences in demographic data between PVD & MTVD groups

- PVD group women were older (7.4 years)
  - PVD group mean age of **50.7 years***
  - MTVD group had a mean age of 43.3 years
- Tertiary educational levels
  - PVD group women 38% (14/37)
  - MTVD group women 72% (26/36)
- Occupations – Managerial, professional, and supervisory roles
  - PVD group women 62% (23/37)
  - MTVD group women 75% (27/36)
- Education/Teaching roles
  - PVD group women 22% (8/37)
  - MTVD group women 42% (15/36)
- Any experience of sexual abuse in their lifetime
  - PVD group women 43% (16/37)
  - MTVD group women 19% (7/36)
- Mother or Father deceased
  - PVD groups women were more likely to have lost both parents
- Median age of women when parent died
  - Mother – PVD and MTVD group women – **50 years***
  - Father – PVD women, 41 years – MTVD women, 34 years

(Baker, Ben-Tovim, Butcher, Esterman, & McLaughlin, 2013)

References

Akagi, H., & House, A. (2001). Epidemiology of conversion hysteria. In P. W. Halligan, C. Bass & J. Marshall (Eds.), *Contemporary approaches to the study of hysteria.* Oxford: Oxford University Press.

American Speech-Language-Hearing Association. (2008). Incidence and prevalence of speech, voice, and language disorders in the United States. Available at http://www.asha.org/research/reports/speech_voice_language.htm [Accessed September 4, 2013]

Andersson, K., & Schalen, L. (1998). Etiology and treatment of psychogenic voice disorder: Results of a follow-up study of thirty patients. *Journal of Voice, 12*(1), 96–106.

Angelillo, M., Di Maio, G., Costa, H., Angelillo, N., & Barillari, U. (2009). Prevalence of occupational voice disorders in teachers. *Journal of Preventative Medicine and Hygiene, 50*(1), 26–32.

Aronson, A. E. (1990). Psychogenic voice disorders. In A. E. Aronson, *Clinical voice disorders: An interdisciplinary approach.* (3rd ed., pp. 116–159). New York: Thieme.

Aronson, A. E., & Bless, D. M. (2009). *Clinical voice disorders* (4th ed.). New York: Thieme.

Aronson, A. E., Peterson, H. W., & Litin, E. M. (1964). Voice symptomatology in functional dysphonia and aphonia. *Journal of Speech and Hearing Disorders, 28,* 367–380.

Baker, J. (1991). *How much am I bid for this exquisite little dysphonia: The money or the witness box?* Paper presented at the Inaugural Voice Symposium of Australia, Adelaide.

Baker, J. (1998). Psychogenic dysphonia: Peeling back the layers. *Journal of Voice, 12*(4), 527–535.

Baker, J. (2002a). Persistent dysphonia in two performers affecting the singing and projected speaking voice: A report on a collaborative approach to management. *Logopedics Phoniatrics Vocology, 27,* 179–187.

Baker, J. (2002b). Psychogenic voice disorders-heroes or hysterics? A brief overview with questions and discussion. *Logopedics Phoniatrics Vocology, 27,* 84–91.

Baker, J. (2003). Psychogenic voice disorders and traumatic stress experience: A discussion paper with two case reports. *Journal of Voice, 17*(3), 308–318.

Baker, J. (2008). The role of psychogenic and psychosocial factors in the development of functional voice disorders. *International Journal of Speech-Language Pathology, 10*(4), 210–230.

Baker, J., Ben-Tovim, D. I., Butcher, A., Esterman, A., & McLaughlin, K. (2007). Development of a modified diagnostic classification system for voice disorders with inter-rater reliability study. *Logopedics Phoniatrics Vocology, 32,* 99–112.

Baker, J., Ben-Tovim, D. I., Butcher, A., Esterman, A., & McLaughlin, K. (2013). Psychosocial risk factors which may differentiate between women with functional voice disorder, organic voice disorder, and control group. *International Journal of Speech-Language Pathology, 15*(6), 547–563.

Barker, P. (1991). *Regeneration* London: Penguin.

Bhatia, M. S., & Vaid, L. (2000). Hysterical aphonia – an analysis of 25 cases. *Indian Journal of Medical Sciences, 54*(8), 335–338.

Bickford, J., Coveney, J., Baker, J., & Hersh, D. (2012). Living with the altered self. *International Journal of Speech-Language Pathology, 15*(3), 324–333.

Brodnitz, F. S. (1969). Functional aphonia. *Annals of Otolaryngology, (St Louis), 78,* 1244–1253.

Butcher, P., & Cavalli, L. (1998). Fran: Understanding and treating psychogenic dysphonia from a cognitive-behavioural perspective. In D. Syder (Ed.), *Wanting to talk.*: Whurr.

Butcher, P., Elias, A., & Raven, R. (1993). *Psychogenic voice disorders and cognitive behaviour therapy.* San Diego: Singular Publishing Group.

Butler, J. E., Hammond, T. H., & Gray, S. D. (2001). Gender-related differences of hyaluronic acid distribution in the human vocal fold. *The Laryngoscope, 111*, 907–911.

Carding, P. N. (2003). Voice pathology in the United Kingdom. *British Medical Journal, 327*(7414), 514–515.

Connor, N. P., Cohen, S. B., Theis, S. M., Thibeault, S. L., Heatley, D. G., & Bless, D. M. (2008). Attitudes of children with dysphonia. *Journal of Voice, 22*(2), 197–209.

de Jong, F. I. C. R. S., Kooijman, P. G. C., Thomas, G., Huinck, T. G., Graamans, K., & Schutte, H. K. (2006). Epidemiology of voice problems in Dutch teachers. *Folia Phoniatrica et Logopaedia, 58*(3), 186–198.

Dietrich, M., Verdolini Abbott, K., Gartner-Schmidt, J., & Rosen, C. L. (2008). The frequency of perceived stress, anxiety, and depression in patients with common pathologies affecting voice. *Journal of Voice, 22*(4), 472–487.

Folks, D. G., Ford, C. V., & Regan, W. M. (1984). Conversion symptoms in a general hospital. *Psychosomatics, 25*, 285–295.

Gerritsma, E. J. (1991). An investigation into some personality characteristics of patients with psychogenic aphonia and dysphonia. *Folia Phoniatrica, 43*, 13–20.

House, A., & Andrews, H. B. (1987). The psychiatric and social characteristics of patients with functional dysphonia. *Journal of Psychosomatic Research, 31*, 483–490.

House, A., & Andrews, H. B. (1988). Life events and difficulties preceding the onset of functional dysphonia. *Journal of Psychosomatic Research, 32*(3), 311–319.

Hunter, E. J., Smith, M. E., & Tanner, K. (2011). Gender differences affecting vocal health of women in vocally demanding careers. *Logopedics Phoniatrics Vocology, 36*(3), 128–136.

Jain, A., Verma, K. K., Solanki, R. K., & Sidana, A. (2000). Is hysteria still prevailing? A retrospective study of sociodemographic and clinical characteristics. *Indian Journal of Medical Sciences, 53*(3), 395–397.

Mathieson, L. (2001). *Greene and Mathieson's: The voice and its disorders.* (6th ed.). London: Whurr.

McHugh-Munier, C., Scherer, K. R., Lehmann, W., & Scherer, U. (1997). Coping strategies, personality, and voice quality in patients with vocal fold nodules and polyps. *Journal of Voice, 11*(4), 452–461.

Morton, V., & Watson, D. R. (1998). The teaching voice: Problems and perceptions. *Logopedics Phoniatrics Vocology, 23*(3), 133–139.

Oates, J. (2000). Voice disorders associated with hyperfunction. In M. Freeman & M. Fawcus (Eds.), *Voice disorders and their management.* London: Whurr.

Oates, J. (2005). *New concepts in occupational voice.* Paper presented at the 7th Voice Symposium of Australia, Sydney.

Pemberton, C. (2010). Voice injury in teachers: Voice care prevention programs to minimise occupational risk. Available at http://www.voicecareaustralia.com.au/Voice%20Injury%20in%20Teachers.pdf [Accessed October 2016]

Pemberton, C., McCormack, C., & Comensoli, J. (2009). *Comprehensive voice care services for teachers: Preliminary report on Wollongong Voice Care Services.* Paper presented at the The Occupational Voice Symposium London.

Ramig, L. O., & Verdolini, K. (1998). Treatment efficacy: Voice disorders. *Journal of Speech, Language, and Hearing Research, 41*, s101.

Rosen, D. C., & Sataloff, R. T. (1997). *Psychology of voice disorders.* San Diego: Singular Publishing Group.

Roy, N., Merrill, R., Gray, S. D., & Smith, E. M. (2005). Voice disorders in the general population: Prevalence, risk factors, and occupational impact. *The Laryngoscope, 115*(11), 1988–1995.

Roy, N., Merrill, R., Thibeault, S., Parsa, R. A., Gray, S. D., & Smith, E. M. (2004a). Voice disorders in teachers and the general population: Effects on work performance, attendance, and future career choices. *Journal of Speech Language and Hearing Disorders, 47*, 542–551.

Roy, N., Merrill, R. M., Thibeault, S., Parsa, R. A., Gray, S. D., & Smith, E. M. (2004b). Prevalence of voice disorders in teachers and the general population. *Journal of Speech Language Hearing Research, 47*, 281–293.

Roy, N., Stemple, J., Merrill, R. M., & Thomas, L. (2007). Epidemiology of voice disorders in the elderly: Preliminary findings. *The Laryngoscope, 117*, 628–633.

Russell, A., Oates, J., & Greenwood, K. (2005). Prevalence of self-reported voice problems in the general population in South Australia. *Advances in Speech-Language Pathology, 7*(1), 24–30.

Russell, A., Oates, J., & Greenwood, K. M. (1998). Prevalence of voice problems in teachers. *Journal of Voice, 4*, 467–479.

Sacks, O. (1985). *The man who mistook his wife for a hat.* London: Picador.

Schalen, L., & Andersson, K. (1992). Differential diagnosis and treatment of psychogenic voice disorder. *Clinical Otolaryngology, 17*, 225–230.

Seifert, E., & Kollbrunner, J. (2005). Stress and distress in non-organic voice disorders. *Swiss Medical Weekly, 135*, 387–397.

Smith, E., Kirchner, H. L., Taylor, M., Hoffman, H., & Lemke, J. H. (1998a). Voice problems among teachers: Differences by gender and teaching characteristics. *Journal of Voice, 12*(3), 328–334.

Smith, E., Verdolini, K., Gray, S. D., Nichols, S., Lemke, J., Barkmeier, J., Dove, H., Hoffman, H. (1996). Effect of voice disorders on quality of life. *Journal of Medical Speech-Language Pathology, 4*(4), 223–244.

Smurthwaite, H. (1919). War neuroses of the larynx and speech mechanism. *Journal of Laryngology and Otolaryngology*, 13–20.

Sokolowsky, R. R. (1944). War aphonia. *Journal of Speech Disorders, 9*, 193–208.

Titze, I. R., Hunter, E. J., & Svec, J. G. (2007). Voicing and silence periods in daily and weekly vocalizations of teachers. *Journal of Acoustical Society of America, 121*(1), 469–478.

Titze, I. R., Lemke, J., & Montequin, D. (1997). Populations in the U.S. workforce who rely on their voice as a primay tool of trade: A preliminary report. *Journal of Voice, 11*, 254–249.

Titze, I. R., & Verdolini Abbott, K. (2012). *Vocology. The science and practice of voice habilitation.* Salt Lake City: National Center for Voice and Speech.

Trewin, D. (2001). Information paper: Census of population and housing: Socio-economic indexes for areas, Australia 2001. Canberra: Australian Bureau of statistics. Available at http://www.abs.gov.au/AUSSTATS/abs@.nsf/DetailsPage/2039.02001?OpenDocument [Accessed October 2014].

U.S. Department of Labor. (2008). Kindergarten and elementary school teachers. Available at http://www.bls.gov/oco/ocos069.htm [Accessed October 2014].

Verdolini, K., & Ramig, L. O. (2001). Review: Occupational risks for voice problems. *Logopedics Phoniatrics Vocology, 26*, 37–46.

Verdolini, K., Rosen, C. A., & Branski, R. C. (Eds.). (2006). *Classification Manual for Voice Disorders – I*. New Jersey: Laurence Erlbaum Associates.

Vilkman, E. (2000). Voice problems at work: A challenge for occupational safety and health. *Folia Phoniatrica et Logopaedia, 52*, 120–125.

White, A., Deary, I. J., & Wilson, J. A. (1997). Psychiatric disturbance and personality traits in dysphonic patients. *European Journal of Disorders of Communication, 32*, 307–314.

Wilson, J. A., Deary, I. J., & MacKenzie, K. (1995). Functional dysphonia. Not 'hysterical' but seen mainly in women. *British Medical Journal, 311*, 1039–1040.

Yiu, E. M.-L. (2002). Impact and prevention of voice problems in the teaching profession: Embracing the consumers' view. *Journal of Voice, 16*(2), 215– 228.

Yiu, E. M.-L. (Ed.). (2013). *International perspectives on voice disorders*. Bristol: Multilingual Matters.

5

Stressful life events and difficulties preceding onset of voice disorders

Introduction

'Through vocal sound we express our physical, psychological, social and spiritual lives, and our voices grow and change with us in the dance of our individual life'. (Shewell, 2009) (p. 4).

One of the predominant hypotheses regarding *psychosocial causal mechanisms* for functional voice disorders (FVD) suggests that these voice problems may develop in response to negative emotions following stressful life events and difficulties, often in close proximity to onset.[1] These stressful incidents may operate primarily as precipitating factors that influence causal pathways and the clinical presentations of FVD, or they may serve to aggravate or perpetuate the FVD and, to some extent, the course and outcomes of some organic voice disorders (OVD).

In this chapter, I discuss the measures typically used in this area of research, with reference to the strengths and limitations of the different approaches. I then report on findings from a recent literature review with respect to stressful life events and difficulties preceding onset of FVD (Baker, 2008). This includes trends in the anecdotal data drawn from single case and group series reports, and

---

1   Please note that I am maintaining the same terminology and acronyms that I have used throughout this text for FVD, which includes and differentiates between the MTVD and PVD sub-groups as defined by Baker et al. (2007). When describing the different studies in this chapter, I use the diagnostic terms and acronyms that have been nominated by the respective authors.

the rather meagre empirical data that we now have from several comparative group studies. I then highlight some of the key evidence from a more recent study that showed that the *number* and *severity* of life events and difficulties occurring in the 12 months prior to onset clearly differentiated between the FVD and OVD, and the control group women (Baker *et al.*, 2013). The data also indicated that the qualitative nature of many stressful events preceding FVD was characterised by *conflict over speaking out (COSO)*, often rendering the person *powerless in the system (PITS)* to which they belonged. Significantly, analysis of the same dimensions failed to differentiate between the FVD sub-groups, muscle tension voice disorders (MTVD), and psychogenic voice disorders (PVD).[2]

This raises fascinating questions regarding how we might think about causal pathways in relation to MTVD and PVD. Is it possible that *stressful life events and difficulties*, while more traditionally associated with the onset of PVD and affiliated disorders, are just as important in contributing to the onset of MTVD? Is there any difference in the qualitative nature of those events and difficulties preceding PVD and MTVD? Is it possible, too, that stressful life events and difficulties may contribute to a *lowering of resilience* in the immune system with a subsequent vulnerability to the development of OVD in some individuals? If the answer to any of these questions is 'yes', what are the implications for our approaches to assessment and management?

The hard questions and then the harder ones

It has been my experience that most patients want to know what may have caused their voice disorder, and naturally ask very searching questions of their treating specialists. This may occur when they present with an OVD, even though it seems to make sense given the pathology identified during laryngoscopy. For most of these patients the explanation of a medical, structural, or neurological anomaly is enough, but the more psychologically-minded individuals may subsequently begin to ask searching questions such as "Why this voice disorder, why me, why now?". These questions interest me too.

Patients presenting with a FVD ask similar questions, possibly out of curiosity to begin with and later, out of more troubled concern. This may be manifest in much more challenging queries because the explanations of 'nothing

---

2   It is acknowledged that many individuals with MTVD may develop their voice problems in response to heavy vocal demands and consequent phonotrauma, but the focus of the review and the discussion here is on possible external psychosocial factors that may be associated with onset.

wrong with your vocal cords' or '*dysregulated vocal behaviours*' fails to reflect their experience of the severity and limitations of their voice problem. I would suggest that these more probing questions reveal a degree of embarrassment because if there is no physiological explanation, it may mean that the treating specialists consider their voice disorder to be essentially stress-related or indicative of a psychological problem. For many people, this carries with it a sense of shame, even stigma. "I have sung this role 14 times and my technique is secure. Why would anything be different now?". "I have taught for 25 years – why would I start having 'dysregulated vocal behaviours' at this point in my career?". "If there is nothing wrong with my larynx or my vocal folds, is it all up here in my head? Do you think that was what the doctor really thought, but did not say? Is that what you think too?"

These incisive and important questions provide excellent opportunities for clinicians to offer explanations that can validate the severity of a dysphonia despite the healthy structures and potential for normal function, and at the same time, can open up dialogue regarding the possibility that psychosocial factors might be relevant – 'And no, this does not necessarily mean you are mad, bad or sad'.

Approaches used for the measurement of stressful situations

As discussed in Chapter 3, it is generally recognised that exposure to stressors in daily life, or over the course of a lifetime, is one of the most critical factors influencing the health and well-being of individuals (Fava & Sonino, 2000; Kessler, 1997). While it has long been predicted that stress is a risk factor for ill health (Selye & Fortier, 1950) it remains unclear as to what types of stress are likely to have the more powerful influences over the onset of particular physical and mental health conditions; this is also true in relation to the different voice disorders. Measurement of stressors seeks to distinguish between the levels of exposure to stressful situations and the different ways in which people react to such incidents. The main areas of research in this area include: *daily hassles*, which are relatively minor threatening situations; *events* that may be physical or psychological in nature and characterised by threat and loss with the capacity to change the patterns of life or arouse very strong positive or negative emotions; and *longer term difficulties*, which are the more chronic adverse life conditions that generate unpleasant feelings over time and lead to more cumulative effects.

Craig (2001) has highlighted several important methodological considerations that need to be taken into account with any approach designed to show a possible association between preceding events and onset of symptoms. He suggests that any valid *measures of life event stress* in relation to a health condition will need to include:

- Both discrete events and chronic difficulties
- Explicit criteria about those experiences to be included
- Attention to the time order in which incidents occur
- Some means of assessing the independence of the event or difficulty from the physical or mental health condition under investigation (i.e., insuring the event or difficulty has not arisen in response to the target disorder).

The main methods of life event measurement are *checklist measures*, which provide essentially quantitative data, and *personal interview measures* that may generate both quantitative and qualitative material.

Checklist measures

Early checklist methods were based on the premise that exposure to an event requires a readjustment of some kind and typically entailed only negative events, since early findings suggested that negative experiences are more likely to predict health status than positive events (Vinokur & Selzer, 1975). Questions in checklists generally pertain to a wide range of recent life changes such as personal, social, occupational, or family events and the respondent answers in a yes/no format. This gives a summary score of the estimated stressfulness of changes experienced over a given time (Horowitz, Wilner, & Alvarez, 1979; Paykel, Prusoff, & Uhlenhuth, 1971). However, scales such as the *Social Readjustment Rating Scale (SRRS)* (Holmes & Rahe, 1967) and in its more recent form, the *Revised Social Readjustment Rating Scale (R-SRRS)* (Hobson & Delunas, 2001), enable ratings for severity of stress from mildly to extremely stressful (1–3) and events that may be positive and negative, as shown in Box 5.1.

Box 5.1 Examples of positive and negative event items from the R-SRRS

- Death of a close family member
- Change in residence
- Changing work responsibilities
- Infidelity of a partner
- Gaining a new family member
- Major disagreement over child support/custody/visitation
- Experiencing a large unexpected monetary gain

(Hobson & Delunas, 2001)

There are, however, a number of criticisms of the checklist approaches (Bowling, 1995; Wethington, Almeida, Brown, Frank, & Kessler, 2001):

- The scales fail to address the meaning of life events to the individual
- There is a low level of accuracy in the recall of life events
- The scales have low test-retest reliability
- Checklists are too vague in the quality of their questions with respect to stressors
- Many include inappropriate events that would normally be considered minor
- They lack attention to memory bias

The literature suggests that checklist scales are one way of measuring the occurrence of life events and their perceived stressfulness to individuals, and they tend to be popular because they are easy and inexpensive to administer. While recognised as being convenient and suitable for rudimentary screening in large epidemiological surveys, they are not highly regarded in the area of psychosocial research (Turner & Wheaton, 1995).

Personal interview methods

Interview methods are more appropriate for those studies where it is important to be precise about the severity of ratings, to pinpoint the timing of the exposure and disease onset, and to establish that the stressful situations are independent of the illness under investigation. In general, interview methods are more comprehensive; they place emphasis on contextual factors as well as the event itself and importantly, provide more information on the meaning of that event to a person. The interview method includes acute and stressful events that may be positive or negative, and generally provides an assessment of chronic stressors that are particularly relevant for assessing risk for some health outcomes, such as heart disease or depression (Wethington *et al.*, 2001).

Life Events and Difficulties Schedule

The most widely used and well documented of the interview methods is the standardised, semi-structured *Life Events and Difficulties Schedule (LEDS)* (Brown & Harris, 1978). It is based upon the premise that social and environmental changes that threaten the most strongly held emotional bonds or commitments are the basis for severe stress and that severe stress threatens health, rather than minor stress as might be determined using other models (Lazarus & Folkman, 1984). The instrument clearly defines the basic units of study in terms of events and difficulties. *Events* are defined as discrete incidents in daily life that may interfere with, or threaten to disrupt, normal life activities that culminate in their impact 10 to 14 days after the start of the event. They may be either physical or psychological in nature, and are identified in terms of their likelihood to produce strong positive or negative emotions. Events are explored across 10 main areas of inquiry that include: education; work; reproduction; housing money or possessions; crime or legal issues; health or accidents; marital and partner relationships; other relationships including children; and miscellaneous events such as unusual world incidents, harm to pets, special ceremonies, or death of close ties. *Difficulties* are described as chronic adverse life conditions that have been occurring for 4 weeks or more and may be of a psychological or a physical nature. They are explored across the same 10 domains of inquiry and are tracked from time of onset for changes in degree of severity during the period of investigation.

Established guidelines in the interview manual provide inclusion criteria for each class of incident that can be considered to be an *event* or a *difficulty*. They also stipulate on whom the events need to be focused, the nature of the close ties that allow or disallow an event to be considered, and the requirement for the events and difficulties to be independent of the research condition under investigation.

LEDS – Contextual versus reported threat

Here, it is relevant to highlight several notable features of the LEDS that serve to distinguish this approach from other checklist and interview approaches. The LEDS clearly distinguishes between *reported* and *contextual threat* (Brown, Harris, & Hepworth, 1995). *Reported threat* refers to the respondent's style of response and feelings expressed in association with the event; these reactions are inevitably offered by the respondent, and rated by the investigator on the basis of both verbal and non-verbal expressions of emotional distress. However, it is the emphasis on the contextual threat that contributes so powerfully in enabling researchers and clinicians to understand the meaning of these incidents as they may impact upon individuals and influence the onset of their various physical or mental health conditions. In the final analysis, it is the *contextual rating* that determines the severity score for each incident (T. Harris, 2000).

The assessment of *contextual threat* requires the investigator to be as objective as possible when considering all the relevant factual information and circumstances surrounding the event, taking into account the person's biographical history and personal situation. This avoids respondent bias due to preferential recall in 'an effort after meaning' (Bartlett, 1932), fall-off in recall of particular types of situations (Brown & Harris, 1982a), and the effects of the person's health condition as this may effect mood, memory, or style of coping (Craig, 2001). Once a particular incident has been included in the analysis, a range of probe questions enable the investigator to establish the sequence of events over time, and to make a judgment regarding the *severity of threat or unpleasantness* based upon the wider contextual meaning for the person (Box 5.2).

Box 5.2 Examples of standard and probe questions that serve to establish contextual meaning as adapted from the LEDS

- 'Has anyone separated from or divorced their husband or wife in the last 12 months?' If involving S, the probe questions may be:
  - When did this happen? (Specific date?)
  - What were the reasons for this?
  - Did you anticipate this happening?
  - Was anyone else involved?
  - When did this become evident? (Specific date?)
  - Has anyone left the family home? (Specific date?)
  - How have the children reacted? How about the family?
  - How has this affected you, your partner, those close to you both?
  - Have you sought legal advice about custody of the children?
  - Is this satisfactory to both you and your partner?

(Brown & Harris, 1978)

LEDS – Qualitative dimensions

In addition to the traditional measures of threat, the LEDS instrument also enables emphasis on specific classes of incidents. For instance, severe events and difficulties associated with loss have been most poignant in the depression studies, where loss may relate to loss of a person but may also include loss of health, a cherished idea, employment and role, or possessions and security (Brown & Harris, 1989a, 1989b). Other classes of severe events involving danger, disappointment, humiliation, or entrapment have been the focus of a number of studies (Brown *et al.*, 1995; Finlay-Jones, 1989). Three further dimensions involving psychological dilemmas, *conflict over speaking out (COSO)* and *powerlessness in the system (PITS)* have been developed and explored with the LEDS team in relation to conditions such as *chronic fatigue syndrome* and FVD in women (Baker *et al.*, 2013; Hatcher & House, 2003; House & Andrews, 1988).

There are also criticisms of the interview method, namely:

- The expense in time and effort required to administer and rate the interviews
- The inevitable risks of *effort after meaning* from respondents
- The possibility of *recall bias* of the respondent

- The interviewer may skew questions and probes to elicit specific types of material
- Concerns that socioeconomic status or other cultural factors could act as confounders in terms of severity ratings

Nevertheless, there seems to be general consensus throughout the literature that while there is no perfect solution to this problem, *semi-structured interview methods* are preferable to self-report checklists. The LEDS is the interview method judged by experienced researchers to fulfil the stringent criteria for a scientifically valid approach (Craig, 2001; Wethington *et al.*, 2001). In a critique of research studies investigating the relationship between life events and psychosocial variables in relation to breast cancer in women, the LEDS was deemed the most thorough and reliable approach (Butow *et al.*, 2000). As argued by Eysenck (1994), one of the world's most widely published psychologists and possibly one who could be relied upon to be blunt:

> 'There is good evidence that investigations carried out by interviewers involving personal contact, the establishment of trust, and the possibility of explaining doubtful points in the questionnaire to the proband, give significantly better results than studies relying solely on questionnaires dished out anonymously and without detailed explanation and motivation' (p. 202).

Broad trends for stressful life events and difficulties and onset of voice disorders

Most of the published literature relating to causal associations between stressful life events and difficulties, and voice disorders, has focused primarily on the broad FVD group of disorders and more specifically, those patients presenting with PVD. There has been surprisingly little emphasis on possible associations between stressful life incidents as causal factors preceding onset of OVD in general, and few studies that have specifically explored the possibility that stressful situations may contribute to an individual's vulnerability to developing OVD, or the exacerbation and/or perpetuation of these conditions.[3]

---

3   It needs to be emphasised here that the diversity in diagnostic terminologies used by respective authors across many of the studies (an issue previously raised in Chapter 1) does make accurate reporting of trends and generalisations somewhat fraught and at best, approximations only.

Significantly too, the focus of most of the life events and difficulties research in relation to voice disorders has been on women and in particular, women with FVD. Where men have been included, this has been on a very small scale, possibly because men present less often with these disorders. The notable exceptions to this have been those single case or case series reports exploring the possible role of stressful life events and difficulties preceding the onset of voice disorders in soldiers during wartime (Barker, 1991; Smurthwaite, 1919; Sokolowsky & Junkermann, 1944), or preceding the development of PVD, such as *mutational falsetto* and *puberphonia* in adolescent and adult males (Aronson & Bless, 2009; Baker, 1998, 2002a; Froese & Sims, 1987; Hartman & Aronson, 1983; Mathieson, 2001). I suggest that if we reflect on the essential nature of the circumstances that precipitate loss of voice in males, this may shed more light on the higher prevalence in females, or it may highlight some core features of those events and difficulties that are fundamental to both genders. If this is the case, we might wonder how and why females are more frequently exposed to such pressures, or whether it is possible that once exposed, they respond in a different manner.

Life events and difficulties: Single case reports

In a review of the literature with respect to nature and severity of stressful life events and difficulties preceding onset of the broad group of FVD (Baker, 2002b, 2008), it has become clear that much of the early 'evidence' was anecdotal and informally derived from case history or psychiatric interview, rather than from any structured or standardised life events questionnaire or inventory. Traditionally, such incidents were expected to be consciously recalled, relatively recent, and considered by both the patient and clinician to 'make sense' in relation to onset of the particular voice problem. However, in many of the single cases reported, those stressful incidents identified by patients were not necessarily those identified as being relevant by clinicians, and some were neither recent nor consciously recalled during the initial interview but came to light later in the therapeutic process during efforts to recover the voice (Baker, 2003).

It is also significant that in a number of cases, no life events or difficulties were identified by either patients or clinicians, and while this may not seem particularly surprising to experienced therapists, it is worthy of discussion. This is because integral to a number of diagnostic classification systems, such as the earlier version of *Diagnostic and Statistical Manual of Mental Disorders (DSM-IV)* (American Psychiatric Association, 1994), the occurrence of a recent stressful event preceding onset was one of the essential criteria for differential diagnosis to categories such as *psychogenic movement* or *somatoform disorders*, which may include 'functional', 'medically unexplained', or 'psychogenic' voice disorders. Furthermore, in a number of diagnostic classification systems for voice disorders where clear operational definitions and guidelines are given, these suggest that identification of stressful life events preceding onset of the voice disorder, such as PVD and/or conversion reaction, is a necessary requirement for such a diagnosis (Aronson, 1990; Butcher, Elias, & Cavalli, 2007).

While it is most often the case that stressful incidents preceding onset can be recognised and seen to be associated with the onset of the voice problem, the fact that there are times when no incidents are recalled raises some interesting questions. Does this mean that there was nothing significant happening? Could it mean that there was something happening but the patient was not consciously aware of it as being relevant at the time of interview? Could it be that there had not been sufficient time in the therapeutic relationship for the development of trust and safety that would allow for more sensitive issues to be discussed? Alternatively, is it possible that as clinicians we may not be asking the right questions or if we are, is it to do with the timing, the words we use, and the manner in which such questions are being asked?

Following on from these clinical questions it is relevant to note that with the most recent changes to the *DSM-V* (American Psychiatric Association, 2013), evidence of a stressful life event preceding onset of *functional neurologic disorders* is no longer an essential component of the diagnostic criteria. Whereas previously it had to be shown that a psychologically stressful event or series of events had preceded onset of 'conversion reaction' pain, paralysis, or movement disorders, this is no longer the case.

Generally, however, in those single case reports where stressful life events and difficulties have been perceived as relevant, the details about the moderately stressful situations and more traumatic events were rich. Furthermore, it is has been fascinating to observe how the essential nature of those incidents described in the very early studies has been mirrored in the subsequent case series and comparative group studies reported. I would suggest that we should not underestimate the importance of these earlier case reports, despite their being somewhat dismissively relegated to the lowest rung of evidence hierarchies such as the *Joanna Briggs Institute Levels of Evidence Hierarchy* (1998). In many respects these more detailed case reports have set the scene for the surprisingly few case series and comparative group studies that have followed.

Single case reports: Upper respiratory tract infections

The onset of FVD in many single cases reported has often been associated with adverse health conditions, primarily upper respiratory tract infection (URTI). Although we might not consider that an URTI constitutes a stressful event, it is probably the most common incident cited by patients as preceding onset of FVD and as being causally related. This is particularly so for those diagnosed with PVD. The trouble is, it is difficult to verify infection retrospectively (House & Andrews, 1987) and since general practitioners do not generally carry out laryngoscopy, which would confirm or refute the presence of an acute viral laryngitis, a provisional diagnosis of URTI is often given. This inevitably confirms in the patient's mind that the onset of the voice problem is probably medical. Schalen and Andersson (1992) suggest that a more accurate diagnosis in such cases might have been PVD, and many clinicians experienced with diagnosing PVD may well agree. However, even if the person does have an URTI prior to onset, this need not exclude psychosocial factors from being causally related. Alternatively, onset of the URTI might reflect the impact of chronic stressful situations on the person's immune system (Butcher *et al.*, 2007; Kinzl, Biebl, & Rauchegger, 1988a). A patient recently diagnosed with psychogenic aphonia that exemplifies these issues is shown in Case example 5.1.

Case example 5.1

S, a 23 year-old woman presented with a 12-week history of psychogenic aphonia with onset in association with a longer-term pattern of medically confirmed URTIs. At the time, she was working shifts in a part-time job where she was very unhappy, and saw no future for herself. She felt frustrated and sad as she watched her friends flourishing, and described herself as feeling 'rather unaccomplished'. As a result of the shift work, poor sleep patterns and concerns about her future, she felt seriously 'run-down' and more prone to infections than usual. It was the impression of S and her therapist that her vulnerability to illness and infections was as much related to her troubled work situation and hopelessness about her future as was the development of her psychogenic aphonia.

Single case reports: Threatening changes and interpersonal communication problems

Stressful life events described in many single case reports of patients with FVD were often related to threatening changes affecting the patient or close family members. These may have occurred following loss of a partner through death perhaps after a prolonged terminal illness and possibly symbolising a delayed grieving reaction (Baker, 1998), following acrimonious separation or divorce (Butcher & Cavalli, 1998), or after estrangement from close family members following conflict and problems with communication (Arnold & Pinto, 1960; Aronson, 1969; Bangs & Freidinger, 1950; Greene, 1938; Macleod & Hemsley, 1985; Neeleman & Mann, 1993; Sapir, 1995; Sapir & Aronson, 1987; Seifert & Kollbrunner, 2005). In several of these cases, longer term difficulties could often be linked to communication problems amongst family members, including those experienced by women in caring roles with elderly parents or ailing spouses whose devotion and self-sacrifice had been taken for granted. Frequent observations made by the clinicians cited above suggested that for many of their female patients, feelings of rising resentment, hostility, or regret had not been fully expressed, partly because they feared offending the ailing relative and partly because they feared further rejection, reprisal, or making matters worse (Butcher, Elias, Raven, Yeatman, & Littlejohns, 1987). On reflection, the meaning of these emergent themes appears to be related to the constructs of conflict over speaking out (COSO) and the *suppression or repression of negative emotion* that have since arisen in subsequent studies, as outlined in the sections below. A woman with MTVD exemplifies these interpersonal dynamics as illustrated in Case 5.2.

Case example 5.2

S, a 62 year-old woman, presented for therapy with a moderate MTVD and small vocal nodules of 4 months' duration. During the 12 months prior to onset of her voice problem she had given up a successful career to care for her husband who was suffering a progressive neurological disease, with increasing loss of mobility, frequent falls, and incontinence. S withdrew from many activities, and their mutual sense of hopelessness about the future was palpable.

During this same period S was also caring for her 95 year-old mother who lived interstate. Supporting her mother, who was now severely deaf and partially sighted, entailed daily phone calls which had become a significant strain on her voice, or flying to see her each month. Her husband had to accompany S on these trips, as he could not be left alone at home, and all of this was proving very expensive, both in terms of time and money. S's mother was fiercely independent, would not buy in help despite her declining health and personal hygiene. Much of S's time during these visits was spent ringing social workers to negotiate a suitable care facility for her mother who had become recalcitrant and belligerent towards S, despite her enormous efforts. On four occasions during this 12 month period, supported care placements were offered to her mother, which she refused. S's overwhelming feeling in the months prior to onset of her *hyperfunctional* voice disorder was one of being totally shackled, unable to speak her mind about these many constraints in her life, and knowing if she did, she risked 'further rejection, reprisal or making matters worse'.

Single case reports: Workplace issues

Events and difficulties related to work were most frequently associated with ambivalence towards the nature of the work, anxiety about the levels of skill required for the particular job, or incidents related to interpersonal problems with authority figures, other staff, or clients being served by the patient (Aronson, 1969; Baker, 1998; Butcher & Cavalli, 1998; Hartman, Daily, & Morin, 1989; Perepel, 1930). Common to all these incidents were the self-reported dilemmas over being assertive, difficulties with the expression of feelings of anger or dissatisfaction, or a sense of having lost control and becoming powerless in being heard in the work environment. The choices made, interestingly in both male and female patients, had been to effectively silence themselves. These issues are so aptly captured by Fred Cress's "Visages" in Fig. 5.1 and are illustrated in the highly stressful longer-term difficulties experienced by a man with an acute onset of PVD in the form of a mutational falsetto, as outlined in Case example 5.3.

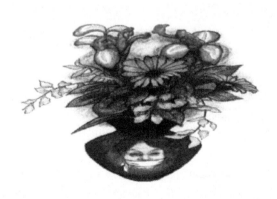

Fig. 5.1 "Visages 18" Fred Cress (2007)

Courtesy Fred Cress Estate.

Case example 5.3

S was a 62 year-old music teacher who presented with a 7 week history of PVD in association with severe URTI. This conservative gentleman was an accomplished organist and an experienced teacher of Latin and Classical Music. Due to the education department requirements that teachers were no longer permitted to stay too long in any one school, S had been transferred six times in the 2 years prior to this illness. In the different schools he was required to teach subjects totally outside his area of expertise, and in the final placement that occurred 2 weeks before his infection, he was moved to a school to teach history, geography, and sex education to 12 and 13 year-olds, rather than classical languages and music to 16 year-olds. Music was of a low priority in this school and here, he was required to offer electives in music when preferences of the students were for 'Heavy Metal'- with the pinnacle of their classical music yearnings on an ambitious day – for Andrew Lloyd Webber. S completely lost control over the behaviour of his pupils and each morning before going to school, he suffered fits of paroxysmal coughing and retching, rendering himself virtually unable to speak. When he did use his voice he was only able to speak in a high-pitched falsetto voice, with little capacity for projection. This disorder appeared to have rendered the gentleman utterly impotent – powerless with his 'Micky-Mouse' voice' as he described it – and powerless in the classroom with no capacity to maintain control of the situation. Resolution to normal phonation took many weeks of intensive voice therapy and counselling by his SLP, and he eventually sought worker's compensation on the basis of stress. S retired early, unable to face the classroom ever again, having been effectively castrated by the system to which he belonged.

Edited excerpt from single case report (Baker, 1998)

Single case reports: Traumatic events

At the extreme end of the continuum, recent and readily recalled *traumatic events* have been documented in a number of single case reports. Such incidents have been perceived as life threatening to the patient or close associates and have taken the form of some violent assault, accident, or health-related condition (Aronson, 1990; Aronson & Bless, 2009; Baker, 2003; Butcher *et al.*, 1987; Case, 1984; Ingals, 1890). (Case example 5.4)

Case example 5.4

A man assaulted a 22 year-old woman, threatening her with a knife and demanding money as she worked late at night in a petrol station. He held the knife to her neck then ran the knife across her throat making a superficial cut to the skin. Although no actual damage was done to her larynx, the woman became aphonic for weeks following this terrifying incident.

Edited excerpt from a single case report (Case, 1984)

In other single case reports, traumatic incidents were recalled either during the consolidation period of the normalised voice, or even some time after resolution of psychogenic aphonia. Such events were neither recent nor readily recalled, and their relevance was not necessarily recognised by the patients as being linked to onset or the ongoing severity of their dysphonia. In these cases, it was during more searching conversations about circumstances in close proximity to onset of the voice problem, and the meaning and emotions associated with the dysphonia, that prompted recall of prior traumatic incidents (Baker, 2003; Baker & Lane, 2009; Matas, 1991). Several of these more complex cases will be discussed in later chapters related to complex PVD.

Life events and difficulties: Descriptive case series

A review of the eight descriptive case series exploring stressful incidents preceding onset of FVD reveals that these too relied upon anecdotal and case history data but again, with a level of detail that is most illuminating (Aronson, Peterson, & Litin, 1964, 1966; Barton, 1960; Brodnitz, 1969; Butcher *et al.*, 1987; Guze & Brown, 1962; Kinzl, Biebl, & Rauchegger, 1988b; Smurthwaite,

1919; Sokolowsky & Junkermann, 1944).[4] The two earlier case series are very interesting because they involved only men, and despite the marked historical and contextual differences, the stressful circumstances preceding their functional voice problems revealed a number of the qualitative characteristics that later epitomised those stressful situations preceding onset of FVD in women.

Wartime experiences involving men

In the first study, Smurthwaite (1919) reported on the circumstances of 260 soldiers where exposure to *traumatic military incidents* was common, and where many of the men were suffering from *war neuroses of the larynx*. This presented as stammering, mutism, or aphonia, with symptoms ranging from 3 to 24 months. The author differentiated between those who had lost their voices from either shell or *gas shock*, with resolution after brief therapy or spontaneous recovery, and those whose aphonia or mutism persisted well after they were sent back to the UK for therapy. In most cases, the original trauma was associated with having been gassed or being involved in the bursting of high explosives, 'being buried under the debris or blown for some distance although with no bodily injury' (p.14). The reflexive response to noxious gassing or to choking under rubble was a sharp laryngeal spasm, with a feeling of tightness in the throat that seemed to persist even after restoration of the voice. The author noted that it was the '*muscle memory*' or mental image of the sensation of being unable to breathe, in association with the emotion of extreme fear, that caused the voice loss well after the original noxious site had been left behind.

The authors observed that the soldiers were not so much afraid of battle but rather, that they were overwhelmed by fatigue and the inevitability of defeat. Pat Barker echoed these same sentiments in her novel *Regeneration* (1991), where she described soldiers returning from the First World War to the psychiatric wards with conversion reaction paralyses and voice loss, reporting an overwhelming sense of futility as they contemplated returning to the front, knowing that if they did, it would make no difference, and that defeat was inevitable.

In the other large case series involving 116 soldiers diagnosed with psychogenic aphonia during the First World War, Sokolowsky and Junkerman (1944) described several different scenarios occurring prior to onset with discerning

---

4 It is relevant to note here that the diagnostic terminology used across these studies was variable and not always clearly defined. The use of the term FVD sometimes included patients with a clinical picture that we would recognise as being either a MTVD or PVD, whereas others seemed to be presenting with a conversion reaction aphonia/dysphonia.

detail and commentary. The physicians found that contrary to other reports where onset of aphonia was invariably related to the traumas of *shell shock* and bombing, many soldiers who attended their medical service developed aphonia after an acute laryngitis, diagnosable on laryngoscopy. Others, too, had no recent experience of bombing, gassing or violent combat, or a diagnosable laryngitis, but seemed to have experienced an event that was so insignificant that it could barely be recognised or was completely missed in the case history taken by the doctor.

These authors observed that the young men were facing numerous changes in relation to their lifestyle, which included separations from their families, living at close quarters with other soldiers with the resulting *interpersonal communication problems* and frictions, and a military work ethos that dictated unconditional subordination to authority figures, often resulting in a *sense of powerlessness* when asserting themselves. They noted that particular men could withstand the extremely unsettling conditions up to a certain point, but once that was reached, even a minor and seemingly innocuous incident could lead to a 'breakdown of his resistance'. They concluded that the psychogenic aphonia represented the expression of 'an abnormal reaction' to the extremely demanding requirements of military life in wartime. With a degree of consternation that we now might find somewhat amusing they concluded:

> '*We thus learned also, that the male psyche, given a certain degree of emnal stress, showed a surprising tendency for functional aphonia*' (Sokolowsky & Junkermann, 1944) (p.197).

Family relationships

In the descriptive case series cited above, the FVD study groups comprised predominantly women, with a small percentage of men in some of the studies. Generally speaking, traumatic life events such as serious threats to personal or family security, separation from close ties, or loss or death of a close family member, were only reported occasionally.

The more typical life events and difficulties for women were those of more moderate severity, related to interpersonal communication problems with partners or members of the family. Marital disharmony invariably involved situational conflicts arising from such issues as infidelity, guilt, and ambivalence, with discomfort over sexual feelings or difficulties in expressing anger (Aronson *et al.*, 1966). In the largest of these early case series, Brodnitz (1969) concluded that the precipitating events were not so much traumatic but related to marital problems as shown in Fred Cress's "Fools 20" (Fig. 5.2).

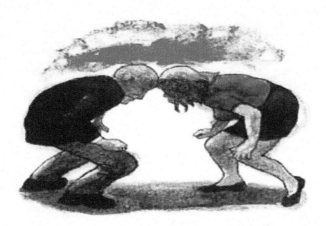

Fig. 5.2 "Fools 20", Fred Cress (2004)

Courtesy Fred Cress Estate.

In his case series of 74 patients with FVD (62 women), he noted that the majority of the women were aged between 40 and 50 years, 'the age of menopause that frequently upsets the emotional balance' (p.1246). The imputation that the physiological state and psychological disposition of middle-aged women might have accounted for the onset of these FVD might seem somewhat dated and offensive from a more modern feminist perspective. However, these pre-emptive observations were not entirely without merit, given the recent trends in the demographic data for a predominance of women with FVD, and the marked spike in the prevalence of voice disorders between 40 and 50 years of age, as discussed in Chapter 4. A more relevant interpretation for the current generation might be that the balancing of heavy vocal demands, full time work, and significant family responsibilities for young and old, tends to peak at this particular age, and to impact on close partner or marital relationships.

Other family issues, although not traumatic, were often experienced as being very stressful and causally related to the FVD by both the patient and therapist. These incidents involved changes to family structures and dynamics, with consequences for tension in relationships and communication. These events included coping with a new baby under trying financial conditions, a child leaving home to take on a new career, or an elderly and dependent relative coming to live with the family. Others entailed more chronic difficulties in communication between parents and their children, with serious conflicts over the setting of boundaries and acceptable behaviours for adolescents transitioning into adulthood (Butcher *et al.*, 2007; Kinzl *et al.*, 1988a). Women often reported that these situations felt 'overwhelming', and that they were reticent to speak out about their frustrations or to seek social support. There was a sense that these women were constantly juggling the priorities of relationships and responsibilities at home and at work against a background of helplessness in effecting change. "Fools 14" by Fred Cress captures elements of this perfectly (Fig. 5.3).

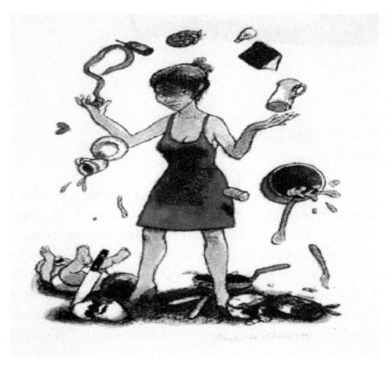

Fig. 5.3 "Fools 14", Fred Cress (1999)

Courtesy Fred Cress Estate.

One cannot help noticing the similarities between the two early case series with men and those described above for women, where onset of FVD may have developed after traumatic events for some, often in association with URTI for others, but more commonly, following stressful events and difficulties in the face of *loss*, *separation*, and ongoing *difficulties with conflict* in their family and work lives. In all these situations involving both men and women, a pattern seemed to be emerging amongst individuals carrying *high levels of responsibility* for others, often in situations where the expression of complex negative emotions was difficult, and where an ongoing *sense of powerlessness* and futility prevailed. These excellent qualitative data and thoughtful analyses of those situations occurring prior to onset of FVD described by the authors above set the scene for the very few comparative group studies into stressful life events and difficulties that have followed.

Life events and difficulties: Comparative group studies

Given this early emphasis on the likelihood that negative emotions in response to stressful life events and difficulties may be associated with onset of the wider range of FVD, it is surprising that until 1998, there have only been five published studies using a comparative group design (Andersson & Schalen, 1998; Friedl *et al.*, 1990; Friedl *et al.*, 1993; House & Andrews, 1988; McHugh-Munier *et al.*, 1997), with one further case-control study conducted more recently (Baker *et al.*, 2013).

Summarising the empirical evidence from the earlier studies is rather difficult because of the differences in instruments used to measure the number and severity of stressful incidents, and a lack of specificity in the time frames for inclusion of incidents preceding onset. For instance, approaches to obtaining life events data ranged from the use of life events checklists, case history interview with grouping of incidents according to a structured inventory, and, in only one study (House & Andrews, 1988), using a standardised semi-structured interview, the Life Events and Difficulties Schedule (LEDS). Research design and methodology showed marked inconsistencies in diagnostic terminologies and classification of patients to study groups (a problem the field continues to face throughout our research literature); uneven distributions of men and women in those studies which included both genders; poorly balanced numbers across study and control groups; and minimal statistical analysis of the data. Taking these limitations into account, however, it is perhaps best to highlight those trends extrapolated from a literature review of the findings emerging from the studies (Baker, 2008), and then to discuss some of the important observations and searching questions posed by these authors that influenced the directions and focus of subsequent studies (Box 5.3).

Box 5.3 Trends for life events data derived from comparative group studies

- Traumatic or severe incidents included death, loss, separation and threat to personal or family safety – reported, but infrequently
- Moderate incidents involved changes in family and work situations, and difficulties in resolving conflicts in relationships – commonly reported
- Studies including comparisons between FVD, OVD and controls, showed a greater number of incidents, and with higher levels of strain reported in the FVD group, **but those with OVD experienced more stressful events than the controls**
- When stressful incidents were commonly reported, they were not necessarily construed as being causally related by patients
- Incidents characterised by dilemma over the expression of negative emotions especially anger were typically reported
- Individuals with a lack of assertiveness, reticence to seek social support and sense of powerlessness in effecting change – frequently observed
- Unsatisfactory ways of coping frequently reported and observed

(Andersson & Schalen, 1998; Friedl, Friedrich, & Egger, 1990; Friedl, Friedrich, Egger, & Fitzek, 1993; House & Andrews, 1988; McHugh-Munier, Scherer, Lehmann, & Scherer, 1997)

Observations and searching questions arising from these early studies

In the seminal study by House and Andrews (1988), the authors noted that rather than traumatic or severe incidents preceding onset of FVD, moderate situations related to family and work issues, and unresolved conflicts in relationships were more likely. They commented upon the preponderance of women with FVD as opposed to men, and suggested that the women they saw were often overly involved in their wider social network in a way that left them both over-committed and relatively powerless. They observed that although the conflicts these women experienced could be described in contextual terms, it was also evident that they had contributed in a significant way to their own context. This was not expressed in a way to imply blame but rather, to raise questions about the nature of their early experiences that might have led to this overly-devoted style in relationships. They went on to suggest that exploration into the nature of personal vulnerability to FVD and other somatisation disorders could be a useful direction for future research.

Their findings also reflected the strong anecdotal details from previous reports which suggested that FVD often arose in situations of interpersonal conflict and difficulty in expressing negative emotions, particularly anger. On the basis of these observations, they developed a new dimension to explore the specific nature of the stresses that might be operating in those patients with FVD. They called this new measure *conflict over speaking out* (COSO), which was operationally defined with two essential criteria. The first gave emphasis to a person having some sense of responsibility and longer-term emotional investment in the relationship continuing, such as a marriage, as a caregiver, as an employee, or as a pivotal member of a family group. The second criterion stressed that COSO events and difficulties were not just situational dilemmas about speaking out but more importantly, that *serious consequences* for speaking out could be recognised, and equally, the very real consequences for not speaking out. It was this *triad of considerations* that helped these investigators to identify, quantify, and rate COSO incidents with attention to the contextual features for each person, and with a reliable degree of objectivity. The tensions inherent in COSO issues that take place in close relationships are shown most vividly in Fred Cress's "Fools 2", (Fig. 5.4).

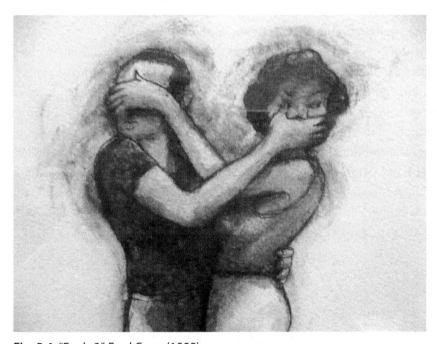

Fig. 5.4 "Fools 2", Fred Cress (1998)

Courtesy Fred Cress Estate and BMGART Gallery South Australia

When reflecting upon their results for the high number of COSO events or difficulties preceding FVD in many patients, they concluded that there was a need for a clear formulation to explain the way in which COSO incidents may be mediated by psychophysiological variables to result in voice disorder. The results from their companion study into psychiatric and social characteristics did not suggest that mood disorder or psychiatric illness was likely to be a primary mediator between COSO events and difficulties and FVD (House & Andrews, 1987). However, they suggested that it would be helpful if we understood how certain responses to COSO situations might contribute to the development of the laryngeal muscle tension patterns so often associated with FVD.

In a similar vein, Andersson *et al.* (1998) observed that patients with PVD often demonstrated patterns of helplessness and difficulties in being assertive, as expressed in comments such as: 'I always get swept aside', 'Nobody listens to me', 'I see no way out' (p. 99). The women in their study mentioned difficulty in expressing themselves verbally, or in formulating their feelings in a distinct and appropriate manner, which led these authors to suggest that PVD might reflect a predisposing personality with diminished capacity to adapt to and cope with conflicts, and a disturbed capacity for emotional expression. They did not go so far as to suggest that some of the patients had *alexithymia*, a psychiatric diagnosis for individuals with a marked difficulty in the verbal expression of emotions, but their observations raised the possibility that some patients with PVD may well present in a clinically similar manner.

They also proposed that in the development of PVD there seems to be a disturbance in the reciprocal interactions between *emotional awareness*, laryngeal perception and *central motor control over phonation*. These ideas echoed those of authors cited in the preceding sections. In a sense they also pre-empted further publications and studies on the understanding of the complex interactions between the emotional, psychological and neurophysiological processes under-pinning FVD (Aronson & Bless, 2009; Baker *et al.*, 2013; Butcher *et al.*, 2007; Dietrich, Andreatta, Jiang, Joshi, & Stemple, 2012; Freeman, 2000; O'Hara, Miller, Carding, Wilson, & Deary, 2011; Rammage, Morrison, & Nichol, 2001; Roy, 2003; van Mersbergen, 2011).

Life events and difficulties: Case control study

Drawing upon these previous findings and helpful insights, my colleagues and I undertook an investigation into a number of psychosocial factors previously identified in the literature (Baker *et al.*, 2013). We used a non-random case-control design with 194 women, aged between 18 and 80 years of age, with a recently diagnosed FVD (n = 73) or OVD (n = 55) and a control group (n = 66) with perceptually normal voices. The LEDS was administered to investigate the number and severity of life events and difficulties experienced by these women during the 12 months preceding onset of their voice disorder, or before interview for control group women. The incidents were rated along traditional lines for threat, unpleasantness, or loss, and by definition they had to involve the patient, or close others such as partner, child, parent or trusted confidante. The same incidents were then rated for COSO and for a new dimension developed by ourselves called *powerless in the system (PITS)*. We also explored a range of other variables related to *psychological traits* and *patterns of emotional expressiveness*. These two principal areas of psychosocial enquiry were initially explored as separate entities, and then as they may interact as risk factors for the development of FVD and/or OVD.

A further analysis of all the data was then undertaken to determine whether the same variables might operate as predictors of risk for the FVD sub-groups, MTVD (n = 36) and PVD (n = 37). Key, statistically-significant findings for the part of the study focused on LEDS and COSO incidents are summarised below. While stressful life events and difficulties were reported across all 10 domains of inquiry for the LEDS, the three primary domains in which the most incidents occurred are included (Box 5.4).

Box 5.4 Findings for LEDS & COSO incidents across three primary domains

Women with **FVD** in comparison to **OVD** and **Control** group experienced:

- At least one and a greater number of **severe life events** – some traumatic
  - Health/treatment/accidents
  - Work and Other relationships/including children
  - Marital/Partner relationships
- At least one and a greater number of **major difficulties**
  - Marital/Partner relationships
  - Other relationship/including children
  - Health/treatment/accidents
- At least one and a greater number of **COSO life events**
  - Work and Other relationships/including children
  - Marital/Partner relationships
- At least one and a greater number of **COSO difficulties**
  - Work and Other relationships/including children
  - Marital /Partner relationships
- At least one and a greater number of **COSO + PITS difficulties**
  - Work and Other relationships/including children
  - Marital /Partner and Housing

Women with **MTVD** ($n = 36$) in comparison with **PVD** ($n = 37$) experienced:

- Minimal differences for severe life events or major difficulties
- No differences for COSO events or COSO difficulties

(Baker, Ben-Tovim, Butcher, Esterman, & McLaughlin, 2013)

Observations in relation to severe events and major difficulties

Our findings for more severe events, and even traumatic occurrences, were similar to previous studies using the LEDS to investigate a range of medically unexplained conditions not unlike FVD, where patients complained of marked physiological discomfort and dysfunction in the absence of organic pathology, sufficient to justify the extent and severity of their symptoms. For instance, in studies exploring external factors preceding onset of *functional abdominal pain* (Creed, Craig, & Farmer, 1988), *functional menorrhagia* (T. O. Harris, 1989), *globus pharyngis* (M. B. Harris, Deary, & Wilson, 1996), *chronic fatigue syndrome*

(Hatcher & House, 2003), and mental health disorders such as *anxiety and depression* (Brown & Harris, 1989a; Finlay-Jones, 1989), it has been clearly shown that severe events and major difficulties experienced in the previous 12 months often operate as significant risk for these physical and mental health problems. In the light of these trends, our strong findings for severe events and major difficulties are of particular interest, especially given that the FVD group women also had significantly higher scores for anxiety and depression than the OVD and Control groups.

Another of our findings was that women with OVD were twice as likely to experience severe life events and major difficulties in the 12 months preceding onset than the control group women. These differences only approached statistical significance but considering that 33% (18/55) of the women with OVD had voice disorders associated with thyroid disease and/or surgery, it would not be unreasonable to wonder if stressful incidents might have been associated with the onset of thyroid dysfunction. Of course, this is merely speculation, but previous studies have shown that psychosocial factors might affect the *neuroendocrine and immunosuppressant function*, leaving the person vulnerable to the development of a range of organic conditions (Biondi & Picardi, 1999). Furthermore, in an extensive review of emerging trends in *psychosomatic medicine*, it was concluded that there is now 'a solid base' of evidence for an association between life events and *Graves' Disease* (Fava & Sonino, 2000). Our initial findings, together with the observations above, suggest that this might be an area that merits further exploration.

The greatest number of major difficulties occurred in relation to marital and partner issues. Central to these difficulties were ongoing power imbalances and struggles, feelings of helplessness in effecting change or making situations any better, and an overall sense of *entrapment*. Fred Cress depicts these nuances and vicissitudes of marital harmony and discord most poignantly in his fiery painting "Duets" (Fig. 5.5). As he said in relation to his own work, "My pictures don't let you out – there is nowhere to go". He was right, and in a review of *Duets* the arts critic John Neylon remarked with equally amusing candour:

'*Big Brother House has nothing, absolutely nothing on Fred Cress's theatres of the emotionally baggaged. Slap any one of those brats behaving badly against some of Cress's seasoned troupers and it's no contest. Duets looks like a cartoon catalogue of gender relations. Couples embrace, quarrel or nag one another and so on, but when you spend longer look at Cress's work the power imbalance becomes apparent and menacing notes sound*' (Neylon, 2004) (p.1–2).

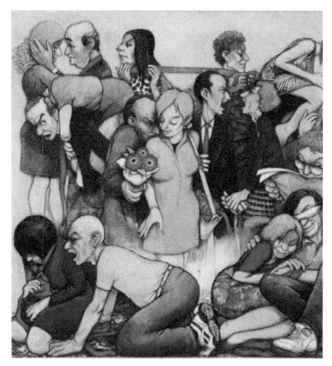

Fig. 5.5 "Duets", Fred Cress (2004)

Courtesy Fred Cress Estate

Observations in relation to conflict over speaking out and powerlessness

The COSO phenomenon as operationally defined by House *et al.* (1988) has been cited as one of the most likely psychosocial factors to be associated with the onset of FVD, and the construct has obvious face validity and strong clinical appeal. In our study, this was the first time the construct has been explored further, either with another group of women with FVD or by including another group with OVD in addition to a control group with normal voices.

The findings showed that women with FVD were more likely to have experienced a significantly greater number of COSO incidents than OVD and Control group women in the 12 months prior to onset. (There were no differences for COSO incidents between the OVD and Control group). These COSO situations occurred primarily across the domains of work, other relationships including children and, to a lesser extent, in marital and partner relationships. The results affirmed the frequent anecdotal observations made in the previous studies, where incidents preceding onset were related to interpersonal conflicts in which the patient felt unable or ambivalent about speaking out for fear of making matters worse, while also reticent to seek social support. Significantly, the results of this current study confirmed the empirical findings with respect to the COSO dimension and suggest that this may be a helpful and valid construct for clinicians to take into account when considering causal pathways for FVD.

As mentioned above, it was in response to so many ongoing COSO difficulties that we developed our new dimension called *powerless in the system (PITS)*. This was operationally defined as a COSO situation where the person had to persevere whether they had spoken out or not, and where there was a clear interaction between a sense of powerlessness, futility in soldiering on, and the inevitability of defeat. Women with FVD were more likely to experience these COSO incidents characterised by PITS than the OVD or Control group women.

This frequently occurred in acrimonious marital relationships where a violent partner threatened a woman with further assault if she asserted herself or threatened to leave. It was common for women in service industries, such as health fund or social service departments, where they had high levels of contact with the public, and when they were delivering information or dealing with enquiries where customers were often angry, frustrated or belligerent. Remaining polite and calm under these trying circumstances was often exceedingly difficult, with serious consequences if they failed to do so. Many COSO situations with PITS were described by schoolteachers when the education system dictated where they would teach, the subjects that they would teach and to whom, with little recourse to choice or negotiation. A number of recurring themes emerged in a more qualitative analysis of these COSO difficulties with PITS as reported by teachers, and these same contextual features were noted in relation to the family lives and occupations of other women with FVD.

Low job control and mastery of the environment

The first was related to *low job control* exacerbated by a lack of permanency and job security. At that time, teachers in public state schools could only stay in any one school for 10 years, resulting in them being required to accept temporary placements anywhere the Education Department had a vacancy. This often meant that they would have a term in one school and then have to change to a different school the following term, and so on. They were often placed in the outer suburbs or the country, requiring them to travel or move to locations well away from their home, with unsettling implications for their families.

The second related to a *loss of mastery over their working environment*, which led many women with FVD to report a loss of self-esteem and confidence in their ability to perform their job properly. This was often associated with a lack of experience in working with students from different socio-demographic areas, learning to manage students in different age groups, or being required to teach in subject areas outside their expertise. These difficulties contributed to a continual sense of being ill-prepared, which led to serious problems in the management of student behaviour. Many teachers lamented that they were no longer teachers but authoritarian custodians of recalcitrant students who did not seem interested in learning. Overwhelmingly, they reported feeling ill-equipped in the area of behaviour management. They also attributed their sense of failure and ineptitude in coping to a lack of support from the larger system, where the rights of the student, the parents, and the school council, seemed to prevail over their own.

It is most interesting to consider these current qualitative findings in the light of the famous Whitehall II studies, and recent studies with indigenous peoples in both Canada and Australia (Daniel, 2006; Marmot, 2008), which have shown that *low job control* and *loss of mastery over one's environment* can have serious implications for increased risk of mortality and a range of physical and mental health conditions. This places our findings into a wider socio-cultural context, and may shed further light on to the meaning of the stressful and COSO incidents as psychosocial factors that contributed to the onset of FVD in this cohort of women as represented in the sculpture "Spiral Woman" by Louise Bourgeois (Fig. 5.6).

This remarkable bronze sculpture captures these sentiments of powerlessness, ambivalence, and difficulty in coping most vividly. And how confronting, too, that in discussing her sculpture on a documentary film about her work by Camille Guichard (2008), she also raises the question about women's possible culpability or contribution to their current situation.

'This small but powerful bronze piece hangs from the ceiling, once again representing ambivalence and doubt. The spiral is my attempt to control the chaos. My woman is bound with thick coil forever trapped and spinning in a constant state of dizzying indecision. Is she a victim of her own making?' (Personal communication 2008)

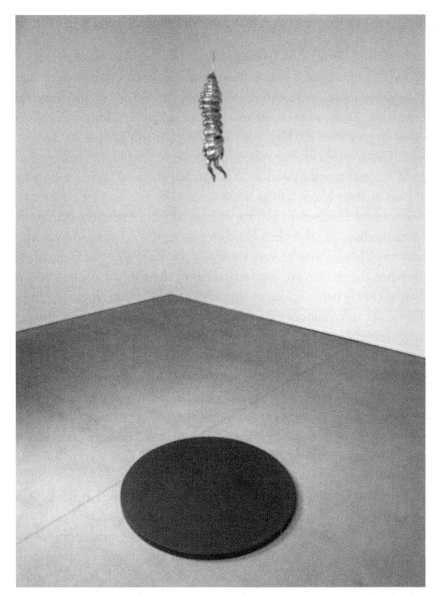

Fig. 5.6 Louise Bourgeois "Spiral woman" (1984)

Bronze and slate disc – Bronze: 48.2x10.1x13.9 cm. Slate disc: 3.17x 86.3cm diameter
Collection The Easton Foundation Photo Allan Finkelman, © The Easton Foundation/Licensed
by Viscopy, Sydney

Emotional labour, compassion fatigue and professional burnout

The third recurring feature that typified many COSO difficulties characterised by PITS was the emotional cost associated with high levels of personal contact, interpersonal communication, and responsibility or care for others. This was the scenario for many women facing demanding family situations, and in occupations ranging from the higher levels of management to those lower down the hierarchy such as teaching or service industries to the public. These women often described events and difficulties that typically required the more invisible facets of work that are referred to as *emotional labour*.

As proposed by Hochschild (1990), emotional labour requires workers to deal with the feelings of others in addition to the regulation of their own. Also, while emotional labour may be very satisfying for many (K. Erickson, 2004), especially when the worker can meet the needs of the self or the job, Erickson and Wharton (1997) have also shown that where there is a discrepancy between the authentic self and emotions that have to be manufactured for others, the cost can be high, leading to distress or even *professional burnout*.

There is now empirical evidence showing that high levels of emotional labour and *compassion fatigue* are associated with service jobs, or with occupations related to education, mental and physical health (Figley, 2002). Moreover, where there are conflicts between the individual and their role identity, this may, over time, lead to professional burnout with the tell-tale signs of emotional exhaustion, depersonalisation and sense of reduced personal accomplishment (Adams, 2006).

These constructs of emotional labour and burnout have been explored from a slightly different perspective by Scheid (2004). She maintains that central to emotional labour is the notion of *self-concept* or *identity*, and that under the administrative regimes of so many institutions for health and education it is difficult for workers to hold on to their sense of self or professional identity. Scheid argues that losing one's prerogative to go about one's work in a way that fits one's image of themselves or their professional role, and *not* being allowed to offer the emotional labour required, can also lead to professional burnout. She suggests that when a worker is prevented from making a meaningful investment of the self in his/her work, this is critical, and it is the *failure of emotional labour* that matters. On the basis of our data, this appeared to be happening with many women with FVD, especially those in teaching positions and service to the public.

Summary and some further questions

In our study, women with FVD in comparison with those in the OVD and Control Groups experienced more severe LEDs and COSO situations prior to onset, against a background of work with high levels of emotional labour and low job control. It seems that many women with FVD had become both vocally and emotionally burnt out, having lost their physiological voice, and 'their voice' in the larger systems to which they belonged. These findings now offer some empirical support for the many excellent earlier studies that provided the strong foundations for this area of psychosocial inquiry.

Women with OVD experienced more stressful life events and difficulties than control group women, (but not COSO incidents), and it is clinically relevant to wonder whether these stressful situations might have contributed to a lowering of resilience in the immune system and vulnerability to the OVD in some individuals?

Significantly, too, further analysis of the same dimensions between the two FVD sub-groups, MTVD and PVD, failed to predict voice disorder group membership. Although women in both groups experienced a high number of severe events and difficulties, including those imbued with COSO and PITS, there were no statistically significant differences for these measures. This was a surprising result, given that 35% (13/37) of PVD group women were totally aphonic. From a clinical point of view, this is often judged as indicating a more 'severe' clinical presentation, with the presumption, rightly or wrongly, that such a voice disorder may have been preceded by a more traumatic incident or a greater number of severe events, major difficulties or COSO situations.

The strong LEDS and COSO data suggest that this may be a helpful way of thinking about the context in which FVD in women develops. The fact that these dimensions did not differentiate between the PVD and MTVD sub-groups raises fascinating questions about how we might seek to understand causal pathways for these disorders. It may be relevant to consider whether sudden and/or total loss of voice necessarily means that this has arisen as a response to a more threatening event. Are stressful life events and difficulties, while more traditionally associated with the onset of PVD and affiliated disorders, just as important in contributing to the onset of MTVD? Is it possible that PVD and MTVD rightfully belong together within the larger diagnostic classification of FVD, but somewhere along a continuum? Is it possible that given a particular set of circumstances, the particular responses to stressful life events and COSO situations, and the clinical presentations of the voice disorder, are determined more by the dispositional vulnerabilities of a person? Certainly some of the recent studies exploring a range of *psychological correlates* related to *personality traits, emotional expressiveness* and *coping styles* bear this out, and these will now be considered in Chapter 6.

References

Adams, R. E., Boscarino, J.A., & Figley, C. R. (2006). Compassion fatigue and psychological distress among social workers: A validation study. *American Journal of Orthopsychiatry, 76*(1).

American Psychiatric Association. (1994). *Diagnostic and statistical manual of mental disorders DSM-4.* (4th ed.) Arlington: American Psychiatric Association.American Psychiatric Association. (2013). *Diagnostic and statistical manual of mental disorders DSM-5* (5th ed.). Arlington: American Psychiatric Association.

Andersson, K., & Schalen, L. (1998). Etiology and treatment of psychogenic voice disorder: Results of a follow-up study of thirty patients. *Journal of Voice, 12*(1), 96–106.

Arnold, G. E., & Pinto, S. (1960). Ventricular dysphonia: New interpretation of an old observation. *Laryngoscope, 70,* 1608–1627.

Aronson, A. E. (1969). Speech pathology and symptom therapy in the interdisciplinary treatment of psychogenic aphonia. *Journal of Speech and Hearing Disorders, 34*(4), 321–341.

Aronson, A. E. (1990). Psychogenic voice disorders. In A. E. Aronson, *Clinical voice disorders: An interdisciplinary approach.* (3rd ed., pp. 116–159). New York: Thieme.

Aronson, A. E., & Bless, D. M. (2009). *Clinical voice disorders* (4th ed.). New York: Thieme.

Aronson, A. E., Peterson, H. W., & Litin, E. M. (1964). Voice symptomatology in functional dysphonia and aphonia. *Journal of Speech and Hearing Disorders, 28,* 367–380.

Aronson, A. E., Peterson, H. W., & Litin, E. M. (1966). Psychiatric symptomatology in functional dysphonia and aphonia. *Journal of Speech and Hearing Disorders, 31,* 115–127.

Baker, J. (1998). Psychogenic dysphonia: Peeling back the layers. *Journal of Voice, 12*(4), 527–535.

Baker, J. (2002a). Persistent dysphonia in two performers affecting the singing and projected speaking voice: A report on a collaborative approach to management. *Logopedics Phoniatrics Vocology, 27,* 179–187.

Baker, J. (2002b). Psychogenic voice disorders – heroes or hysterics? A brief overview with questions and discussion. *Logopedics Phoniatrics Vocology, 27,* 84–91.

Baker, J. (2003). Psychogenic voice disorders and traumatic stress experience: A discussion paper with two case reports. *Journal of Voice, 17*(3), 308–318.

Baker, J. (2008). The role of psychogenic and psychosocial factors in the development of functional voice disorders. *International Journal of Speech-Language Pathology, 10*(4), 210–230.

Baker, J., Ben-Tovim, D. I., Butcher, A., Esterman, A., & McLaughlin, K. (2007). Development of a modified diagnostic classification system for voice disorders with inter-rater reliability study. *Logopedics Phoniatrics Vocology, 32*, 99–112.

Baker, J., Ben-Tovim, D. I., Butcher, A., Esterman, A., & McLaughlin, K. (2012). Psychosocial risk factors which may differentiate between women with Functional Voice Disorder, Organic Voice Disorder, and Control group. *International Journal of Speech-Language Pathology*. doi: 10.310-/17549507.2012.721397

Baker, J., Ben-Tovim, D. I., Butcher, A., Esterman, A., & McLaughlin, K. (2013). Psychosocial risk factors which may differentiate between women with Functional Voice Disorder, Organic Voice Disorder, and Control group. *International Journal of Speech-Language Pathology, 15*(6), 547–563.

Baker, J., & Lane, R. D. (2009). Emotion processing deficits in functional voice disorders. In K. Izdebski (Ed.), *Emotions in the human voice* (Vol. 3, pp. 105–136). San Diego: Plural Publishing.

Bangs, J. L., & Freidinger, A. (1950). A case of hysterical dysphonia in an adult. *Journal of Speech and Hearing Disorders, 15*, 316–323.

Barker, P. (1991). *Regeneration* London: Penguin.

Bartlett, F. (1932). *Remembering: A study of experimental and social psychology*. Cambridge: Cambridge University Press.

Barton, R. T. (1960). The whispering syndrome of hysteric dysphonia. *Annals of Otolaryngology Rhinology and Laryngology, 69*, 156–164.

Biondi, M., & Picardi, A. (1999). Psychological stress and neuroendocrine function in humans: The last two decades of research. *Psychotherapy and Psychosomatics, 68*, 114–150.

Bowling, A. (1995). *Measuring disease*. Buckingham: Open University Press.

Brodnitz, F. S. (1969). Functional aphonia. *Annals of Otolaryngology, (St Louis), 78*, 1244–1253.

Brown, G. W., & Harris, T. O. (1978). *Social origins of depression*. London: Tavistock Publications.

Brown, G. W., & Harris, T. O. (1982a). Fall-off in the reporting of life events. *Social Psychiatry, 17*, 23–28.

Brown, G. W., & Harris, T. O. (1989a). Depression. In G. W. Brown & T. O. Harris (Eds.), *Life events and illness* (pp. 49–93). London: The Guilford Press.

Brown, G. W., & Harris, T. O. (1989b). *Life events and illness*. London: The Guilford Press.

Brown, G. W., Harris, T. O., & Hepworth, C. (1995). Loss, humiliation and entrapment among women developing depression: A patient and non-patient comparison. *Psychological Medicine, 25*(1), 7–22.

Butcher, P., & Cavalli, L. (1998). Fran: Understanding and treating psychogenic dysphonia from a cognitive-behavioural perspective. In D. Syder (Ed.), *Wanting to talk*.: Whurr.

Butcher, P., Elias, A., & Cavalli, L. (2007). *Understanding and treating psychogenic voice disorder: A CBT framework*. Chichester: Wiley.

Butcher, P., Elias, A., Raven, R., Yeatman, J., & Littlejohns, D. (1987). Psychogenic voice disorder unresponsive to speech therapy: Psychological characteristics and cognitive-behaviour therapy. *British Journal of Disorders of Communication, 22*, 81–92.

Butow, P. N., Hiller, J. E., Price, M. A., Thackway, S. V., Kricker, A., & Tennant, C. C. (2000). Epidemiological evidence for a relationship between life events, coping style, and personality factors in the development of breast cancer. *Journal of Psychosomatic Research, 49*, 169–181.

Case, J. L. (1984). Psychogenic (nonorganic) voice disorders. *Clinical management of voice disorders.* (pp. 197–234). Maryland: Aspen Publications.

Craig, T. K. J. (2001). Life events: meanings and precursors. In P. W. Halligan, C. Bass & J. C. Marshall (Eds.), *Contemporary approaches to the study of hysteria* (pp. 88–101). Oxford: Oxford University Press.

Creed, F., Craig, T., & Farmer, R. (1988). Functional abdominal pain, psychiatric illness, and life events. *Gut, 1988*(29), 235–242.

Daniel, M., Brown, A., Dhurrkay, J.G., Cargo, M.D. & O'Dea, K. (2006). Mastery, perceived stress and health-related behaviour in northeast Arnhem Land: A cross-sectional study. *International Journal for Equity in Health, 5*(10).

Dietrich, M., Andreatta, R. D., Jiang, Y., Joshi, A., & Stemple, J. C. (2012). Preliminary findings on the relation between the personality trait of stress reaction and the central neural control of vocalization. *International Journal of Speech-Language Pathology, 14*(4), 377–389.

Erickson, K. (2004). To invest or detach? Coping strategies and workplace culture in service work. *Symbolic Interaction, 27*, 549–572.

Erickson, R. J., Wharton, A.S. (1997). Inauthenticity and depression: Assessing the consequences of interactive service work. *Work and occupation, 24*, 188–213.

Eysenck, H. J. (1994). Cancer, personality and stress: Prediction and prevention. *Behaviour Research and Therapy, 16*, 167–215.

Fava, G. A., & Sonino, N. (2000). Psychosomatic medicine: Emerging trends and perspectives. *Psychotherapy and Psychosomatics, 69*(4), 184.

Figley, C. R. (Ed.). (2002). *Treating compassion fatigue.* New York: Brunner-Routledge.

Finlay-Jones. (1989). Anxiety. In G. W. Brown & T. O. Harris (Eds.), *Life events and illness* (pp. 95–112). London: The Guilford Press.

Freeman, M. (2000). Psychogenic, psychological and psychosocial issues in diagnosis and therapy. In M. Freeman & M. Fawcus (Eds.), *Voice disorders and their management.* (pp. 137–155). London: Whurr.

Friedl, W., Friedrich, G., & Egger, J. (1990). Personality and coping with stress in patients suffering from functional dysphonia. *Folia Phoniatrica, 42*, 13–20.

Friedl, W., Friedrich, G., Egger, J., & Fitzek, T. (1993). Psychogenic factors in the etiology of functional voice disorders. *Folia Phoniatrica, 45*, 10–13.

Froese, M. D., & Sims, P. (1987). Functional dysphonia in adolescence: Two case reports. *Canadian Journal of Psychiatry, 32*(5), 389–392.

Greene, J. S. (1938). Psychiatric therapy for dysphonia: Aphonia, psycho-phonasthenia, falsetto. *Archives of Otolaryngology, 28*, 213–221.

Guichard, C. (Writer). (2008). Louise Bourgeois, *Facets Video*. USA.

Guze, S. B., & Brown, O. L. (1962). Psychiatric disease and functional dysphonia and aphonia. *Archives of Otolaryngology, 76*, 84–87.

Harris, M. B., Deary, I. J., & Wilson, J. A. (1996). Life events and difficulties in relation to the onset of globus pharyngis. *Journal of Psychosomatic Research, 40*, 603–615.

Harris, T. (Ed.). (2000). *Where inner and outer worlds meet. Psychosocial research in the tradition of George Brown*. London: Routledge.

Harris, T. O. (1989). Disorders of menstruation. In G. W. Brown & T. O. Harris (Eds.), *Life events and illness*. London: The Guilford Press.

Hartman, D. E., & Aronson, A. E. (1983). Psychogenic aphonia masking mutational falsetto. *Archives of Otolaryngology, 109*, 415–416.

Hartman, D. E., Daily, W. W., & Morin, K. N. (1989). A case of superior laryngeal nerve paresis and psychogenic dysphonia. *Journal of Speech and Hearing Disorders, 54*, 526–529.

Hatcher, S., & House, A. (2003). Life events, difficulties and dilemmas in the onset of chronic fatigue syndrome: A case-control study. *Psychological Medicine, 33*, 1185–1192.

Hobson, C. J., & Delunas, L. (2001). National norms and life-event frequencies for the revised social readjustment rating scale. *International Journal of Stress Management., 8*(4), 299–314.

Hochschild, A. (1990). Ideology and emotion management: A perspective and path for future research. In T. D. Kemper (Ed.), *Research agendas in the sociology of emotions* (pp. 117–142). Albany: SUNY Press.

Holmes, T. H., & Rahe, R. H. (1967). The Social Readjustment Scale. *Journal of Psychosomatic Research, 11*, 213–218.

Horowitz, M. J., Wilner, N., & Alvarez, W. (1979). Impact of event scale: A measure of subjective stress. *Psychosomatic Medicine, 41*(3), 209218.

House, A., & Andrews, H. B. (1987). The psychiatric and social characteristics of patients with functional dysphonia. *Journal of Psychosomatic Research, 31*, 483–490.

House, A., & Andrews, H. B. (1988). Life events and difficulties preceding the onset of functional dysphonia. *Journal of Psychosomatic Research, 32*(3), 311–319.

Ingals, E. F. (1890). Hysterical aphonia. *Journal of the American Medical Association, 15*, 92–95.

Joanna Briggs Institute for Evidence Based Nursing and Midwifery. (1998). Available at http://www.joannabriggs.edu.au/ [Accessed October 2016]

Kessler, R. C. (1997). The effects of stressful life events on depression. *Annual Review of Psychology, 48*, 191–214.

Kinzl, J., Biebl, W., & Rauchegger, H. (1988a). Functional aphonia: A conversion symptom as defensive mechanism against anxiety. *Psychotherapy and Psychosomatics, 49*, 31–36.

Kinzl, J., Biebl, W., & Rauchegger, H. (1988b). Functional aphonia: Psychosomatic aspects of diagnosis and therapy. *Folia Phoniatrica, 40*, 131–137.

Lazarus, R. L., & Folkman, S. (1984). *Stress appraisal and coping*. New York: Springer.

Macleod, C., & Hemsley, D. R. (1985). Visual feedback of vocal intensity in the treatment of hysterical aphonia. *Journal of Behavioural and Experimental Psychiatry, 16*(4), 347–353.

Marmot, M., Friel, S., Bell, R., Houweling, T.A.J., & Taylor, S. (2008). Closing the gap in a generation: Health equity through action on the social determinants of health. *Lancet, 372*, 1661–1669.

Matas, M. (1991). Psychogenic voice disorders: Literature review and case report. *Canadian Journal of Psychiatry, 36*, 363–365.

Mathieson, L. (2001). *Greene and Mathieson's: The voice and its disorders.* (6th ed.). London: Whurr.

McHugh-Munier, C., Scherer, K. R., Lehmann, W., & Scherer, U. (1997). Coping strategies, personality, and voice quality in patients with vocal fold nodules and polyps. *Journal of Voice, 11*(4), 452–461.

Neeleman, J., & Mann, A. H. (1993). Treatment of hysterical aphonia with hypnosis and prokaletic therapy. *British Journal of Psychiatry, 163*, 816–819.

Neylon, J. (2004). A Hotel California for art lovers. *The Adelaide Review: Archives* (November).

O'Hara, J., Miller, T., Carding, P., Wilson, J., & Deary, V. (2011). Relationship between fatigue, perfectionism, and functional dysphonia. *Otolaryngology-Head and Neck Surgery, 144*(6), 921–926.

Paykel, E. S., Prusoff, B. A., & Uhlenhuth, E. H. (1971). Scaling of events. *Archives of General Psychiatry, 25*, 340–347.

Perepel, E. (1930). On the physiology of hysterical aphonia and mutism. *International Journal of Psychoanalysis*, 185–192.

Rammage, L., Morrison, M., & Nichol, H. (2001). *Management of the voice and its disorders.* San Diego: Singular Publishing Group.

Roy, N. (2003). Functional dysphonia. *Current Opinion in Otolaryngology and Head and Neck Surgery, 11*(3), 144–148.

Sapir, S. (1995). Psychogenic spasmodic dysphonia: A case study with expert opinions. *Journal of Voice, 9*(3), 270–281.

Sapir, S., & Aronson, A. E. (1987). Coexisting psychogenic and neurogenic dysphonia: A source of diagnostic confusion. *British Journal of Disorders of Communication, 22*, 73–80.

Schalen, L., & Andersson, K. (1992). Differential diagnosis and treatment of psychogenic voice disorder. *Clinical Otolaryngology, 17*, 225–230.

Scheid, T. L. (2004, 14th August). *The commodification of care: Consequences for emotional labour and burnout.* Paper presented at the Annual American Sociological Association.

Seifert, E., & Kollbrunner, J. (2005). Stress and distress in non-organic voice disorders. *Swiss Medical Weekly, 135*, 387–397.

Selye, H., & Fortier, C. (1950). Adaptive reaction to stress. *Psychosomatic Medicine, 12*(3), 149–157.

Shewell, C. (2009). *Voice work: Art and science in changing voices.* Chichester: Wiley-Blackwell.

Smurthwaite, H. (1919). War neuroses of the larynx and speech mechanism. *Journal of Laryngology and Otolaryngology*, 13–20.

Sokolowsky, R. R., & Junkermann, E. B. (1944). War aphonia. *Journal of Speech Disorders*, *9*, 193–208.

Turner, R. J., & Wheaton, B. (1995). Checklist Measurement of Stressful Life Events. In M. E. Cohen, R. C. Kessler & L. U. Gordon (Eds.), *Measuring Stress* (pp. 29–58). Oxford: Oxford Univ. Press.

van Mersbergen, M. (2011). Voice disorders and personality: Understanding their interactions. In T. L. Eadie (Ed.), *Perspectives on voice and voice disorders* (Vol. 21, pp. 31–38). Rockville: ASHA.

Vinokur, A., & Selzer, M. L. (1975). Desirable versus undesirable life events: Their relationship to stress and mental disease. *Journal of Personality and Social Psychology*, *32*, 329–337.

Wethington, E., Almeida, D., Brown, G. W., Frank, E., & Kessler, R. C. (2001). The assessment of stressor exposure. In A. Vingerhoets (Ed.), *Assessment in behavioural science.* (pp. 113–134). Hove: Brunner-Routledge.

6

Personality traits, emotional expressiveness, and psychiatric disorder

'Exploring the characteristics of the "person" behind the voice may be as fruitful as studying the structure that produces it' (Roy et al., 2000b) (p.766)

Introduction

There are two further areas of inquiry with respect to psychosocial factors and voice disorders. One group of studies has explored possible *causal associations* between dispositional and psychological correlates that may contribute to an individual's vulnerability to the development, exacerbation, and/or perpetuation of particular voice disorders. Others have focused on the *psychosocial impact* of voice disorders on individuals, noting changes to their quality of life, participation in wider social systems, and overall sense-of-self and identity. (This research will be discussed in Chapter 7.) These interrelated areas offer essential insights about those individuals we seek to help, with powerful implications for our comprehensive clinical management of voice disorders.

In this chapter I refer to several underlying preconceptions about the psychological correlates and dispositional features frequently attributed to individuals with specific voice disorders. These have been drawn from early single case and descriptive case series reports, and interestingly, from early Victorian medical and fictional literature. It is timely to tease out that which has now been relegated to 'myth', that which has been subjected to more rigorous methodologies, and finally, those issues which still hang in our shared intellectual space, still important but not yet fully resolved.

I then discuss trends in the data that suggest possible *causal associations* between psychosocial factors and some voice disorders, with brief reference to several *theoretical models* that seek to explain the development and maintenance of these conditions. The psychosocial variables explored in recent studies have included: *personality traits*; *emotional expressiveness*, *coping styles* and *reactivity to stress*; *attachment profiles* and *social supports*; vulnerability to *abnormal illness behaviours* and other *medically-unexplained conditions*; and *mood disorders* such as *anxiety* or *depression* that may or may not reach the threshold for psychiatric diagnosis.

Once again, studies have generally focused on women with FVD, variously labelled across different studies as 'conversion reaction', 'psychogenic voice disorder' (PVD), 'functional aphonia or dysphonia' (FD), 'hyperfunctional dysphonia' and 'muscle tension dysphonia' (MTVD). In some studies, patients with *vocal nodules* have been included in the FVD study groups and in others, they have been differentiated as vocal nodule (VN) groups or even classified as having an organic voice disorder (OVD). It is a welcome development that FVD groups have been compared with other disorders such as *paradoxical vocal fold dysfunction (PVFD)*, acquired neurological conditions such as *spasmodic dysphonia (SD)* or *unilateral vocal fold paralysis (UVFP)*, or more general OVD groups.

Please note that while I am maintaining the same terminology and acronyms that I have used throughout this text for FVD, which both includes and differentiates between the MTVD and PVD sub-groups, when describing the different studies in this chapter, I use the diagnostic terminology and acronyms that have been nominated by the respective authors. A glossary of terms and acronyms for this particular chapter is shown below.

Diagnostic terminologies and acronyms as operationally defined for this text

FVD: Functional voice disorder, which includes both MTVD and PVD:

MTVD: Muscle Tension Voice Disorder (includes those with no pathology and those with minor benign lesions such as vocal nodules)

PVD: Psychogenic Voice Disorder

OVD: Organic Voice Disorder

(Baker *et al.*, 2007)

Diagnostic terminologies and acronyms as used by the authors in relation to specific studies discussed in this chapter

FD: Functional Dysphonia
PVFD: Paradoxical Vocal Fold Dysfunction
VN: Vocal Nodules
SD: Spasmodic Dysphonia
UVFP: Unilateral Vocal Fold Paralysis
URTI: Upper Respiratory Tract Infection

Early single case and descriptive case series reports

'The evidence is scanty and primarily impressionistic. This is not to demean the role of impressionistic deduction; impressions based on previous observations and experience have definitive value' (Aronson et al., 1968) (p.218).

At the turn of the 20th century, the primary focus for the single case and descriptive case series reports was on female patients diagnosed with a range of non-organic health conditions. These included 'functional voice disorders' such as 'hysterical aphonia/dysphonia' 'conversion reaction', or 'psychogenic voice disorders'. Aronson and Bless (2009) have recently emphasised that the specialties of neurology, psychiatry and psychology were essentially in their infancy at that time, and it is evident in reviewing these early reports, that many conclusions were based upon rather meagre data, clinical observations and conjecture (Baker, 2008).

However, I agree with Aronson that we should not demean these processes. The specialists, including those from otolaryngology and speech pathology, were resolute in their efforts to understand the way in which personality traits, patterns of emotional expression in the face of traumatic or situational conflicts, and associated psychiatric disturbances may contribute to the causal mechanisms underlying these functional conditions, and how they may have supported or contradicted prevailing aetiologic theoretical models. While some early 'impressionistic deductions' have been shown to be unfounded, others have set the foundations for more rigorous studies and are now incorporated into our current clinical understanding.

It is well known that the ancient Greek physicians labelled psychogenic voice loss or the *'globus phenomenon'* as 'hysterical', based upon the widely accepted proposition that these symptoms occurred most frequently in women and that they represented the wandering of the womb (derived from the Greek word for uterus, *hystera*). The stresses being experienced by these women were thought to cause the womb to travel to their throats, hence causing the feeling of a large foreign object in the throat on swallowing, or to block the passage of air for the utterance of speech. And while it is easy to smile at this fanciful conjecture, it is important to acknowledge that here was a very real attempt to understand both the neurophysiology of this phenomenon and the possible conscious or unconscious symbolic meaning attached to the development of the symptom. Ironically, although loss of speech and voice was frequently noted in men who had been 'struck dumb', 'deprived of utterance', or 'aphonic' under traumatic conditions of war and extreme fear (Charcot, 1887; Janet, 1920), none had been referred to as hysterics. Moreover, no parallel explanations regarding aspects of their anatomy travelling to their throats during these more heroic circumstances of combat have ever been offered (Baker, 2002).

As previously highlighted (Baker, 2003, 2008), much of the earlier medical and psychiatric literature in relation to the FVD and other medically-unexplained conditions has been considered in the light of Freud's *unacceptable impulse theory* and his model for the *hysterical conversion reaction* (1962/1896a). *Conversion reaction* referred to the psychological processes whereby repressed or unconscious energy associated with unbearable ideas related to sexual or aggressive instincts were converted into physical symptoms. This conversion or 'transmutation of energy' was thought to block the normal functioning of the sensory motor pathway, and to serve the psychological purpose of enabling the patient to deny or avoid awareness of emotional conflict or personal failure that might otherwise have proven emotionally unbearable to face directly. The symptom or the voice disorder was thought to provide *primary gain* by assisting a woman to extricate herself from the difficult situation, and when the symptom persisted, the attention and illness behaviours were thought to provide *secondary gains*, thus maintaining and reinforcing the conversion reaction. In medicine, psychiatry and speech pathology, a clinical picture unduly biased towards a disease model was adopted, with the psychopathology located firmly in the neurotic minds and personalities of women inevitably suffering from unresolved sexual and aggressive urges. While perspective about the psychological processes involved has now shifted, we should not lose sight of the fact that the speculation with respect to different levels of activation in the neural substrates of the brain was neither fanciful nor irrelevant.

Freud's psychodynamic framework underpinned the early attitudes and approaches of medical and psychiatric practitioners to the management of many functional health conditions, and it is evident that his notion of the hysterical conversion reaction has been more influential than any other in shaping our early understandings of the aetiology of the broad group of FVD, both those with MTVD and PVD (Butcher, Elias, & Cavalli, 2007). The model has also served, rightly or wrongly, to perpetuate a number of myths about the people with functional health conditions, including those with voice disorders. For example, it was implicit that those diagnosed with conversion reaction symptoms would be women, and that these individuals would invariably present with a *hysterical personality profile*. According to Briquet (1859), this meant that she would be seductive and flirtatious; sometimes of a hostile or manipulative disposition; immature in the management of her emotions, especially anger and other negative feelings; invariably suggestible, dependent, shallow, theatrical and often, extravert. She denied the presence of emotional distress and was likely to portray *la belle indifference*, one of the hallmark features of the true conversion reaction.

As extrapolated from the early reports cited in a previous review paper (Baker, 2008), many women with these functional and conversion reaction voice disorders were described as exhibiting: an excessive sensitivity to life's situations; a pattern of tense, restless, and apprehensive affect; a tendency to insomnia, despondency, and extreme or continual tiredness; a range of other functional medical symptoms; heightened degrees of subjectivity, egocentricity, or aloofness as defense mechanisms against feelings of inadequacy or inferiority; and an immature, dependent, and histrionic personality inclined to role-playing and suggestibility. These features often culminated in a range of psychiatric disorders characterised by neurotic anxiety or phobias, fluctuating melancholy or chronic depression, and sometimes, with schizophrenic or psychotic processes.

In those rare cases where males were diagnosed with *conversion reaction voice disorders*, apart from those arising in relation to combat in times of war as described in Chapter 5, their dysphonia often presented in the form of an abnormally high-pitched falsetto phonation, or *puberphonia*. However, as with the soldiers, these men were not described as having an hysterical personality but with dispositional features such as: 'a delicate or feeble look'; 'a marked want of vitality', 'general debility and 'lack of robust appearance'; and 'a tendency to nervousness or uneasiness'. It was observed that they were more than normally embarrassed by general systemic changes, including the voice, and that they demonstrated a very real and determined preoccupation with financial compensation issues in relation to their loss of voice.

In her scholarly book *Passion and Pathology in Victorian Literature*, Jane Wood (Wood, 2001) highlights the parallels between the writings of the highly respected patriarchal medical fraternity in Victorian England and the novelists of the day. She shows how many of these novelists perpetuated similar ideas about the non-organic or medically-unexplained conditions such as *hysteria* and *neurasthenia* being the exclusive domain of women who were often described as 'nature's invalids'. In this riveting treatise she shows how female characters in Victorian literature were depicted as being subject to any or all of those dispositional characteristics outlined above, and inclined to respond to life's stresses in an emotionally volatile or labile manner, rather than with mature, measured and reasoned approaches as generally modelled by their male counterparts in these novels. These dispositional frailties prepared the women to fulfil their quintessential roles as 'the angels in the house', or to suffer the vicissitudes of female psychosomatic illnesses signifying 'social, moral or sexual-political transgression' (Wood 2001, p.16). Fortunately, Jane Wood goes on to show how novelists such as Jane Austen and Charlotte Bronte challenged these prejudices, giving their key female characters some spine and louder voices. It is fascinating to see how these medical and psychiatric perceptions were being replicated and reinforced in the most widely read fictional literature of the times.

Influential foundation studies

In the field of speech pathology, Arnold Aronson has been recognised as one of the most influential clinicians and writers, seeking, for over 40 years now, to understand the psychological and dispositional features of patients presenting with FVD. In his early studies he included MTVD, or '*habitual dysphonias*' as described by Heaver (1958), under his classification of PVD, but he also maintained that many of the functional cases he encountered fulfilled the diagnostic criteria for a conversion reaction disorder (Aronson *et al.*, 1968; Aronson, Peterson, & Litin, 1964, 1966). He challenged the fundamental notion of psychic energy related to unconscious libidinal or aggressive instincts being transformed into physical symptoms. Rather, he adopted an alternative interpretation of conversion reaction symptoms as representing a symbolic expression of an internal conflict or threatening idea in response to emotionally laden and stressful events, as proposed by Ziegler *et al.* (1962). Inevitably, these symptoms would also provide some immediate primary gain by enabling the person to avoid facing or dealing with the immediate dilemma and conflict. Furthermore, they may lead to secondary gains associated with solicitousness and attention from others, or fewer expectations in their work and family settings.

Ziegler and colleagues urged practitioners to distinguish carefully between the theoretical explanation of those psychological processes underpinning the conversion reaction, and the personality profiles frequently attributed to these patients. They found that less than half of the patients that presented with conversion reaction symptoms had a *hysterical personality profile*, a term which they criticised as being 'scattered in its constellation of personality traits', unnecessarily pejorative in its connotations of 'emotional incontinence', and 'a term we could graciously relinquish to the laity altogether' (Ziegler & Imboden, 1962, p. 906). With a command of language such as this, these authors might have won a regular spot on Stephen Fry's QI panel.

They also noted that while personality traits such as emotional immaturity, dependency, and a propensity for over-dramatisation were sometimes seen in association with conversion reaction symptoms, these histrionic traits were not a necessary condition for a diagnosis of conversion reaction disorders.

Similarly, in the seminal studies by Aronson *et al.* (1966) which drew upon data from the *Minnesota Multiphasic Personality Inventory (MMPI)*, standardised questionnaires and psychiatric interview of patients with 'functional aphonia or dysphonia', many were diagnosed with a conversion reaction disorder but did not necessarily reveal a hysterical personality. In some cases, the dysphonia developed after extremely stressful and traumatic situations, but many patients reported onset following what appeared to be an *upper respiratory tract infection (URTI)*, feelings of intense *fatigue or exhaustion*, and *stressful situations* that were described as emotionally disturbing, often related to conflicted interpersonal relationships. Invariably, *difficulties in the expression of negative emotions* and in particular, a *conflict over expressing angry feelings*, were reported. Furthermore, despite traits of suggestibility, an excessive preoccupation with bodily symptoms, and a propensity for neurotic anxiety and low-level depression, very few suffered from a verified psychiatric disorder.

Of equal significance at this time, Aronson and his colleagues (1968) challenged the previously held notion that all clinical presentations of what was then termed '*spastic dysphonia*' were of psychoneurotic origin. In a study using data from standardised questionnaires and detailed psychiatric interview, they compared the vocal, neurological signs and *psychosocial profiles* of patients with 'spastic dysphonia', PVD, and a general medical group. While there were some commonalities between groups, several key differences emerged. In addition to clear neurological signs observed in the 'spastic dysphonia' group, a number of biographical and psychological correlates differentiated them from the patients with PVD, as shown in Box 6.1.

Box 6.1 Psychosocial profile for patients with 'spastic dysphonia'

- An almost equal distribution of men and women
- Little evidence of stressful events, emotional trauma or interpersonal conflicts preceding onset
- Personality traits suggesting perfectionism, rigidity and introversion
- Preference to suppress angry feelings in the face of interpersonal conflicts
- Psychiatric profile suggesting more pessimism
- Less likely to seek social interactions, and depressed
- Lower scores on the hypochondriasis and emotional maturity scales, and higher on the depression scale as measured by MMPI

(Aronson, Brown, Litin, & Pearson, 1968)

The authors cautioned that some of these psychosocial factors were no more exclusive to individuals with 'spastic dysphonia' than patients with other health conditions, and that the psychiatric conditions of depression and lack of optimism could well have arisen as a result of the voice disorder. They proposed that patients presenting with both neurological and psychiatric findings may have a basic predisposition or 'instability of innervation' within the motor system, and a 'susceptibility to reactivity' in the face of stressful life events in combination with their particular dispositional traits. They stressed that these hypotheses were speculative, and that associations between prior experiences and psychosocial profiles of patients who developed these functional and neurological voice disorders required further substantiation from neurophysiological, psychological and psychiatric studies. These foundation studies set the tenor for the research that has followed.

Comparative group studies

During the last four decades, researchers have generated empirical evidence to support many of the observations and hypotheses outlined above. There is still controversy over those *neuropsychological processes* thought to be operating within the conversion reaction disorders, and some practitioners have distanced themselves from psychodynamic constructs in favour of more contemporary theoretical models that may explain the development of FVD. These models have been based upon findings showing associations between a range of psychological correlates in relation to specific voice disorders, and these will be discussed in more detail, along with current models for conversion reaction disorders, in Chapter 8. In the sections below I discuss the empirical findings in relation to personality traits, concomitant psychiatric disorders, and a range of *dispositional factors*.

Personality traits, psychiatric disorder, and other dispositional features

A number of trends in the findings can be extrapolated from the many case series and comparative case-control studies cited in the previous extensive literature review by Baker (2008).[1]

Contrary to psychodynamic formulations, the hysterical personality profile with its typical features of emotional immaturity, seductive or manipulative disposition, and bland indifference to symptoms, was rarely reported, with prevalence figures of less than 4–5% for all cases of with FVD, including those diagnosed with conversion reaction voice disorder.

When extrapolating from these many studies, although it is evident that there were consistent findings for psychiatric disturbance in relation to FVD, very few individuals were formally diagnosed with psychosis, schizophrenia, or personality disorder. Women with FVD, some of whom who were diagnosed with PVD or MTVD (described as functional dysphonia with or without pathologies such as vocal nodules in some studies), often presented with co-existing psychiatric disorders such as depression, anxiety, and somatization disorders, or general states of *emotional maladjustment*. Bland indifference was not often reported and most women showed a genuine concern and curiosity about the possible psychological factors underlying their voice disorders. Overwhelmingly, these women revealed personality profiles reflecting high levels of reactivity to stress, social anxiety, and depressive affect, but not necessarily of such severity to reach

---

1   This review included reference to studies by the following authors: (Andersson & Schalen, 1998; Aronson et al., 1968; Aronson et al., 1966; Butcher, Elias, Raven, Yeatman, & Littlejohns, 1987; I. J. Deary, Wilson, Carding, & MacKenzie, 2003; Friedl, Friedrich, & Egger, 1990; Gerritsma, 1991; Goldman, Hargrave, Hillman, Holmberg, & Gress, 1996; Gunther, Mayr-Graft, Miller, & Kinzl, 1996; House & Andrews, 1987; Kinzl, Biebl, & Rauchegger, 1988; Lauriello, Cozza, Rossi, DiRienzo, & Tirelli, 2003; McHugh-Munier, Scherer, Lehmann, & Scherer, 1997; Millar, Deary, Wilson, & MacKenzie, 1999; Mirza, Ruiz, Baum, & Staab, 2003; Roy et al., 2000a, 2000b; Roy et al., 1997; Schalen & Andersson, 1992; White, Deary, & Wilson, 1997; Willinger, Volkl-Kernstock, & Aschauer, 2005; Yano, Ichimura, Hoshino, & Nozue, 1982).

the threshold for clinical diagnosis of frank mood disorder. The most common dispositional qualities as extrapolated from these studies are summarised in Box 6.2.

Box 6.2 Dispositional attitudes, behaviours and coping styles in women with FVD as extrapolated from case reports and comparative group studies

- Emotional maladjustment and poor levels of adaptive functioning
- Elevated levels of state and trait anxiety
- Vulnerability to tensional or somatic symptoms
- Low self-esteem
- Tendency to withdrawal or wish to escape in stressful situations
- Fatigue and preoccupation with somatic complaints
- Sense of futility or powerless in effecting change
- Lack of assertiveness
- Perfectionism and a strong sense of propriety/shame at violation of norms
- Assuming the brunt of responsibilities but often feeling over-loaded

(Baker, 2008; Baker *et al.*, 2013)

These features have been captured in two remarkable sculptures by Louise Bourgeois shown at an exhibition in the Hirshorn Gallery of Modern and Contemporary Art in Washington DC, in 2009. The international *Psychogenic Movement Disorder Conference* was being held in Washington at the same time, and how remarkable that the very first item in this exhibition was this stunning sculpture of the *Arch of Hysteria* (Fig. 6.1). The highly polished bronze depicts a person in a state of 'hysterical torsion' suspended from the ceiling. Such a precarious placement in space always represented states of ambivalence and doubt for this artist. In the accompanying video she acknowledged that although it was usually women who were diagnosed with functional or conversion reaction disorders, this sculpture illustrated that men could also experience the same conditions. She wanted to demonstrate how the physical, psychological, and mental states are merged, in this case reflecting the physical and emotional stress of 'having too much to cope with in life', 'always trying to do one's best', or 'bending over backwards'.

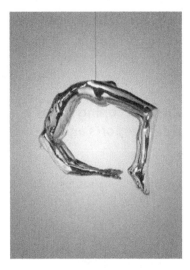

Fig. 6.1 Louise Bourgeois "Arch of Hysteria" (1993)

Bronze, polished patina, hanging piece
83.8 x 101.6 x58.4 cm
Collection Hakone Open-Air Museum,
Kanagawa-Perfecture, Japan
Photo: Christopher Burke, © The Easton
Foundation/Licensed by Viscopy, Sydney

On display at the same exhibition was another of her creations, a second rendition of the *Arch of Hysteria* (Fig. 6.2). Again, the person was suspended from the ceiling but this time, was described as 'a lumpen and awkward body of a woman, roughly stitched together from sections of pink cloth that have been over-stuffed so as to force the feeling of anxiety and tension', a particularly apt description as we reflect upon the dispositional profiles of a range of women with FVD, as described in the earlier studies above.

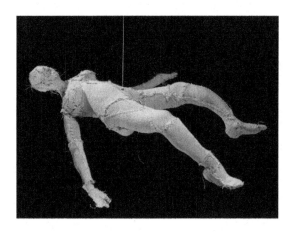

Fig. 6.2 Louise Bourgeois "Arch of Hysteria" (2000)

Pink fabric hanging piece
13.9 x 44.4 x 27.9 cm
Collection Claudia and
Karsten Greve. Photo:
Christopher Burke © The
Easton Foundation/Licensed
by Viscopy, Sydney

Key studies supporting the development of a Theory for the Dispositional Bases of Functional Dysphonia and Vocal Nodules

In arguably two of the most robust studies in terms of methodology and statistical analyses, Roy and colleagues explored the possible role of personality in contributing to onset and outcome in four different voice disorder groups. These included women with a diagnosis of: functional dysphonia (FD); vocal nodules (VN); spasmodic dysphonia (SD); unilateral vocal fold paresis (UVFP); and an otolaryngology control group with no voice disorders (Controls) (Roy & Bless, 2000a, 2000b; Roy *et al.*, 2000a, 2000b). The studies were based upon the premise that personality reflects a set of relatively stable traits that develop early in life, and that these will shape the attitudes, cognitions and behaviours of individuals as they may both seek to influence or respond to their environment. A brief summary of the psychology of personality and trait theory, relevant to our understanding and clinical management of voice disorders, has been subsequently presented in two excellent review papers. Some of the key tenets underpinning the psychology of personality are listed below (Roy, 2011; van Mersbergen, 2011).

1. Personality comprises complex, organised, heritable, and interrelated characteristics that influence how individuals are likely to respond to different situations over time; this will determine an individual's overall functioning in relation to the environment, both physical and interpersonal.
2. Personality represents the three higher order globally recognised personality constructs of *Extraversion vs. Introversion (E)*, *Neuroticism vs. Stability (N)*, and *Constraint vs. Disinhibition (CON)*.
3. Personality traits are relatively stable and as such, may render a person vulnerable to the development and recurrence of particular kinds of symptoms.
4. Personality traits may be linked to particular psychophysiological processes and neurobiological substrates.

In the first of two companion studies, the authors used the *Eysenck Personality Questionnaire (EPQ)* (Eysenck & Eysenck, 1975), which is designed to generate 'the big three' superfactor constructs of *Extraversion vs. Introversion (E)*, *Neuroticism vs. Stability (N)*, and *Psychoticism or Constraint vs. Disinhibition (CON)*. In a companion study with the same participants, they used the *Multidimensional Personality Questionnaire (MPQ)* (Tellegen, 1982). This is designed to elicit the three superfactors and their lower-order constituents accordingly: Extraversion or Positive Emotionality (E/PEM) – *well being, social potency, achievement and social closeness*; Neuroticism or Negative Emotionality (N/NEM) – *stress reaction, alienation, aggression*; Psychoticism, since referred to as Constraint (CON) – *control, harm avoidance and traditionalism*. Other measures included the *State Trait Anxiety Inventory-Trait Scale (STAI-Trait)* (Spielberger, Gorusch, Lushene, Vagg, & Jacobs, 1983), the *Beck Depression Inventory (BDI)* (Beck & Steer, 1993), and the *Voice Handicap Profile (VHP)* (Adapted from the ASHA Special Interest Division 3 Voice and Voice Disorders). Features that characterise these higher-order traits are summarised in Box 6.3.

Box 6.3 The 'Big Three' superfactor personality traits

Extraversion or Positive Emotionality (E/PEM) vs. Introversion

* Positive emotionality, affiliation and dominance, willingness to actively engage in the physical and social environment
    * *Introversion* – more passive and careful, socially quiet and distant, more reluctant to actively engage in the social environment

Neuroticism (N) or Negative Emotionality N/NEM vs. Stability

* Negative emotionality related to anxiety, depression, tension
* Emotional reactivity or sensitivity to threatening environmental stimuli
* Engagement with others unpleasant, stressed by actions, attitudes of self and others
* Tendency to worry, to feel victimised and resentful
    * *Not to be confused with psychodynamic notion of psychoneurosis*

Psychoticism or Constraint (CON) vs. Disinhibition

* Relates directly to impulse control and perfectionism
* Cautious, plans carefully before acting, restrained from risky adventures
* Controlled by implications of behaviour and societal conventions
    * *Disinhibited* – more inclined to be impulsive, adventurous, reject conventional restrictions, more disagreeable and aggressive

(Extrapolated from Roy & Bless, 2000a, 2000b; Roy, Bless, & Heisey, 2000a, 2000b)

The principal findings showed significant temperamental differences between the functional dysphonia (FD) and vocal nodule (VN) groups in comparison to the other three groups, with higher overall scores on Neuroticism and Negative Emotionality (N/NEM). The FD group in comparison to the VN group showed significantly higher scores on the constructs of N/NEM, with more reactivity to stress. The FD group was also more likely to be introverted, and the CON personality dimension distinguished it from the VN group. The FD group showed more emotional turmoil typically with more *behavioural restraint*, and they seemed to be more socially alienated and unhappy as revealed by having less satisfaction with themselves and their lives. Overall, they were more likely to report a lower threshold for emotional upset, and were prone to emotional reactivity.

The VN group on the other hand, while also reactive to stress, did not present with such elevated scores on the N/NEM scale, but were more extravert, socially dominant, impulsive, and aggressive. The VN group also scored higher than any of the others on the lower-order trait of 'social potency', which Roy suggests is not merely a matter of enjoying being with others and social affiliation, but reflects a propensity to 'take charge', to assume leadership, and to enjoy being the centre of attention (Roy, 2011). Here, he has stressed that although such a quality can be construed as positive, the associated high levels of impulsivity and *disinhibition* may also have a 'toxic' element, with implications for therapeutic strategies that emphasise restraint.

No significant differences were found for the personality profiles or on measures of anxiety and depression between the spasmodic dysphonia (SD) and unilateral vocal fold paralysis (UVFP) groups, or between these two groups and the controls. This confirmed the authors' hypothesis that personality was not likely to be aetiologically significant in the acquired neurological conditions of SD and UVFP. In addition, the levels of anxiety, depression, and well-being as rated on the other questionnaires were not related to the degree of self-reported voice impairment or length of time suffering from the voice disorder. As such, there was no support for the *disability hypothesis* proposing that dispositional differences may have developed as a consequence of the particular health condition under consideration.

These results confirmed earlier speculations that particular trait-like qualities may constitute 'a persistent vulnerability for the development of tensional and somatic symptoms when under conditions of psychological distress' (Roy *et al.*, 1997) (p. 449), a conclusion in close agreement with that of Aronson some 30 years before (Aronson *et al.*, 1968). They thought that their study provided strong evidence to suggest that personality traits may contribute to the onset of FD and

VN, supporting their *Theory of the Dispositional Bases of Functional Dysphonia and Vocal Nodules* (Roy & Bless, 2000a, 2000b), which will be discussed in more detail in Chapter 8.

Other studies showing personality differences with specific voice disorders

Subsequent studies have provided further support for the personality profiles proposed by Roy and colleagues, while others have revealed differences with some challenging caveats to their findings.[2]

Generally speaking, individuals with FVD in association with vocal nodules have been shown to be vulnerable to increased stress reactivity and high levels of anxiety but in particular, they are more likely to be extraverted and impulsive, and inclined to hostility or aggression, than those diagnosed with FVD and no pathology (Abeida *et al.*, 2013; Ban *et al.*, 2007; Ratajczak, Grzywacz, Wojdas, Rapiejka, & Jurkiewicz, 2008).

However, a somewhat different trend was noted in a rigorous study conducted by Dietrich and colleagues (2008). They compared the *perceived stress*, state anxiety, and depressive mood between four groups of patients: vocal nodules (VN); MTD (suggested by the authors as being synonymous with psychogenic, functional or non-organic dysphonia); paradoxical vocal fold dysfunction (PVFD); and glottal insufficiency. They used the *Hospital Anxiety Scale and Depression Scale (HADS)*, which refers to generalised state anxiety and depression as construed by a loss of pleasure, and the *Perceived Stress Scale PSS-10*, which provides a measure of global perceived stress that addresses issues related to the feelings of life being somewhat unpredictable and out of control, accompanied by a sense of being overloaded in life.

---

2   (Abeida et al., 2013; Ban, Lee, & Jin, 2007; Dietrich & Verdolini Abbott, 2012; Dietrich, Verdolini Abbott, Gartner-Schmidt, & Rosen, 2008; Gassull, Casanova, Botey, & Amador, 2010; Husein et al., 2008; O'Hara, Miller, Carding, Wilson, & Deary, 2011; Seifert & Kollbrunner, 2005; Sinkiewicz et al., 2013; Siupsinskiene, Razbadauskas, & Dubosas, 2011; Van Houtte, Van Lierde, & Claeys, 2009; van Mersbergen, Patrick, & Glaze, 2008).

One of the key findings revealed that those with PVFD had the highest scores across all three dimensions of perceived stress, state anxiety, and depression. This is of interest given the ongoing controversy over the primary aetiology of this troubling voice disorder thought to be of psychological origin but which is often seen as 'an airway problem' in association with asthma, or in relation to symptoms of gastroesophageal reflux. It may also be confused with spasmodic dysphonia. These results are not dissimilar to those of Husein *et al.* (2008), who found that in many cases, but not all, PVFD is associated with the typical *'conversion V profile'* as generated by the MMPI-2, suggesting to these authors that it may be construed as a conversion reaction disorder, representing underlying psychological conflicts.

Another interesting finding was that those with VN reported elevated scores on state anxiety but to a lesser extent on perceived stress and depression than the other groups, and contrary to the findings of Roy and colleagues, the VN group members were more anxious than the MTD group. In seeking to explain this somewhat surprising difference, the authors suggested that it might be accounted for by the anxiety measures used, which focused on recent *state anxiety* rather than *trait anxiety* as in the previous studies. They speculated that the higher anxiety, perceived stress, and low mood scores may have reflected current concerns about having lesions such as vocal nodules, and how this might impact upon their future. In this sense, the more recently experienced anxiety was construed not only as a dispositional factor contributing to onset but possibly also as an outcome of the voice disorder. Overall, these results contribute to their *Psychobiological Framework for studying Psychological Stress and its Relation to Voice Disorders* (Dietrich & Verdolini Abbott, 2008). This theoretical model will be discussed in Chapter 8.

Constraint as reflected in perfectionism and extreme fatigue

Additional support for the personality profiles of individuals with functional dysphonia (FD) as proposed by Roy *et al.* (2000a, 2000b) is highlighted in two further studies and although very different in their apparent emphasis, they both tap into the constructs inherent in the higher-order personality trait related to *Constraint (CON)*.

The first study explored the possible role of *fatigue* and associated *perfectionism* as dispositional factors that may contribute to the onset and maintenance of functional dysphonia (FD) (O'Hara *et al.*, 2011). These authors defined FD as 'a dysphonia or aphonia where there was no detectable organic pathology or where what was detectable was not commensurate with the degree of vocal dysfunction' (p. 921). Fatigue and perfectionism as expressed by 'bending over backwards to do one's best' were implicit in a number of the earlier studies cited.

These features have also been recognised in individuals presenting with *abnormal illness behaviours* and *medically-unexplained conditions* such as *chronic fatigue syndrome* and *irritable bowel syndrome* (Chaturvedi, Desai, & Shaligram, 2006; V. Deary, Chalder, & Sharpe, 2007), and it has been suggested by these authors that there may be some similarities in the clinical profiles of individuals with FD. In the recent study by O'Hara *et al.* (2011), men and women with FD were compared with controls who had no voice problems on measures for fatigue and perfectionism. The authors emphasised that whereas *healthy perfectionism* may encourage a person to do things well and can be positively construed as conscientiousness, *unhealthy perfectionism* is characterised by self-criticism and dissatisfaction with one's performance, and is typically associated with the personality trait of neuroticism and negative emotionality (N/NEM).

The key findings showed that the FD group reported significantly *higher levels of fatigue* than the control group, not as high as expected for patients with conditions such as chronic fatigue syndrome, but higher than for the normal population. The FD group were also more likely to be *perfectionistic* than the control group in general perfectionism (both positive and negative), but negative perfectionism was not found to be statistically significant for the FD group. The authors suggested their research, interpreted in the light of the *Bio-psychosocial Model of Medically Unexplained Physical Symptoms* (V. Deary *et al.*, 2007), may add to our understanding of the processes underlying the development and maintenance of functional voice disorders. This model will be discussed in Chapter 8.

A second very interesting study by van Mersbergen *et al.* (2008) also focused upon the notion of dispositional constraint (CON). In this study, which was conducted under experimentally controlled conditions, individuals with functional dysphonia (FD) but no pathology, as excluded by laryngoscopy, were compared with those with social anxiety (SA) and a group of healthy controls on a battery of psychometric tests (personality, psychopathology, and voice handicap) and *psychophysiological measures* taken before, during, and after exposure to a series of spoken scripts of aversive, neutral, and positive mental imagery scenarios.

Those with FD were more *behaviourally constrained*, despite indications for higher levels of arousal as measured by increased heart rate in response to both positive and negative stimuli. The FD group demonstrated higher scores for the psychometric measures, self-reported difficulties with voice, and more autonomic activation than the SA and control groups. However, those with FD also showed *reduced muscular activation* of the speech and voice muscles following imagery of emotional communication, leading the authors to suggest 'that the underlying cause of FD may be a discrepancy between the subjective experience and motivation to engage the muscles of speech' (p.1420).

The finding that individuals with FD responded to emotional stimuli with *reduced behavioural expression*, which is typically associated with the personality trait of behavioural constraint (CON), lends support to the findings from many of the earlier studies involving individuals with 'functional', 'psychogenic' and/or 'conversion reaction' voice disorders, and is consistent with the personality trait theory in relation to individuals with FD as described by Roy and colleagues (2000a, 2000b).

Coping styles, emotional expressiveness, suppression, and repression

This personality construct of constraint (CON), and the analysis by Mersbergen *et al.* (van Mersbergen, 2011; van Mersbergen *et al.*, 2008), is particularly relevant as we now consider the commonly held notion that individuals with FVD, especially those variously diagnosed as 'conversion reaction', 'psychogenic voice disorder' or 'functional aphonia and dysphonia', are more inclined to *suppress* or *repress negative emotions* under stressful conditions. These psychological processes are thought to shape a person's *general coping style*, and to contribute to the development of the voice disorders. (Here I am distinguishing between other studies that have investigated ways of coping *in response to voice disorders* that will be discussed in Chapter 7.) The empirical evidence for coping style as a dispositional trait is surprisingly meagre and somewhat contradictory.

For instance, in one study, those with FVD reported an *anxious coping style*, not a *repressive coping style* as anticipated, indicating that the participants were able to recognise and acknowledge their anxiety or negative emotions rather than repress them (Friedl *et al.*, 1990). In another study, individuals with FVD reported an *emotion focused coping style* with a preference for controlling emotional reactions, implying the suppression or repression of emotional reactions (McHugh-Munier *et al.*, 1997). The authors suggested that these heightened emotions might lead to increased levels of tension in the muscles of phonation, explaining to some extent the subsequent development of small vocal lesions in some of their cohort.

On the basis of these earlier studies there was insufficient evidence to make generalisations about emotional expressiveness and coping styles that clearly predispose individuals to develop FVD or any other voice disorder (Baker, 2008). Other authors have since cautioned that the suppression and repression of negative emotion may not provide the full answer and that other factors, such as life stresses and concurrent fatigue and illness so often prevalent in individuals with FVD, may provide a different perspective (O'Hara *et al.*, 2011). We might ask at this point if we really know whether the *suppression* or *repression of negative emotion* in response to stressful situations is any more potent as an aetiological factor for FVD than the *awareness and expression of negative emotions* in response to these same stressful experiences. I am not convinced that we know the answer to this yet.

The suppression or repression of emotion has continued to be a fundamental construct underpinning several theoretical causal models for FVD. These are: the *Freudian Model for Conversion Reaction* with its emphasis on repression of feelings arising from unconscious conflicts (Breuer & Freud, 1955/1893– 1895); the *Reformulated Psychoanalytic and Psychosocial Model* which proposes the suppression of negative emotions in response to recent life events and interpersonal conflicts (Butcher *et al.*, 2007); the *Physiological Model* which seeks to relate elevated levels of laryngeal muscular tension to stressful situations, including interpersonal conflicts (Morrison & Rammage, 1994); the *Dispositional Trait Theory Model*, in which the authors propose a conflict between laryngeal motor inhibition and activation that has its origins in different personality traits and dispositional behaviour driven by nervous system functioning (Roy & Bless, 2000a); and the *Emotion Processing Deficits Model* (Baker & Lane, 2009).

These models will be discussed in Chapter 8.

Dispositional profiles and patterns of emotional expressiveness: Case-control study

In addition to our investigation of stressful incidents preceding onset of FVD and OVD, we also explored a range of psychological correlates such as anxiety, anger, depression, attachment style, social support, and optimism, and dispositional qualities reflecting emotional expressiveness and control (Baker *et al.*, 2013). In particular, we were interested in determining whether those with FVD revealed a *repressive coping style* or attitudes and behaviours suggesting *ambivalence over emotional expression*. Questionnaires used are listed in Box 6.4.

Box 6.4 Instruments and self-report questionnaires used in relation to psychosocial traits and emotional expression

- Demographic Data and Diagnostic Classification of Voice Disorders
  - (Baker, Ben-Tovim, Butcher, Esterman, & McLaughlin, 2007)
- **Semi-structured Interview**
  - Life Events and Difficulties Schedule (LEDS) and Social Supports
    - (Brown & Harris, 1978)
  - Attachment Style Interview (ASI)
    - (Bifulco, Lillie, Ball, & Moran, 1998b)
- **Self-Report Questionnaires**
  - Self-Assessment Questionnaire-Nijmegen (SAQ-N)
    - (Van der Ploeg, 1989a)
  - Repressive Coping style
    - Manifest Anxiety Scale (BMAS)
    - Marlowe Crowne Social Desirability Scale (MC)
    - (Bendig, 1956; Crowne & Marlowe, 1960)
  - Ambivalence over Emotional Expression Questionnaire (AEQ)
    - (King & Emmons, 1990)
  - Family of Origin Expressive Atmosphere Scale (FOEAS)
    - (Yelsma, Hovestadt, Anderson, & Nilsson, 2000)

(Baker *et al.*, 2013)

Observations in relation to psychological traits and emotional expression

The study demonstrated that the FVD group reported dispositional differences to those with OVD and the control groups related to coping style, anxiety, emotional expressiveness, and insecure attachment.

In view of the previous literature, we had anticipated that women with FVD, and then those in the PVD sub-group, might have been more prone to difficulties in the expression of emotions and, in particular, the *repression of negative emotions*. As originally construed, repression is a process which involves turning something away and keeping it at a distance from the conscious mind (Freud, 1962/1896a). Freud used the terms repression and suppression interchangeably to denote 'an effortful struggle not to know', with the purpose of repression being to avoid anxiety. I would suggest, however, that it is now generally accepted that mental health practitioners and even the lay public differentiate between suppression of emotion as being a conscious or even subconscious process, and repression as an unconscious process. We wanted to explore whether women with different voice disorders were able to acknowledge a preference for suppressing the expression of negative emotions, or whether this might be revealed in a *repressive coping style*.

Repressors have been defined as individuals who score low on self-report measures of trait anxiety but high on defensiveness, with associated findings of behavioural and physiological responses indicative of anxiety (Weinberger, 1990). Weinberger identifies the interactions between these measures as four different coping styles referred to as *Low-Anxious*, *High-Anxious*, *Defensive High-Anxious*, and *Repressive Coping*. There is now substantial literature reporting studies on *repressive coping style*. *Repressors* see themselves as coping very well with a tendency to answer questions in an overly optimistic fashion, likely to recall fewer negative memories, stating that they prefer a more rational approach in the case of threat or challenge, and revealing a stoical self concept, believing that they are not upset despite evidence to the contrary. It is this discrepancy in the disavowal of anxiety and the physiological and behavioural responses indicative of that anxiety that has led researchers to suggest that the repressive coping style has consequences for health (Myers & Derakshan, 2004; Vingerhoets, Nyklicek, & Denollet, 2008).

Our key findings showed that FVD group women most commonly reported a *high-anxious coping style*, which has been operationally defined as a tendency to interpret one's own behaviour as being more anxious than it really is; a capacity to identify personal distress; and an emotional rather than a rational approach to solving problems (Derakshan & Eysenck, 2001). Our results were in agreement with the former study mentioned above, where these same measures for coping style had been used (Friedl *et al.*, 1990). Interestingly, the OVD group reported a *repressive coping style* more than any of the other coping styles and somewhat ironically, the control group women were the most likely to report a *repressive coping style*.

Certainly, our findings provided little evidence for '*la belle indifference*', or even the unconscious repression of negative affect, as we might have expected. Rather, there seemed to be a strong trend towards anxiety and the more conscious suppression of negative emotion or behavioural constraint, as noted by other researchers exploring these constructs in relation to different study groups within the FVD classification (Butcher *et al.*, 2007; Roy & Bless, 2000a, 2000b; van Mersbergen *et al.*, 2008). With respect to the other measures, the FVD group women could admit to being more generally anxious, and they also reported more anger, a vulnerability to depressive symptoms, and lower levels of optimism. Their family-of-origin data showed that emotional expression was not encouraged, that they preferred to direct negative emotions inwards, and that they felt more ambivalent about the expression of both positive and negative emotions. These findings are summarised in Box 6.5.

Box 6.5 Statistically significant findings for psychological correlates, emotional expression, attachment style, sexual abuse, violence, and/or strangulation

Women with FVD (*n* = 73) vs. OVD (*n* = 55) and Controls (n = 66) revealed:

- Greater vulnerability to anxiety, anger, and depression
- Lower levels of optimism and fewer social supports
- An insecure attachment style with fewer social supports
- Attitudes and behaviours reflecting a fearful attachment profile
- More lifetime experiences of sexual abuse, violence, or strangulation
- A High-Anxious coping style – not a Repressive coping style
- A pattern of emotional *expression-in* reflecting suppression of feelings
- Lower levels of emotional expressiveness in family-of-origin
- Higher ambivalence over expression of positive and negative emotion

NB: Multivariate analysis showed that the LEDS and COSO data were the strongest predictors of group status, while traits were more like moderator variables

Women with PVD (*n* = 37) vs. MTVD (*n* = 36) revealed:

- Insecure attachment style, fearful attachment profile, fewer social supports
- More lifetime experience of sexual abuse
- A pattern of emotional *expression-in* reflecting suppression of feelings

NB: Multivariate analysis showed that neither the LEDS and COSO nor traits data distinguished between PVD and MTVD groups

(Baker, Ben-Tovim, Butcher, Esterman, & McLaughlin, 2013)

Questions arising from these findings

These findings raise some further questions. Does repressive coping as determined by these particular measures really tap into repression as originally construed by Freud? Given the findings for the control group who scored highest of all on repressive coping, is repressive coping style necessarily detrimental to the physical or mental health of an individual? Is unconscious repression of negative emotions a causal factor when considering the large heterogeneous FVD classification? Is the repression of negative emotion the primary psychological process that differentiates the different clinical FVD sub-groups, MTVD and PVD?

Observations in relation to attachment style and social supports

Much of the life events research has also explored how personal relationships might play a part in predisposing some individuals to the development of certain physical and mental health conditions. In a review of a number of studies using the LEDS, Craig (2001) identified several trends in the more qualitative aspects of the events and difficulties data. These were related to difficulties in relationships where humiliation, entrapment, or rejection was paramount, or where there was an inherent COSO. Craig suggested that 'the next generation of studies would need to take into account wider issues concerning the quantity and quality of personal relationships' (p. 99), and for these reasons a preliminary exploration of attachment style in close relationships and behaviours related to social support was included with our LEDS and other dispositional traits measures.

The *Attachment Style interview (ASI)*, as cited above, has been used in a number of studies relating to *attachment style, social support*, and vulnerability to depression (Andrews & Brown, 1988; Harris & Bifulco, 1991). It gives a global measure of a respondent's ability to form and maintain intimate relationships with a partner and close support figures, and attachment style is initially rated as either standard/secure or non-standard/insecure. It also provides a measure for five operationally-defined *attachment profiles*: secure, fearful, dismissive, isolated, and *preoccupied/enmeshed*. Social support is thought to contribute to an individual's overall sense of well-being and includes feelings of intimacy, belonging, social acceptance, and approval, as well as feeling able to depend on others for help (Bowling, 1995). The ASI seeks details about the numbers of social supports, the frequency of contacts with emphasis on the availability of trusted others in whom the individual might confide or seek help, and the individual's ideas about the quality and meaning of those relationships in their lives.

Our findings showed that women with FVD had fewer social supports, and described attitudes and behaviours reflecting an *insecure attachment style* and a *fearful attachment profile*, which by definition reflects fear and mistrust of others, high levels of social anxiety, and concerns about being rejected or let down (Bifulco *et al.*, 1998b). This same pattern was shown for PVD group women in comparison with those with MTVD, once again showing some dispositional distinctions between the two FVD sub-groups. These findings, albeit with a different emphasis, were consistent with the other features showing a proneness to elevated levels of general anxiety, an anxious coping style, and lower levels of optimism as shown in Box 6.5, and as reported in some of the studies previously cited.

During the ASI interview, many women commented spontaneously that had they been asked the same questions at a different time, such as prior to their current marriage or partnership, job or recent situation with family members, they may well have answered differently. This was especially with respect to issues related to trust, and seeking of social support from confidantes. This raises interesting questions about whether or not attachment style in adult relationships is sufficiently stable to be thought of only as a 'trait', as originally conceived by Bowlby (1969). Our findings were similar to those of others who have suggested that attachment behaviour may also be construed as 'a state' phenomenon contingent upon current relationships and interpersonal experiences (Maunder & Hunter, 2001). The results of our study showing that so many women with FVD experienced stressful incidents and interpersonal conflicts that then influenced their pattern of seeking social support, affirm the suggestion by Bifulco *et al.*, (2002) that 'attachment style may involve a more dynamic relationships to an adverse social environment than is generally documented or acknowledged' (p.56).

Observations in relation to prior experience of sexual abuse, violence or strangulation

Inquiries were also made about any lifetime experience of *sexual abuse, violence* or *strangulation*. Traumatic incidents such as these have often been linked with other conversion reaction symptoms, including loss of voice (Roelofs, Keijsers, Hoogduin, Näring, & Moene, 2002), and I was also interested to investigate whether sexual abuse or strangulation might have been an issue, especially for those with PVD.

Our findings showed that the FVD group women were more likely to report experiences of sexual abuse, violence or strangulation in their lifetime, and comparisons between the PVD and MTVD sub-groups showed that more PVD group women reported sexual abuse than those with MTVD. Some of these incidents had occurred in the individual's formative years and for others, in the 12 months prior to onset of the voice disorder. It is not intended to overstate the significance of these preliminary findings, but it is reasonable to wonder if these prior experiences might have contributed in some way to the more insecure and fearful attachment profiles of the FVD group women. A similar question arises for the PVD group when compared with the MTVD women, especially in view of previous studies which have demonstrated a more anxious and introverted personality amongst women with FD and no pathology (Roy *et al.*, 2000a).

To our knowledge, this was the first time that the quality of attachment in adult relationships, and information in relation to the experience of violence, sexual abuse, or strangulation, had been formally investigated with any voice disordered population other than in isolated individual case reports (Baker, 2003; Baker & Lane, 2009; Freud, 1905/1962). In the light of the interesting work which has focused on suppression of negative emotion and behavioural constraint as these may affect vocal function, it is suggested that further exploration of this sensitive area may contribute to our understanding of why *some* individuals may be more vulnerable to elevated levels of anxiety, introversion, and behavioural constraint, and more prone to the development of particular voice disorders such as FVD that includes the MTVD and PVD sub-groups.

Observations in relation to the interaction between LEDS and traits data

As highlighted in Chapter 5, and as mentioned in Box 6.5 above, regression analysis showed that the number and severity of stressful and COSO incidents preceding onset of voice disorder were the most potent factors in differentiating the FVD group women from the OVD and control groups. Surprisingly, the *dispositional traits data* were shown not to be key predictors of risk. The fact that the traits did not remain in the statistical models was puzzling, especially in the light of the strong results for the measures when examined independently. This may have been due to similarities in a number of measures used, which may have weakened their predictive power. Alternatively, the LEDS data were so strong that in groups of this size, there was insufficient power to demonstrate the more subtle effects of the traits data. We concluded that perhaps the traits such as anxiety, ambivalence over emotional expression and insecure attachment may have operated to influence or moderate the strength of these women's responses to the stressful life event and difficulties, and COSO incidents.

Analysis of the interaction effects for these dimensions between the PVD and MTVD sub-groups showed that neither the LEDS data nor the dispositional data distinguished between the two groups. Women with PVD were more prone to report an insecure and anxious attachment profile, fewer social supports, a preference for the suppression of negative emotions, and a previous lifetime experience of sexual abuse. However, in the more stringent regression analysis, these features did not operate as predictors of voice disorder group membership. Perhaps the measures used in relation to emotional expressiveness were not sufficiently discerning, and that more traditional measures related to personality traits would have been more revealing. Alternatively, although it is contrary to my clinical experience, is it possible that PVD and MTVD sub-groups are not as aetiologically different as we may have assumed? Or asked another way, is it possible that different psychological processes are operating that will only be revealed by further neurophysiological studies? I would predict that is where the answers may lie.

Issues and questions remaining in relation to dispositional profiles

In drawing the findings from this chapter together, it would be ideal to embrace the proposal by Roy *et al.* (2000a) that there are typical 'personological resumés' for different voice disorder groups. Certainly within the context of their dispositional trait theory that identifies personality as a contributor to voice pathology, with FD patients being more introverted and behaviourally constrained and those with VN being more extraverted, such a proposal would seem very reasonable. It would also be tempting to conclude that the experience of negative emotions in response to stressful and COSO incidents preceding the onset of the full range of FVD may well predispose some individuals to the development of a FVD, and that the way in which individuals express, suppress, or repress their emotions may account for those who present with PVD as opposed to MTVD, and then those who go on to develop vocal nodules.

As suggested by the above authors, and keeping in mind our own recent findings and the cautions from others (Dietrich & Verdolini Abbott, 2008; Husein *et al.*, 2008), although some clear group trends have been identified across many studies, numerous exceptions have been noted where participants *did not* have abnormal scores on the various measures and *did not conform* to the personality typologies. These different research teams concede that although personality has been shown to be an important consideration in the development of FVD, including those with PVD and MTVD, personality differences 'do not meet the requirement of necessary or sufficient causal status' (Roy *et al.*, 2000b) (p. 762).

Perhaps the answers to some of our remaining questions may be found in *functional brain imaging studies* which could give further confirmation for the notion that the personality trait of *constraint (CON)* relates to 'the degree of activation of behavioural inhibition observed in the pre-frontal cortex' (van Mersbergen, 2011) (p.34). In a study by Aybek *et al.* (2013), *neurological substrates* that may underpin the *repression of emotions* in patients with conversion reaction symptoms and other psychogenic movement disorders have recently been identified. Furthermore, in other laboratory and functional Magnetic Resonance Imaging (fMRI) studies, neural substrates that may be differentially activated during phonation when responding to stressful situations with introverted and extraverted individuals have been located (Dietrich, Andreatta, Jiang, Joshi, & Stemple, 2012; Dietrich & Verdolini Abbott, 2012). The implications for these promising new developments in support of hypotheses related to the non-expression of emotion and behavioural constraint, and the way in which these psychosocial processes may contribute to the different theoretical models underpinning FVD, will be discussed in Chapter 8.

Summary and concluding comments

The evidence suggests that FVD can be considered as a spectrum of conditions, with those referred to as conversion reaction, psychogenic voice disorder (PVD) or functional dysphonia (FD) towards one end of the continuum, and those referred to as hyperfunctional dysphonia or muscle tension voice disorder (MTVD) who may go on to develop vocal nodules (VN), lying at the other end (Baker *et al.*, 2007; Dietrich *et al.*, 2008; Goldman *et al.*, 1996). Rather than these disorders being construed as having fundamentally different causal pathways, it is reasonable to speculate whether factors such as the personality traits of introversion and extraversion, or the different degrees of constraint or impulsivity, may operate to influence the way one person responds to stress by withdrawing and closing down, or another chooses a more impulsive, energetic and hyperfunctional approach.

I would agree with the many authors cited in this chapter that we need to be wary of making assumptions or overestimating psychological involvement in all cases of FVD. If there is a causal relationship, such as in relation to stressful or COSO events preceding onset, or predisposing personality traits, other factors such as individual physiological and vocal differences, and the influences of high vocal demands in different situational contexts, also need to be taken into account (Dietrich *et al.*, 2008; Roy, 2011; van Mersbergen, 2011). In addition, I suggest that we should not underestimate the fact that stressful incidents often precede onset of OVD as well, and that dispositional factors of individuals with OVD should not be dismissed as irrelevant.

The considerable empirical findings from these many studies should encourage practitioners across disciplines to recognise that different personality traits and dispositional features may predispose individuals to particular voice disorders. These factors are also likely to colour the way in which individuals react to their vocal problems, and to influence the impact that such a condition will have on that person and those in their wider social network. These issues are now discussed in Chapter 7.

References

Abeida, M. E. U., Liesa, R. F., Verala, H. V., Campayo, J. G., Gormedino, P. R., & Garcia, A. O. (2013). Study of the influence of psychological factors in the etiology of vocal nodules in women. *Journal of Voice, 27*(1), 129.e115–129.e120. doi: 10;1016/j.jvoice.2011.08.012

Andersson, K., & Schalen, L. (1998). Etiology and treatment of psychogenic voice disorder: Results of a follow-up study of thirty patients. *Journal of Voice, 12*(1), 96–106.

Andrews, B., & Brown, G. W. (1988). Social support, onset of depression and personality: An exploratory analysis. *Social Psychiatry and Psychiatric Epidemiology*, 99–108.

Aronson, A. E., & Bless, D. M. (2009). *Clinical voice disorders* (4th ed.). New York: Thieme.

Aronson, A. E., Brown, J. R., Litin, E. M., & Pearson, J. S. (1968). Spastic dysphonia I. Voice, neurologic, and psychiatric aspects. *Journal of Speech and Hearing Disorders, 33*, 203–218.

Aronson, A. E., Peterson, H. W., & Litin, E. M. (1964). Voice symptomatology in functional dysphonia and aphonia. *Journal of Speech and Hearing Disorders, 28*, 367–380.

Aronson, A. E., Peterson, H. W., & Litin, E. M. (1966). Psychiatric symptomatology in functional dysphonia and aphonia. *Journal of Speech and Hearing Disorders, 31*, 115–127.

Aybek, S., Nicholson, T. R., Zelaya, F., O'Daly, O. G., Craig, T. K., David, A. S., & Kanaan, R. A. (2013). Neural correlates of recall of life events in conversion disorder. *JAMA Psychiatry*. doi: doi:10.1001/jamapsychiatry.2013.2842

Baker, J. (2002). Psychogenic voice disorders – heroes or hysterics? A brief overview with questions and discussion. *Logopedics, Phoniatrics, Vocology, 27*, 84–91.

Baker, J. (2003). Psychogenic voice disorders and traumatic stress experience: A discussion paper with two case reports. *Journal of Voice, 17*(3), 308–318.

Baker, J. (2008). The role of psychogenic and psychosocial factors in the development of functional voice disorders. *International Journal of Speech-Language Pathology, 10*(4), 210–230.

Baker, J., Ben-Tovim, D. I., Butcher, A., Esterman, A., & McLaughlin, K. (2007). Development of a modified diagnostic classification system for voice disorders with inter-rater reliability study. *Logopedics Phoniatrics Vocology, 32*, 99–112.

Baker, J., Ben-Tovim, D. I., Butcher, A., Esterman, A., & McLaughlin, K. (2013). Psychosocial risk factors which may differentiate between women with functional voice disorder, organic voice disorder, and control group. *International Journal of Speech-Language Pathology, 15*(6), 547–563.

Baker, J., & Lane, R. D. (2009). Emotion processing deficits in functional voice disorders. In K. Izdebski (Ed.), *Emotions in the human voice* (Vol. 3, pp. 105–136). San Diego: Plural Publishing.

Ban, J. H., Lee, K. C., & Jin, S. M. (2007). Investigation into psychological correlates of patients with vocal nodules using the Symptom Checklist-90-Revision. *The Journal of Otolaryngology, 36*(4), 227–232.

Beck, A. T., & Steer, R. A. (1993). *Beck Depression Inventory manual*. San Antonio: The Psychological Association.

Bendig, A. W. (1956). The development of a Short Form of the Manifest Anxiety Scale. *Journal of Consulting Psychology, 20*(5).

Bifulco, A., Lillie, A., Ball, C., & Moran, P. (1998b). *Attachment Style Interview (ASI). Training manual*. London: Royal Holloway, University of London.

Bifulco, A., Moran, P., Ball, C., & Lillie, A. (2002). Adult attachment style II: Its relationship to psychosocial depressive vulnerability. *Social Psychiatry and Psychiatric Epidemiology, 37*, 60–67.

Bowlby, J. (1969). *Attachment and loss*. (Vol. 1). New York: Basic Books.

Bowling, A. (1995). *Measuring disease*. Buckingham: Open University Press.

Breuer, J., & Freud, S. (1955/1893–1895). Studies on hysteria. In J. Strachey (Ed.), *The standard edition of the complete works of Sigmund Freud*. (Vol. 2, pp. 1–305). London: Hogarth Press.

Briquet, P. (1859). *Clinical and therapeutic treatise on hysteria*. Paris: Balliere.

Brown, G. W., & Harris, T. O. (1978). *Social origins of depression*. London: Tavistock Publications.

Butcher, P., Elias, A., & Cavalli, L. (2007). *Understanding and treating psychogenic voice disorder: A CBT framework*. Chichester: Wiley.

Butcher, P., Elias, A., Raven, R., Yeatman, J., & Littlejohns, D. (1987). Psychogenic voice disorder unresponsive to speech therapy: Psychological characteristics and cognitive-behaviour therapy. *British Journal of Disorders of Communication, 22,* 81–92.

Charcot, J. M. (1887). *Lessons on the illnesses of the nervous system.* Paris: Delahaye, A., Lecrosnie, E.

Chaturvedi, S. K., Desai, G., & Shaligram, D. (2006). Somatoform disorders, somatization and abnormal illness behaviour. *International Review of Psychiatry, 18*(1), 75–80.

Craig, T. K. J. (2001). Life events: Meanings and precursors. In P. W. Halligan, C. Bass & J. C. Marshall (Eds.), *Contemporary approaches to the study of hysteria* (pp. 88–101). Oxford: Oxford University Press.

Crowne, D. P., & Marlowe, D. (1960). A new scale of social desirability independent of psychopathology. *Journal of Consulting Psychology, 24*(4), 349–354.

Deary, I. J., Wilson, J. A., Carding, P. N., & MacKenzie, K. (2003). The dysphonic voice heard by me, you and it: Differential associations with personality and psychological distress. *Clinical Otolaryngology, 28,* 374–378.

Deary, V., Chalder, T., & Sharpe, M. (2007). The cognitive behavioural model of medically unexplained symptoms: A theoretical and empirical review. *Clinical Psychology Review, 27,* 781–797.

Derakshan, N., & Eysenck, M. W. (2001). Manipulation of focus of attention and its effects on anxiety in high-anxious individuals and repressors. *Anxiety, Stress and Coping., 14,* 177–191.

Dietrich, M., Andreatta, R. D., Jiang, Y., Joshi, A., & Stemple, J. C. (2012). Preliminary findings on the relation between the personality trait of stress reaction and the central neural control of vocalization. *International Journal of Speech-Language Pathology, 14*(4), 377–389.

Dietrich, M., & Verdolini Abbott, K. (2008). Psychobiological framework of stress and voice. In K. Izdebski (Ed.), *Emotions in the Human Voice: Volume 2* (pp. 159–178). San Diego: Plural Publishing.

Dietrich, M., & Verdolini Abbott, K. (2012). Vocal function in introverts and extraverts during a psychological stress reactivity protocol. *Journal of Speech, Language and Hearing Research, 55,* 973–987.

Dietrich, M., Verdolini Abbott, K., Gartner-Schmidt, J., & Rosen, C. L. (2008). The frequency of perceived stress, anxiety, and depression in patients with common pathologies affecting voice. *Journal of Voice, 22*(4), 472–487.

Eysenck, H. J., & Eysenck, S. B. G. (1975). *Manual for the Eysenck Personality Questionnaire.* London: Hodder and Stoughton.

Freud, S. (1905/1962). Fragment of an analysis of a case of hysteria. In J. Strachey (Ed.), *The complete works of Sigmund Freud* (Vol. 9, pp. 229–234). London: Hogarth Press.

Freud, S. (1962/1896a). Heredity and the aetiology of the neuroses. In J. Strachey (Ed.), *The standard edition of the complete psychological works of Sigmund Freud.* (Vol. 3, pp. 141–156). London: Hogarth Press.

Friedl, W., Friedrich, G., & Egger, J. (1990). Personality and coping with stress in patients suffering from functional dysphonia. *Folia Phoniatrica, 42,* 13–20.

Gassull, C., Casanova, C., Botey, Q., & Amador, M. (2010). The impact of the reactivity to stress in teachers with voice problems. *Folia Phoniatrica et Logopaedia, 62*, 35–39. doi: 10.1159/000239061

Gerritsma, E. J. (1991). An investigation into some personality characteristics of patients with psychogenic aphonia and dysphonia. *Folia Phoniatrica, 43*, 13–20.

Goldman, S. L., Hargrave, J., Hillman, R. E., Holmberg, E., & Gress, C. (1996). Stress, anxiety, somatic complaints, and voice use in women with vocal nodules: Preliminary findings. *American Journal of Speech-Language Pathology, 5*, 44–54.

Gunther, V., Mayr-Graft, A., Miller, C., & Kinzl, H. (1996). A comparative study of psychological aspects of recurring and non-recurring functional aphonias. *European Archives of Otorhinolaryngolgy., 253*(4–5), 240–244.

Harris, T. O., & Bifulco, A. (1991). Loss of parent in childhood, attachment style and depression in adulthood. In C. Murray-Parkes, J. Stevenson-Hinde & P. Marris (Eds.), *Attachment across the life-cycle.* London: Routledge.

Heaver, L. (1958). Psychiatric observations of the personality structure of patients with habitual dysphonia. *Logos, 1*, 21–26.

House, A., & Andrews, H. B. (1987). The psychiatric and social characteristics of patients with functional dysphonia. *Journal of Psychosomatic Research, 31*, 483–490.

Husein, O. F., Husein, T. N., Gardner, R., *et al.* (2008). Formal psychological testing in patients with paradoxical vocal fold dysfunction. *The Laryngoscope, 118.*

Janet, P. (1920). *The major symptoms of hysteria.* New York: Hafner.

King, L. A., & Emmons, R. A. (1990). Conflict over emotional expression: Psychological and physical correlates. *Journal of Personality and Social Psychology, 58*(5), 864–877.

Kinzl, J., Biebl, W., & Rauchegger, H. (1988). Functional aphonia: A conversion symptom as defensive mechanism against anxiety. *Psychotherapy and Psychosomatics, 49*, 31–36.

Lauriello, M., Cozza, K., Rossi, A., DiRienzo, L., & Tirelli, G. C. (2003). Psychological profile of dysfunctional dysphonia. *ACTA Otorhinolaryngologica Italica, 23*, 467–473.

Maunder, R. G., & Hunter, J. J. (2001). Attachment and psychosomatic medicine: Developmental contributions to stress and disease. *Psychosomatic Medicine., 63*(4), 556–567.

McHugh-Munier, C., Scherer, K. R., Lehmann, W., & Scherer, U. (1997). Coping strategies, personality, and voice quality in patients with vocal fold nodules and polyps. *Journal of Voice, 11*(4), 452–461.

Millar, A., Deary, I. J., Wilson, J. A., & MacKenzie, K. (1999). Is an organic/functional distinction psychologically meaningful in patients with dysphonia? *Journal of Psychosomatic Research, 46*(6), 497–505.

Mirza, N., Ruiz, C., Baum, E. D., & Staab, J. P. (2003). The prevalence of major psychiatric pathologies in patients with voice disorders. *Ear Nose and Throat Journal, 82*(10), 808–812.

Morrison, M. D., & Rammage, L. (1994). *The management of voice disorders.* San Diego: Singular Publishing Group.

Myers, L. B., & Derakshan, N. (2004). The repressive coping style and avoidance of negative affect. In I. Nyklicek, L. Temoshok & A. Vingerhoets (Eds.), *Emotional expression and health* (pp. 169–184). Hove and New York: Brunner-Routledge.

O'Hara, J., Miller, T., Carding, P., Wilson, J., & Deary, V. (2011). Relationship between fatigue, perfectionism, and functional dysphonia. *Otolaryngology-Head and Neck Surgery, 144*(6), 921–926.

Ratajczak, J., Grzywacz, K., Wojdas, A., Rapiejka, P., & Jurkiewicz, D. (2008). The role of psychological factors in pathogenesis of disturbance of voice caused by vocal nodules. *Otolaryngologica Polska (Polish Otolaryngology), 62*(6), 758–763.

Roelofs, K., Keijsers, G. P. J., Hoogduin, K. A. L., Näring, G. W. B., & Moene, F. C. (2002). Childhood abuse in patients with conversion disorder. *American Journal of Psychiatry, 159*(11), 1908–1913.

Roy, N. (2011). Personality and voice disorders. In T. L. Eadie (Ed.), *Perspectives on voice and voice disorders* (Vol. 21, pp. 17–23). Rockville, ML: ASHA.

Roy, N., & Bless, D. M. (2000a). Toward a theory of the dispositional bases of functional dysphonia and vocal nodules: Exploring the role of personality and emotional adjustment. In R. D. Kent & M. J. Ball (Eds.), *The handbook of voice quality measurement.* (pp. 461–481). San Diego: Singular Publishing Group.

Roy, N., & Bless, D. M. (2000b). Personality traits and psychological factors in voice pathology: A foundation for future research. *Journal of Speech, Language, and Hearing Research, 43*, 737–748.

Roy, N., Bless, D. M., & Heisey, D. (2000a). Personality and voice disorders: A multi-trait-multidisorder analysis. *Journal of Voice, 14*, 521–548.

Roy, N., Bless, D. M., & Heisey, D. (2000b). Personality and voice disorders: A super-factor trait analysis. *Journal of Speech, Language and Hearing Research, 43*, 749–768.

Roy, N., McGory, J. J., Tasko, S. M., Bless, D. M., Heisey, D., & Ford, C. (1997). Psychological correlates of functional dysphonia: An investigation using the Minnesota Multiphasic Personality Inventory. *Journal of Voice, 11*(4), 443–451.

Schalen, L., & Andersson, K. (1992). Differential diagnosis and treatment of psychogenic voice disorder. *Clinical Otolaryngology, 17*, 225–230.

Seifert, E., & Kollbrunner, J. (2005). Stress and distress in non-organic voice disorders. *Swiss Medical Weekly, 135*, 387–397.

Sinkiewicz, A., Jaracz, M., Mackiewicz-Nartowicz, H., et al. (2013). Affective temperament in women with functional aphonia. *Journal of Voice, 27*(1), 129.e111–129.e114.

Siupsinskiene, N., Razbadauskas, A., & Dubosas, L. (2011). Psychological distress in patients with benign voice disorders. *Folia Phoniatrica et Logopaedia, 63*, 281–288.

Spielberger, C. D., Gorusch, R. L., Lushene, R., Vagg, P., & Jacobs, G. A. (1983). *Manual for the State-Trait Anxiety Inventory (Form Y Self-Evaluation Questionnaire).* Palo Alto: Consulting Psychologists Press.

Tellegen, A. (1982). *A brief manual for the Multidimensional Personality Questionnaire* Unpublished manuscript. University of Minnesota, Minneapolis.

Van der Ploeg, H. M. (1989a). *Self-Assessment Questionnaire-Nijmegen (SAQ-N).* Lisse: Swets and Zeitlinger.

Van Houtte, E., Van Lierde, K., & Claeys, S. (2009). Pathophysiology and treatment of muscle tension dysphonia: A review of the current knowledge. *Journal of Voice, 25*(2), 202–207.

van Mersbergen, M. (2011). Voice disorders and personality: Understanding their interactions. In T. L. Eadie (Ed.), *Perspectives on voice and voice disorders* (Vol. 21, pp. 31–38). Rockville: ASHA.

van Mersbergen, M., Patrick, C., & Glaze, L. (2008). Functional dysphonia during mental imagery: Testing the trait theory of voice disorders. *Journal of Speech, Language, and Hearing Research, 51*, 1405–1423.

Vingerhoets, A., Nyklicek, I., & Denollet, J. (Eds.). (2008). *Emotion regulation: Conceptual and clinical issues*. New York: Springer.

Weinberger, D. A. (1990). The construct validity of the repressive coping style. In J. L. Singer (Ed.), *Repression and dissociation: Implications for personality theory, psychopathology, and health.* (pp. 337–386). Chicago and London: The University of Chicago Press.

White, A., Deary, I. J., & Wilson, J. A. (1997). Psychiatric disturbance and personality traits in dysphonic patients. *European Journal of Disorders of Communication, 32*, 307–314.

Willinger, U., Volkl-Kernstock, S., & Aschauer, H. N. (2005). Marked depression and anxiety in patients with functional dysphonia. *Psychiatry Research, 134*(1), 85–91.

Wood, J. (2001). *Passion and pathology in Victorian literature.* New York: Oxford University Press.

Yano, J., Ichimura, K., Hoshino, T., & Nozue, M. D. (1982). Personality factors in pathogenesis of polyps and nodules of vocal cords. *Auris, Nasus, Larynx (Tokyo), 9*, 105–110.

Yelsma, P., Hovestadt, A. J., Anderson, W., & Nilsson, J. (2000). Family-of-origin expressiveness: Measurement, meaning, and relationship to Alexithymia. *Journal of Marital and Family Therapy, 26*(3), 353–363.

Ziegler, F. J., & Imboden, J. B. (1962). Contemporary conversion reactions II: A conceptual model. *Archives of General Psychiatry, 6*, 279–287.

7

Psychosocial impacts of vocal impairment on individuals

"People who live with a painful gap between who they have been and who they are now, of who they dreamt themselves to be and who they still long to be, are living with chronic sorrow" (Weingarten, 2012) (p.440).

Introduction

Further research efforts have focused on the *psychosocial impacts* that impairment of the voice may have for individuals and those close to them,, for groups with specific voice disorders, and the implications of these problems for the wider social system. Many of these studies have revealed that voice impairment can lead to changes in overall *quality of life (QOL)* as reflected in general and voice-related health, sense-of-self and identity, communication with others and interpersonal relationships, and participation in work and leisure activities.

In this chapter I refer to a number of quantitative and qualitative approaches that provide some measure of changes to QOL for voice disorder groups and individuals. It is suggested that while quantitative self-report questionnaires are helpful in identifying obvious changes, attention to qualitative methodologies such as the *International Classification of Functioning, Disability and Health (ICF)* (World Health Organization, 2001), and those that draw upon in-depth interviews or other creative forms of expression, may enable the more subtle and significant meanings associated with loss of voice to emerge. It is proposed that information gleaned from both of these approaches will provide a more stable foundation for helping clients to deal with the impact of their vocal impairment.

I then present an overview of the primary psychosocial domains of people's lives affected by vocal impairment, highlighting the clinical and empirical evidence for the impact on individuals with a range of functional and organic voice disorders, including those adjusting to total laryngectomy, or transgender individuals undertaking sexual reassignment. The implications of vocal impairment on the psychological and emotional well-being of individuals or patient groups are discussed, and attention is drawn to the fact that the perceived severity and impact of a voice disorder on a person is a very individual phenomenon. This is especially so for professional voice users, where seemingly minor changes to their vocal function may lead to a profound sense of loss with significant implications for current and future career prospects.

The empirical evidence suggests that while the consequences of voice problems on individuals rely to some degree on external factors such as the professional help and social supports available, the greater impacts depend upon internal factors such as the *sense of loss* and grief associated with changes to a person's identity, limitations on maintaining communication in close relationships, and reduced capacity to sustain roles and status in society through work and leisure activities.

Enduring dispositional traits and different coping styles have been shown to influence the way in which some individuals deal with the consequences of their voice disorders in the short term. However, other studies indicate that where a person is required to manage adverse responses of others to their condition, or where the voice disorder is likely to recur, become chronic, deteriorate progressively, or lead to permanent disability, alternative coping strategies and patterns of resilience may be required. It is proposed that we need to be vigilant in our understanding of the different degrees of loss and grief associated with vocal impairment and disability, and that an *altered sense-of-self* may render people vulnerable to the development of abnormal illness behaviours and somatisation disorder, or symptoms of anxiety and depression. In these situations, additional psychological or psychiatric support over and above the traditional voice therapy and counselling offered during speech pathology intervention may be required.

So much to say
But no one to hear
Strangled with pain,
Trying to speak.
There is no breath
My throat on fire
Choked by invisible hands
Cracked, broken sound
Then only a whisper
Voiceless
No mode of expression
Silence descends
Smothered in despair
Shall I ever be heard?

Reproduced with kind permission, Margaret Jacobs (2011).

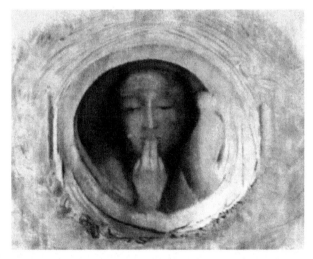

Fig. 7.1 SILENCE (LE SILENCE), Odilon Redon (c. 1911)

The significance of voice in our everyday lives

'The voice is integral to our spoken and sung communication, and the importance of the voice cannot be overstated (Sataloff, 1991) (p.1).

The voice may be used in an attempt to express a range of pre-verbal noises and powerful emotions such as crying, laughing, squeaking, grunting, groaning, whimpering, yelling, or screaming. Alternatively it may be used for the higher functions of expressing thought through speech and song, where consciously motivated meaning is conveyed. Modifications to our vocal quality, pitch, intensity, and intonation enable us to influence the emotional states of others by commanding attention, persuading, motivating, and inspiring, or even repelling and actively driving somebody away (Aronson & Bless, 2009; Baker, 2010; Colton, Casper, & Leonard, 2006; Oates, 2011). It has now been clearly established that in many Western countries, employment requires the use of the voice as a primary tool of trade, and that 'an effective and reliable voice has become one of the keys to economic and vocational success' (Oates, 2011) (p. 243).

The voice readily gives clues about a person's age and gender, and may be an early indicator of changes to an individual's physical or mental health. It reflects our mood, providing an outlet for the cathartic expression of intense emotions, which is thought to contribute to a person's psychological equilibrium (Aronson & Bless, 2009). In addition to supporting verbal communication with others where an ostensible message is intended, the voice, above all other paralinguistic features, may suggest aspects of meaning or more deeply nuanced emotions, which at times are more potent than the verbal content itself (Mathieson, 2001). It is this discrepancy between the spoken words and the meaning gleaned from the voice during interpersonal conflicts that may lead people to remark with conviction "It was not *what* she said but *how she said it* that mattered!" This brings to mind parallel distinctions in relation to transformational grammar, which distinguishes between the more obvious surface structures of spoken language and the deeper structures of meaning underpinning such utterances (Chomsky, 2006).

Over the centuries the voice has often been described as the mirror of the soul, or as a reflection of the inner self, and experienced clinicians stress that in learning about the voice, we need to understand not only how it functions mechanically but also, how much it reveals about the speaker (Colton & Casper, 1990). As suggested by Mathieson (2001), our vocal behaviour is closely tied up with our total image, and it is one of the primary means by which our personality may be projected and revealed. Implicit in these observations are the axiomatic notions that *voice and emotion*, and *voice and self*, are inextricably linked, and that impairment of the voice may impact upon the quality of life for individuals and for those close to them.

Impact of vocal impairment across the human life cycle

The consequences of vocal impairment or disability are experienced broadly across the human life cycle. For instance, when occurring in children, voice disorders have been associated with developmental and behavioural problems, with implications for peer relationships, communication with teachers, and participation in the classroom (Connor *et al.*, 2008; Ramig & Verdolini, 1998). These difficulties may lead to self-consciousness because their unusual voices draw adverse attention from peers, a loss of self-esteem and frustration at the difficulties they may have in expressing themselves, and very real consequences associated with participation in classroom activities that are expected of them. When persisting into adolescence, vocal difficulties may lead to embarrassment, with subtle behavioural strategies reflected in withdrawal or isolation from peers and school activities (Baker, 2002). In adults, voice problems often affect relationships with immediate and extended family members, work colleagues, and community relationships. For some people, a voice disorder may lead them to withdraw from their normal social activities and for others, it can compromise their capacity to carry out their work. For those adults who rely on their voices as a primary tool of trade, such as teachers, or for those who depend on the excellence of their voices for artistic performance, such as singers, a voice disorder can be emotionally traumatic with serious implications for health, employment, and financial security. In more extreme cases it may mean the end of their chosen career (Baker, 1998; D. C. Rosen & Sataloff, 1997; Titze & Verdolini Abbott, 2012). It has been estimated that a quarter of the adults who seek professional help for their voice problems are over 65 years-of-age, and the capacity to communicate effectively with others remains a primary concern for this age group. Roy *et al.* (2007) have shown that voice disorders in the elderly affect QOL due to 'increased effort and discomfort, combined with increased anxiety and frustration and the frequent need to repeat'(p. 633). Other findings suggest that the elderly report grave concerns when vocal impairment prevents them from singing, or when it leads to diminished social interactions, with implications for their overall physical and mental health (Etter, Stemple, & Howell, 2013).

As emphasised by many of the authors cited above, the severity of loss and impact of voice impairment on an individual is not necessarily commensurate with the severity of the voice disorder as judged by others, including expert opinion by the otolaryngologist and speech pathologist. Rather, the impact of a voice problem has been shown to rely on factors such as a person's age and gender, the level of dependence on voice as the primary tool of trade for work or creative performance, how aware a person may be about their voice disorder and the effect it is having on others, or socio-cultural factors that may influence how others view the person and their voice, and respond to them (Oates, 2011). Consequently, some individuals with no vocal fold pathology and a relatively minor vocal impairment may consider the impact as highly significant, while others with vocal fold lesions and what may be judged to be a more severe disorder of the voice, may not experience it as very troubling at all (Smits, Marres, & de Jong, 2012). As recently suggested by Ingo Titze and confirmed with some amusement by clinicians at a scientific meeting of the Australian Voice Association (personal communication, July 13, 2013), one only has to listen to the voices of adolescents in our respective nations, with their monotonous, low energy utterances grinding along from one glottally-fried syllable to the next, to appreciate that judgments about the existence or severity of a voice disorder are definitely not only in the ear of the listener. Essentially, the severity of the impact has been shown to depend on how much the vocal impairment compromises the person's life at the time.

However, it is alarming to note that when the impact of a voice problem is experienced as being severe, the psychosocial effects on many individuals have been shown to be similar or even worse than those reported by patients with more life-threatening illnesses (Smith *et al.*, 1996; Yiu, 2002). These broad psychosocial and economic ramifications have been recognised for some time, and they are now of sufficient magnitude to confirm that disorders of the voice are a significant public health issue (Roy, Merrill, Gray, & Smith, 2005; Russell, Oates, & Greenwood, 2005; Titze & Verdolini Abbott, 2012; Vilkman, 2000).

Approaches to the measurement of the impact of vocal impairment

Quantitative measures

In a comprehensive overview of the different research efforts carried out to measure or quantify the impact on QOL in association with vocal impairment or disability, Jennifer Oates (2011) has highlighted a number of issues in relation to the nature of the instruments and methodologies used in many of the earlier studies conducted prior to the late 1990s. These included: the use of questionnaires that had been designed for particular studies by the researchers with little input from participants; a predominance of scales that emphasise general or health-related QOL; questions that lead to the reporting of symptoms of anxiety or depression that may have contributed to onset or that may have developed as outcomes; and the fact that most of the questionnaires failed to focus specifically on impairment of the voice. Oates (2011) suggests that while there was some evidence for restrictions to levels of activity and participation across work-related and social domains, with commonly reported symptoms of stress and anxiety, depression and somatisation, there were insufficient data 'to allow robust conclusions about the impact of specific types of voice disorders or the impacts on specific groups of occupational voice users' (p. 247).

She also reports that since the late 1990s there has been a strong and welcome emphasis on the development and psychometric evaluation of several other self-report questionnaires designed specifically to measure the impact of voice impairment. Most of these instruments are designed for use across a range of voice disorders, but some have been tailored to specific voice disorder groups. These were for dysphonia following vocal fold paralysis (Gliklich *et al.*, 1999), *vocal problems of the singing voice* (Cohen *et al.*, 2007), and male to female clients during *transgender transition* (Dacakis *et al.*, 2013; Hancock *et al.*, 2011). Oates (2011) suggests that findings derived from studies using these *voice-specific QOL instruments* reflect those from the earlier health-related QOL studies, with moderate levels of psychosocial impact across the domains of physical, mental, vocational, and social functioning. However, she also argues that these findings do not adequately reflect the highly complex impacts of voice impairment on individuals, and, along with other authors, she proposes that further research efforts need to be placed within the context of conceptual frameworks such as the ICF (2001). She also advocates that researchers should draw upon qualitative methodologies to enable a deeper understanding of the meaning of the vocal disability to the person (Baylor, Yorkston, & Eadie, 2005; Baylor *et al.*, 2009; Eadie *et al.*, 2006).

Several other papers reviewing the psychometric features of some of these scales have highlighted the strengths and considerable limitations of the instruments, with the strong caveat that while many do serve a useful function in identifying the more obvious consequences of vocal impairment for individuals and patient groups, greater specificity and sensitivity in the various scales is needed (Branski *et al.*, 2010; Franic, Bramlett, & Cordes Bothe, 2005; Zraick & Risner, 2008). These authors recommend that in the development of such instruments, scales need to reflect the input from participants, and that all scales should be developed with improved psychometric properties that would meet appropriate reliability and validity standards. It is proposed that this would enhance the clinical relevance of these instruments in providing more effective pre- and post- therapy assessment, and would offer improved insights for clinicians when planning therapeutic interventions. Some of the more widely used self-report questionnaires, and others that have attempted to address some of the criticisms above while also enabling more input from the participant, are shown in Box 7.1.

Box 7.1 Instruments measuring the impact of voice disorders in adults

- Quality of Life Questionnaire (Smith *et al.*, 1996)
- Voice Handicap Index (VHI) (Jacobson *et al.*, 1997)
- Voice-Related Quality of Life Questionnaire (V-RQOL) (Hogikyan & Sethuraman, 1999)
- Voice Activity and Participation Profile (VAPP) (Ma & Yiu, 2001) derived from the ICF (2001)
- Voice Symptoms Scale (VoiSS) (Deary, Wilson, Carding, MacKenzie, & Watson, 2010; Deary, Wilson, Carding, & MacKenzie, 2003)
- Short Form-Voice Handicap Index (VHI-10) (C. A. Rosen, Lee, Osborne, Zullo, & Murry, 2004)
- Voice Outcome Survey (VOS) (Gliklich, Glovsky, & Montgomery, 1999)
- Singing Voice Handicap Index (SVHI) (Cohen *et al.*, 2007)
- Communicative Participation Item Bank (Baylor, Yorkston, Eadie, Miller, & Amtmann, 2009)
- Transgender Self-Evaluation Questionnaire (TSEQ) (Hancock, Krissinger, & Owen, 2011)
- The Transsexual Voice Questionnaire for Male to Female Transsexuals (TVQ^{MtF}) (Dacakis, Davies, Oates, Douglas, & Johnston, 2013)

One example, where closer attention to participant perception has been incorporated into the ongoing development of the instrument, is the *Communication Participation Item Bank* (Baylor *et al.*, 2009). Intended as an outcome measure that would have applications for clinical trials and clinical practice across a range of communication disorders, it provides a more explicit measure of an individual's levels of participation in communication activities. It achieves this, in part, by placing the emphasis on *levels of satisfaction* that the person reports about their capacity to participate, and by tapping into *latent traits* 'such as self-perceived interference with participation' (p.1303).

In another study that has enabled greater input from the *'participant's voice'*, Deary *et al.* (2010) recently re-examined their *Voice Symptom Scale (VoiSS)* by applying a 'Mokken scaling procedure' to the items. One objective of the study was to determine whether there is a *phenomenological hierarchy* to vocal symptoms experienced by people with a range of voice disorders and if so, would this suggest further associations between vocal and psychosocial impairments. A further objective was to establish 'whether there is a place on a reliable continuum of voice-related complaints where reports of dysphoric phenomena appear' (p. 68).

The findings showed a clear hierarchy of voice-oriented difficulties at the less severe end, progressing from practical problems, to disturbances of social relationships, and lastly, to effects on mood or *dysphoria* at the more severe end. The authors emphasised that the psychosocial factors related to alterations in mood were reported only after individuals had attempted the more practical solutions, and that the psychosocial sequelae of voice pathology, such as low mood, embarrassment, and loneliness tend to occur at the 'far end' of the experience. They cautioned that in those cases where a vocal impairment becomes chronic, additional psychological or psychiatric interventions may be required.

Although these authors considered that one of the strengths of their study was the inclusion of patients across a spectrum of disorders, I would suggest that it would be fascinating to explore these hierarchical patterns for specific voice disorder groups, and to ascertain whether symptoms such as anxiety or low mood are reported earlier along the continuum for some disorders and later for others.

Qualitative approaches

More recent efforts have been devoted to the use of *qualitative methodologies* that draw upon *semi-structured interviews* in which a person is able to recount their thoughts, feelings, beliefs, and attitudes about the impact of a particular disorder as it affects them directly, those close to them, and their wider social network. Outside the constraints of structured questionnaires, semi-structured interviews can provide the time and scope for participants, in collaboration with researchers, to select the information that they consider to be relevant and to prioritise those issues that matter most. They may also generate explanations for the ways in which external and internal factors have been interacting with one another to shape the lived experience of a particular condition for that individual. There are many texts on the theoretical foundations underpinning different approaches to qualitative research interviewing and the methodologies for the systematic gathering and thematic analyses of the data. However, for the purposes of this discussion, two approaches that have been used in relation to the impacts of health and impairment of the voice are mentioned briefly in the sections below.

One of these is *phenomenological inquiry*. This is a both a philosophical discipline and a research method (Heidegger, 1962; Husserl, 1970). The primary tenet is that phenomenology seeks to describe and understand the lived experience of individuals with a particular condition. In an excellent and readily accessible discussion paper focused upon biopsychosocial perspectives on nursing care, Wojnar and Swanson (2007) highlight several core concepts of phenomenology and provide lucid descriptions of two different approaches to phenomenological inquiry.

Underpinning the first *descriptive approach* is the premise that the meaning of lived experience from the first person point of view can only be discovered through a one-to-one interaction between researcher and participant, and that through the processes of 'attentive listening, interaction and observation' (p.173), more refined perceptions and understandings of reality can be co-constructed.

The crux of the second *hermeneutic* or *interpretive approach* is the search for meaning, but always within the context of an individual's socio-cultural and political context. Therefore, when extrapolating this to the possible impact of vocal impairment, the experience for a person is understood in the context of family traditions, community values, and the broader socio-political context. I would suggest that these key tenets are remarkably similar to the processes underpinning all effective models of psychotherapy and counselling that may be used in helping patients to resolve different voice disorders.

The other qualitative methodologies have emerged from *grounded theory*. Influenced by the philosophical theory of *symbolic interactionism* (Blumer, 1969; Mead, 1962), the grounded theory methodologies of in-depth interviewing, and the gathering and comparing thematic analyses of data across interviews, were originally developed by Glaser and Strauss (1967). They have since been refined further by Charmaz *et al.* (1990, 2003; 2012).

As explained by Charmaz (2012), the *in-depth interview* and *directed conversation* enables particular experiences of the person's life to be explored. Throughout this process it is acknowledged that more than one reality exists;

the data that emerge holds notions generated by both participant and researcher, and the researcher joins the participant's world to the extent that he or she is affected by it. The conversations and thematic analyses of data enable the impact of adverse experiences, such as health conditions or a voice disorder, to be understood through the thoughts, feelings, and behaviours expressed by the person involved. It is then possible to appreciate the way in which such a condition has impacted upon an individual's 'self-esteem', 'personal identity', or 'sense-of-self'.

It is not within the scope of this book to debate the philosophies related to the emergence of the self with the depth that this topic deserves, but it is, however, relevant to consider the nature of the self and how this may be altered through the experience of losing one's voice or vocal impairment. In his most fascinating treatise *Concepts of the Self*, Anthony Elliott (2008) discusses notions related to 'the self', 'selfhood', and 'self-identity'. Drawing upon the philosophical foundations of *symbolic interactionism* as originally proposed by Mead (1962), Elliott explains that the experience of the self cannot be sufficiently understood 'in terms of psychological dispositions or inner depth, because of the *shared symbolic meanings* that define day-to-day social life' (p.163), and that 'the central dilemma of personal identity is that of balancing the multiple demands of society and culture on the self with inner definitions of identity' (p.163).

Therefore, one of the fundamental constructs underpinning *symbolic interactionism* is that the self is essentially social in nature (Charmaz, 1983), and that this perspective 'permits examining the ways in which changes in self-concept occur throughout the life cycle' (p.170). This notion is developed further by Elliott (2008). He challenges the commonly held assumption that 'selfhood' necessarily means 'sameness' over time, and argues that it is an unrealistic expectation that 'I am the same self as I was yesterday' (p.15). He highlights the ongoing tensions between notions of a 'fixed selfhood' that remains unchanged, and a 'psychologically flexible or pliable' sense-of-selfhood that is influenced by day-to-day living and challenging experiences over time.

These philosophical constructs in relation to *the self* and *personal identity* may seem somewhat esoteric and possibly far removed from the demands of quantifiable and empirical evidence. I would suggest however, that they offer crucial insights into many anecdotal and clinical reports, and the more recent empirical data emerging from studies using both qualitative and quantitative methodologies. From all of these sources it is clear that the impact of vocal impairment on an individual is often experienced as much more than loss of one's physiological voice. It may also entail a loss of one's personal voice, one's psychological voice, one's voice in close interpersonal relationships, in relation to employment and performance, and in the wider sociocultural network. At the more severe or chronic end of the continuum, it may precipitate a *'loss of self'* (Charmaz, 1983) (p.168).

Creative approaches to exploring the perceived nature of a voice disorder

In addition to self-report questionnaires and in-depth interviews designed to explore the impact of vocal impairment on individuals, the use of *guided drawing* and *expressive art* can also provide a fascinating window into the different ways in which patients perceive their voices, how they would like it to be, and how their voice problems may have impacted upon them (Baker, 1981; D. C. Rosen & Sataloff, 1997).

In my own earlier work, when undertaking psychotherapeutic training and supervised practice in *transactional analysis*, I had the opportunity to run ongoing medical problem-solving groups with doctors and clinical psychologists who were also fascinated by the speech pathologist's perspectives on communication and voice. Patients coming to these psychotherapy groups presented with long-standing unresolved medical problems, some of which were related to the voice and others to specific medical conditions. During the course of some of these sessions patients were invited to draw their voice as construed now, and then as visualised in the future. This provided an excellent way of initiating conversations about how the voice works, how they experienced their voice, how others perceived it, and how they envisaged it might be. Interestingly, too, during these conversations issues often emerged which related to their other health concerns, albeit quite unconsciously, and in a way that enabled the person to consider them from a new perspective.

For instance, a 34 year-old woman came to the group primarily to help resolve issues related to her long-term problems with fertility and difficulties in conceiving. She also expressed interest in improving her voice, which was typical of a hyperfunctional muscle tension voice disorder, characterised by a strained hoarseness in vocal quality, and a tendency to deteriorate into low-pitched glottal fry phonation towards the end of utterances. As she drew and described her voice, she referred to it as being 'tight to the core', 'a somewhat tangled web', with 'real roughness around the edges'. The image of her *idealised voice* was drawn to reflect 'warmth and well roundedness with resonance and colour'. As she reviewed her evocative images that were ostensibly in relation to her voice, she became very still and her eyes filled with tears. She immediately recognised its significance in the light of her problems in striving to conceive, likening the first image to her twisted and tangled fallopian tubes, and the second to healthy ovaries ripe for conception. What is so interesting in reflecting on these images is that when we *look* at each picture we *hear* her voice, both real and metaphorical (see Figs 7.2a and 7.2b).

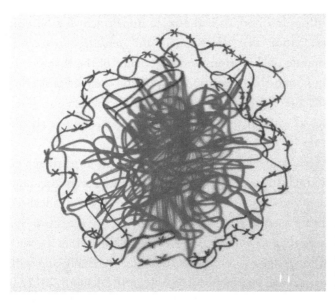

Fig. 7.2a Woman's image showing her current perception and experience of her voice

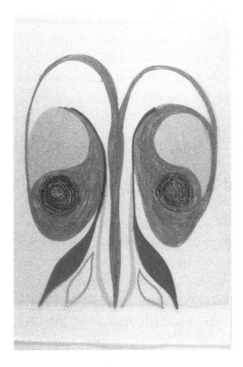

Figure 7.2b Woman's image showing her idealised voice

Rosen and Sataloff (1997) provide an excellent theoretical rationale for their work in which they use guided drawings as a component of their assessment of professional voice users with vocal problems. Here, the emphasis is on how the person perceives the impact of their voice loss on their personal identity, and how they cope with the grief associated with their vocal impairment. Patients are also invited to provide drawings that represent how they perceive themselves once their voice problem has resolved, or if the voice impairment has become permanent. The authors caution that the value in this *projective artwork* is closely tied to the appropriate qualifications and experience of the therapist in interpreting such drawings, and that practitioners must be wary of projecting their own psychological issues onto the images drawn by the patient. Each image should be approached without any preconceived agenda, and one should always 'listen to the picture' (p. 190).

These creative approaches to exploring the impact of vocal impairment on individuals may not seem mainstream, and some readers may be sceptical about the idea of inviting patients to create drawings of their perceived or idealised voice, or images symbolising themselves with or without their voice. However, for decades the *symbolic significance of art* has been recognised in therapy with terminally-ill children who are unable to express themselves verbally, and with adults with a range of physical and mental health problems (Malchiodi, 2012). It is not suggested that this activity should replace the more empirically validated quantitative or qualitative approaches to measurement of impact of voice loss, or that it should become a substitute for traditional voice therapies and appropriate counselling. Rather, as shown so effectively by Rosen *et al.* (1997), I would agree that it is a powerful tool that may provide further insights for patients and practitioners into the nature of a voice problem, the way in which it impacts on a person's life, and how he or she may learn to cope and to develop resilience while coming to terms with these changes.

Psychosocial domains affected by vocal impairment or disability

A review of the literature reveals a number of key *psychosocial domains* most commonly affected by vocal impairment for individuals, their families, and society (Aronson & Bless, 2009; Benninger, Ahuja, Gardner, & Grywalski, 1998; Epstein, Hirani, Stygall, & Newman, 2009; Etter *et al.*, 2013; Krischke *et al.*, 2005; Mathieson, 2001; Oates, 2011; Pemberton, 2010; Rammage, Morrison, & Nichol, 2001; Roy *et al.*, 2004; Roy *et al.*, 2007; Royal College of Speech and

Language Therapists, 2009; Smith *et al.*, 1996; Titze & Verdolini Abbott, 2012; Yiu, 2002). They are shown in Box 7.2.

Box 7.2 Psychosocial domains affected by vocal impairment or disability

* Individual or Group
  * Socio-demographic factors – gender and age
  * Physical health, both general and specific to voice
  * Mental health as reflected in psychological and emotional well-being
* Interpersonal communication
  * Social interactions and relationships with close others
  * Communication and intelligibility with others in wider social system
* Participation in social, cultural and religious activities
  * Hobbies, sports and creative pursuits
  * Religious practices and involvement with cultural activities
* Employment and work
  * Capacity to carry out normal work
  * Implications for current and future career prospects
* Societal implication
  * Economic, loss of skills, productivity
  * Healthcare costs to societies

Although there appear to be explicit boundaries between areas, in reality, most individuals describe experiences and consequences that merge across the different domains. Moreover, as suggested by Etter *et al.* (2013), when participants are invited to talk about 'any changes to your quality of life', they may not even recognise that many of the changes in their daily living and activities do, in fact, constitute an alteration to their QOL. This makes it all the more important that in addition to standardised voice-related QOL questionnaires, practitioners and researchers need to probe more deeply. It has been suggested that this is best achieved through in-depth interviews, with an emphasis on qualitative methodologies and with close reference to frameworks such as the (ICF) (2001), both for voice disorders in general and for specific voice disorder groups (Eadie, 2007; Ma, Yiu, & Verdolini Abbott, 2007).

Evidence for impact of voice impairment across mixed voice disorder groups

There are several strong trends within the empirical data where the impacts of vocal impairment on QOL across mixed voice disorder groups have been compared with non-patient groups, or groups of individuals with other medical conditions[1]. In these studies, which have included heterogeneous groups of patients diagnosed with both FVD and OVD, the findings showed that vocal impairment impacted across all the commonly recognised psychosocial domains, as shown in Box 7.2.

Socio-demographic data showed that females were more likely to present with voice disorders than males (except in the study by Etter *et al.*, 2013), and patients ranged from approximately 18 to 90 years-of-age. Interestingly, those in the 65 years and over age group reported the most significant consequences of voice impairment, with concerns about the quality of their interactions with family and friends, and their diminished levels of involvement with leisure and community activities, such as singing.

Findings for health-related QOL showed that overall physical health, sense of vitality, and mental health were generally worse in the voice disorder groups. Participants reported that their voice problems affected their capacity to carry out daily tasks, with substantial limitations in social and work-related roles. *Fatigue* was the most commonly reported health concern associated with the sustained effort required to produce an adequate voice, to project sufficiently, especially over background noise, and to repeat themselves for others. During social communication, voice disorder groups reported feeling embarrassed and concerned that they may be annoying to others, or frustrated during conversations where it was difficult to express their feelings or opinions.

The impact of vocal impairment across voice disorder groups was highly significant for participants in maintaining roles at work, not only for current levels of effectiveness and productivity but also, with serious implications for future employment and longer-term career prospects. For some, the threats to employment and financial security were experienced as being emotionally devastating (Smith *et al.*, 1996), and for those whose communication with close associates was seriously compromised, they chose to avoid or withdraw from social situations, with a lowered overall sense of emotional well-being, and a

---

1 (Benninger *et al.*, 1998; Etter *et al.*, 2013; Krischke *et al.*, 2005; Mirza, Ruiz, Baum, & Staab, 2003; Scott, Robinson, Wilson, & MacKenzie, 1997; Siupsinskiene, Razbadauskas, & Dubosas, 2011; Smith *et al.*, 1996; Wilson, Deary, Millar, & MacKenzie, 2002).

vulnerability to symptoms associated with anxiety and depression (Mirza *et al.*, 2003; Siupsinskiene *et al.*, 2011). An excellent conceptual map of the individual impacts and inter-related consequences of voice disorder on communication behaviours, developed by Mathieson (2001), is shown in Fig. 7.3. The author emphasises that 'each individual responds differently but communication patterns inevitably change according to the speaker's personality and the type of dysphonia' (p. 131).

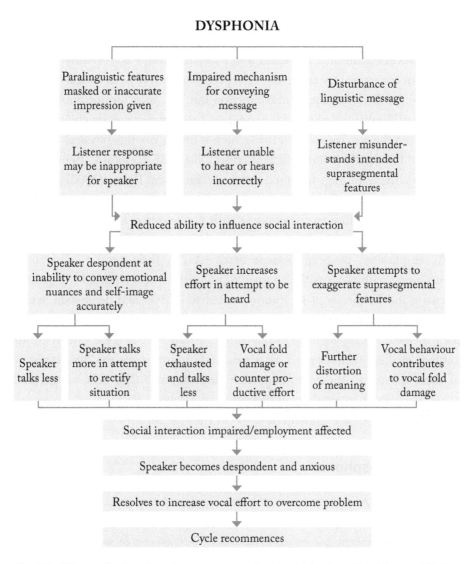

Fig. 7.3 Effects of voice disorder on communication behaviour (Mathieson, 2001)

Kind permission from L. Mathieson © and courtesy Wiley Publishers

Evidence for impact of voice impairment across specific voice disorder groups

Vocal fold paralysis

In two of the studies with mixed voice disorder groups cited above, further analysis of specific voice disorder sub-groups was undertaken (Benninger *et al.*, 1998; Siupsinskiene *et al.*, 2011). Here, patient groups with *vocal fold paralysis* were the most seriously compromised, and those with benign *vocal fold mass lesions* such as nodules or polyps were the least likely to report serious impacts of their vocal conditions. The vocal fold paralysis groups consistently reported significant consequences, rendering their problem equivalent to a vocal disability not only in relation to their vocal function but also, as a serious limitation to their overall health and physical functioning. This was particularly obvious when carrying out the activities of daily living, such as lifting, or other physical exertions that would normally require efficient effort closure of the glottis (Benninger *et al.*, 1998). These findings mirrored those of Murry and Rosen (2000) who also showed that groups of patients with vocal fold paralysis had higher self-reports on voice handicap indices than groups with benign vocal fold lesions or those with laryngopharyngeal reflux.

As emphasised by Siupsinskiene *et al.* (2011), their vocal fold paralysis group, along with those with *laryngeal papillomatosis*, also reported the greatest intensity and frequency of symptoms related to anxiety and depression, which these authors attributed to concerns over life-threatening implications of their medical management, possible complications over surgical interventions, dubious medical or therapeutic outcomes, and in some cases, the chronic nature of these disorders. These are important findings, and they echo suggestions made in earlier chapters that consideration of psychosocial perspectives are just as relevant for the management of OVD as they are for FVD.

Spasmodic dysphonia

> '*These patients prove how considerably important normal voice is to the maintenance of a secure self-image and how alienated we become with ourselves and society when our self-image, epitomized by our voices, is threatened by our own and others' adverse reactions to it*' (Aronson & Bless, 2009) (p.106).

Spasmodic dysphonia (SD) is a troubling voice disorder with significant impacts on the psychological, social and work-related domains of a person's life (Aronson

& Bless, 2009; Aronson, Brown, Litin, & Pearson, 1968). In a number of studies, these psychosocial consequences have been assessed with instruments such as *health-related questionnaires* (Cannito, 1991; Courey *et al.*, 2000; Murry, Cannito, & Woodson, 1994), the *Voice Handicap Index (VHI)* (Benninger, Gardner, & Grywalski, 2001; Courey *et al.*, 2000), and the *Voice-Related Quality of Life (V-RQOL)* (Rubin, Wodchis, Spak, Kileny, & Hogikyan, 2004). However, as suggested by Baylor *et al.* (2005), when these studies are considered within the more recent context of the ICF, much of the emphasis has been placed upon aspects of the framework that assess *levels of impairment* and *restrictions to participation*, with less attention to contextual factors such as *environmental (external)* and *personal (internal)* factors. It is these features that tend to exert the greatest impact and consequences of any given condition.

In order to redress some of these issues, Baylor *et al.* (2005) conducted a phenomenological study, interviewing six patients with SD who had received a minimum of five botox injections. They suggested that in order to gain a deeper understanding of the meaning of the disability of SD, it was also essential to obtain 'the insider's perspective' (p. 397). The aim of their study was to explore the meaning of the lived experience of each person, and to understand any experiences in common. Analysis of their data revealed three pivotal themes related to the *physiologic*, *personal*, and *social* impacts of SD on these individuals. These themes led to the development of a model that maps out the consequences of SD from the *insider's perspective*, with emphasis on the various individual components, and then as these might interact with one another (Fig. 7.4).

The authors claimed that their findings supported those from previous studies using quantitative self-report methodologies. However, the in-depth analysis also highlighted a number of interesting different issues not previously or sufficiently explored.

For instance, one of the most consistent themes under *physiologic factors* was the perception of *vocal dysfunction* with the associated high levels of *physical effort* and *associated fatigue* when using the voice, a problem noted in many previous studies. An additional new finding related to a person's voice being *'undependable'*, *'inconsistent'*, and *'unreliable'*, especially where work or social requirements demanded consistency, and the authors suggested that this issue of inconsistency was an area warranting further exploration.

Apropos of these findings, it has been interesting to note two recent studies highlighting the fact that individuals with SD commonly report a *low health-related locus of control* in comparison to other voice and health conditions, with implications for a person's perception of their capacity to influence their own health and behaviours in a way that makes a difference (Haselden, Powell, Drinnan, &

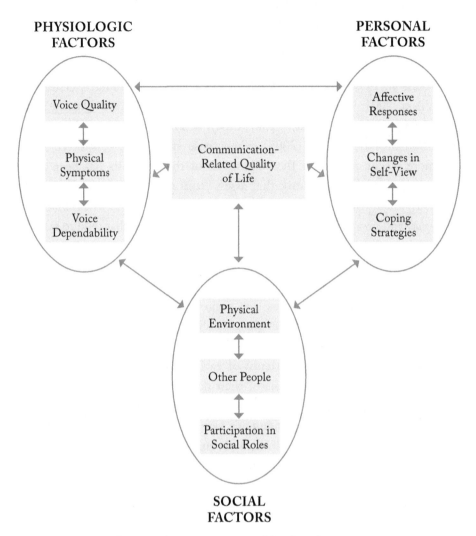

Fig. 7.4 A model of the insider's experiences of SD that shape communication related quality of life (Baylor et al., 2005 – p. 411)

Reproduced with kind permission Baylor et al., and courtesy Elsevier

Carding, 2009; Kaptein, Hughes, Scharloo, Hondebrink, & Langeveld, 2010). Furthermore, as recently emphasised by Rough and Brake (2013), one of the key aspects of assisting patients with SD is to help them improve their sense of control over these troubling unpredictable vocal symptoms.

The second theme identified by Baylor *et al.* (2005) was the individual's *personal experience* of their SD, where patients reported troubling emotional reactions to the experience of living with SD. Participants reported that their voices 'did not represent who they are' (p.407) and led them to feeling 'frustrated, hopeless, embarrassed, and self-conscious' (p.408). These data supported the findings from many of the previous studies cited above, where SD has been shown to lead to significant negative emotions in relation to communication and, in many patients, to *elevated levels of anxiety and depression*. In addition to these emotional reactions, they also commented on how they perceived *changes to their personalities* in response to the disorder, which the authors suggested could be a further area for investigation. These findings raise challenging questions, especially in the light of some previous studies discussed in Chapter 6, where enduring personality traits have been shown to predispose some individuals to the development of particular voice disorders and in others, where dispositional features were construed as current states contingent upon recent life experiences.

Additional findings for the personal experiences of these individuals indicated different ways of coping, with some reporting a preference for *behavioural strategies* such as *avoidance*, especially where situations called for higher levels of communication, while others used *attitudinal coping* such as trying to maintain a positive approach. The authors emphasised that *coping strategies* specifically in relation to SD have not been a focus in previous studies, and that coping as defined by the participant, rather than coping as defined by a particular research paradigm, would be an important next step. (More recent findings in relation to coping with a voice disorder will be discussed later in this chapter.)

The third major theme related to *social issues*, with difficulties in 'communicating in the world around me' (Baylor *et al.*, 2005. p. 410). In terms of the ICF, this refers to external contextual influences, and participants referred to the physical environment where communication was taking place, the effect that other people had on them during interactions, and ways in which SD restricted their ongoing participation in social roles. These included work, leisure or friendships roles. In keeping with the literature, factors such as background noise were commonly identified, with particular challenges during telephone conversations where the symptoms of SD made it difficult to project adequately or to be understood.

The reactions of others had a profound impact on these participants, especially those who did not know the person with whom they were trying to communicate, or others who had no knowledge of the condition SD. This often led to intrusive questions about their general health, assumptions that they may be nervous or lacking in confidence, or that they may not be very intelligent and capable. With respect to restrictions in maintaining social roles, the more serious consequences involved leaving jobs, changing career aspirations, or avoiding active roles in those social and community activities that normally would have been embraced. An apt distinction between *attending* and *participating* was made when individuals reported: 'Truly participating meant achieving some level of involvement or interaction with others, above and beyond merely being present at an event' (p. 407). The model developed by Baylor *et al.* (2005) captures many of the issues highlighted in previous studies, and although it has been derived from interviews specific to SD, I would suggest it would be relevant for other voice disorder groups, with implications for interventions that could be uniquely tailored to 'the insider's perspectives' on the impacts of their vocal impairment.

It is fascinating to observe how these recent qualitative data reflect the poignant comments made during the 100 interviews of SD patients conducted by Aronson some 30 years ago, and as exemplified in several of his conversations from previous case studies (Aronson, 1979; Aronson & Bless, 2009). The emotional pain, sense of loss, and frustration reflected in these early reports is palpable, and is most powerfully captured in this anguished and disembodied sculpture by Louise Bourgeois (Fig. 7.5).

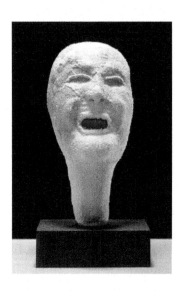

Fig. 7.5 Louise Bourgeois "Rejection" (2001)

Fabric, steel and lead, 63.5 x 33 x 30.5cm.
Private Collection, courtesy Cheim & Read, New York
Photo: Christopher Burke © The Easton Foundation /
Licensed by Viscopy, Sydney

Alaryngeal speech after total laryngectomy

There are some very interesting similarities in the impacts on individuals adjusting to *total laryngectomy* and those dealing with SD. For instance, in a number of studies, quantitative self-report measures such as the VHI and V-RQOL were used to measure the impacts of total laryngectomy on the patient, with the additional consequences of radiotherapy, chemotherapy, and various surgical methods that provide tracheoesophageal speech. Findings viewed once again within the context of the ICF showed that alaryngeal speech production, at the very least, constitutes a vocal impairment for many, and a disability for others, with very real restrictions to the participation in work and socially related activities (Kazi *et al.*, 2006).

Interestingly, in the same way that clinicians working with patients with SD have argued for research methodologies that will enable an insider's perspective, a plea for qualitative approaches has facilitated a number of studies where the deeper meaning of these impacts of total laryngectomy on individuals and their families has been explored.

Key findings from some of these studies suggest that changes to the voice and speech do not necessarily remain as the most commonly reported impact, especially some years after laryngectomy. Rather, there seems to be a predominance of psychosocial consequences, such as *sense-of-loss* due to *reduced self-esteem*, changes to *body image*, and lowered confidence in sexuality, with further social losses related to changes in work, family and societal roles (Eadie, 2003, 2007). Similar consequences have also been found for individuals suffering from head and neck cancer, with practitioners suggesting that if issues related to the distress, anxiety and potential depression of these populations were addressed more actively, it would have a more substantial impact on QOL than focusing solely on issues related to vocal impairment (Lee, 2011).

A number of new issues related to the impact of laryngectomy on individuals and those close to them have emerged from a recent study using a qualitative constructivist grounded theory methodology (as described by Charmaz (2003)). Twelve post-laryngectomy participants were interviewed in order to explore how these patients experienced their *'altered identity'*, and to identify any other key psychosocial factors that may be operating (Bickford, Coveney, Baker, & Hersh, 2013). A coding map showing the different elements that emerged from the analysis is shown in Fig. 7.6.

The core concept emerging from this study related to the participants' continuous process of *'identifying with the altered self after total laryngectomy'* (p.327) and the ways in which they reflected on how they used to be, and how they were now.

"I've lost my voice... I've lost part of my character, part of my personality...and that is very difficult, you know... for a long time I used to dream of still being able to speak properly... that expression has gone, ...it can, ... be very distressing, if I dwell on it" (p. 328).

Three major themes in the data analysis supported this concept of *identifying with the altered self*. These were: the *dynamic multi-level changes* involving communication competence, appearance, swallowing, respiratory functions, social

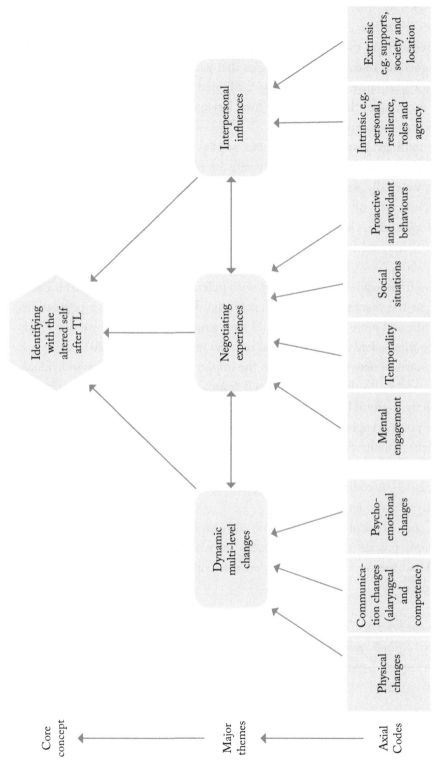

Fig. 7.6 Coding map of analysis levels (Bickford et al., 2013)

Reprinted with kind permission Bickford and colleagues and courtesy Taylor & Francis Publisher for International Journal of Speech-Language Pathology

and emotional well-being; *negotiating experiences*, which included both everyday situations and social interactions; and *interpersonal influences* that reflected issues intrinsic to the individual such as age, gender, and socioeconomic status and factors related to resilience, coping skills and *locus of control.*. Extrinsic factors involved issues related to *social supports*, reactions of others, and sociocultural influences.

The third theme of *interpersonal influences* placed many of the other issues into context for this group of patients and provided the deeper meaning of their condition for each person and those around them. Bickford *et al.* (2013) identified profound impacts from difficulties in communicating during social interactions, and their interpretation through a lens of *symbolic interactionism* highlighted how meaning and self-concept are constructed through language and the *suprasegmental features* of voice.

For instance, female participants expressed their embarrassment and distress at being mistaken for males, especially on the telephone, where they felt the need to mentally brace themselves in preparation for confused listener reactions. Moreover, participants of both genders reported their frustrations with loss of the paralinguistic features that have been shown to be so vital in reflecting a person's gender, identity, personality, emotions, and mood (Laver, 1980). Many noted that since they were less able to convey the more subtle aspects of meaning, other listeners were apt to misjudge or misinterpret their intended meaning. It was this confusion over gender for some, and in grasping the shared meaning of conversations for many, that often led these individuals to choose coping strategies of avoidance which, over time, led to more social isolation, change in social roles, or earlier retirement. These findings are of interest in the light of another recent study conducted by Eadie and Bowers (2012), where *avoidant coping strategies* were found to predict poorer outcomes in QOL for a proportion of their cohort of 67 patients post-laryngectomy. According to these authors, in cancer patients, avoidant coping strategies that involve cognitive and behavioural processes of distancing themselves predict poor QOL outcomes, often leading to increased vulnerability to mood disorders and chronic disease progression, whereas coping strategies, such as optimism, focusing thoughts on the positives, and making efforts to seek out social supports generally lead to more positive QOL outcomes.

Overall, the strong qualitative data emerging from this study supports previous findings for the consequences of changes to communication and personal appearance, and the impact that this has on social interactions for individuals. Of particular interest in these new data were the constructs associated with adjusting to and 'identifying with the altered self'(Bickford *et al.*, 2013) (p.

327), and the interactions between the contextual factors such as a person's *resilience* and *coping skills* with the external factors such as the adverse reactions or supportive responses of others. All of the authors cited in the section above have emphasised that clinicians need to be sensitive to the different ways in which individuals learn to adjust to 'their altered self' and the way in which they adopt different coping strategies, during both the earlier and later phases of their rehabilitation, so that interventions may be targeted if maladaptive coping strategies begin to impact on longer term QOL outcomes.

Voice and communication in the lives of male to female transsexual people

"The problem is that while we know that for many male-to-female transsexuals there are huge psychosocial implications of a gender incongruent voice, there is little published to reflect the anecdotal reports. An otherwise well adjusted human being, whose social presentation does not attract unwanted attention – until they speak – suffers anything from a look of disdain to outright violence and discrimination" (Dacakis, 12 March, 2014, Personal Communication).

In reflecting upon the impact of efforts to change the voice and aspects of communication for transgender clients, especially those transitioning from male to female, it is reasonable to question whether having a voice that is 'non-conforming' or *'incongruent with gender'* is in fact a voice disorder (Hancock *et al.*, 2011; Oates & Dacakis, 2014). It could be argued that an individual making a conscious and concerted effort to alter his gender identity is not the same as having a voice disorder inflicted by structural changes to the larynx following surgery, alterations in pitch due to hormonal changes, or functional aetiologies. However, if we consider the very real impacts for female laryngectomy patients being mistaken for men, as previously reported (Bickford *et al.*, 2013), or the acute embarrassment faced by women who have been administered androgenic hormones for specific medical conditions with resultant lowering of pitch (Baker, 1999; D. C. Rosen & Sataloff, 1997), the answer to the question above would most certainly be "yes".

Recent clinical and empirical evidence indicates that acquiring the voice and communication skills to a level of satisfaction that enables 'passing as female' is one of the most confronting challenges for transgender clients. Until this is achieved, both according to their own perceptions and those of other listeners, their voice continues to influence their sense of identity and QOL (Byrne, 2007;

Dacakis *et al.*, 2013; Hancock *et al.*, 2011; Oates & Dacakis, 2014; Pasricha *et al.*, 2008). Transgender people report problems remarkably similar to those with disorders of the voice such as spasmodic dysphonia, paralysed vocal fold or laryngectomy, where effort and concentration are constantly needed to produce an appropriate voice (in this case with gender-appropriate features) both over time and in different social contexts. Perhaps of even greater significance are the findings that failure to achieve a voice that is congruent with gender places the transsexual at considerable risk of ridicule or rejection, bullying, harassment, or discrimination, and in some social settings may lead to violence. For many, failure to pass as female leads to intense emotions that may result in poor self-image and lowered self-esteem, sometimes progressing to generalised anxiety or vulnerability to depression, *suicidal ideation*, and, in rare cases, to suicidal attempts. As emphasised by Dacakis *et al.* (2013), the overwhelming concerns underlying these intense emotional reactions are that the person's voice does not adequately reflect the 'true self' or 'true identity', a sentiment also expressed by both men and women after laryngectomy. In the light of these data, the authors recommend that in addition to interventions that target achieving an authentic voice, there is 'the ongoing need for psychosocial counselling as part of voice and communication therapy' (p. 319).

Coping with dysphonia

These more recent empirical data from both quantitative and qualitative approaches are now providing support for earlier clinical reports which suggested that altered vocal function, vocal impairment or vocal disability have far-reaching impacts on individuals and on those close to them. This raises issues about how individuals or groups of patients cope with these consequences, and the implications that this may have for clinical management. As discussed previously in Chapter 6, there have been several studies focusing upon personality traits and approaches to coping with stress that might predispose a person to the development of particular voice disorders. However, it still remains a challenge to differentiate explicitly between *coping styles* that might be construed as 'dispositional features', and those *coping strategies* that may have arisen in response to a vocal impairment.

It is interesting to note therefore that there have been relatively few studies specifically focused upon how people cope with the stress and experience of having a voice disorder, and as practitioners, we need to be able to identify those approaches to coping that may help individuals to achieve healthy outcomes, to come to terms with residual vocal impairment, and, in some cases, to adjust to 'their altered self'. Significantly, we also need to be able to recognize which coping styles may intensify and perpetuate the sense-of-loss, delay or prolong the processes of grieving, or render a person more vulnerable to additional mental health sequelae such as abnormal illness behaviours and somatisation disorder, or symptoms of anxiety and depression as a result of their voice disorder (Baker, Oates, Leeson, Woodford, & Bond, 2014; Lauriello, Cozza, Rossi, DiRienzo, & Tirelli, 2003; Willinger, Volkl-Kernstock, & Aschauer, 2005).

It is a welcome development that several studies have recently addressed questions related to coping with dysphonia. Several of these have focused on the coping strategies of particular occupational groups such as teachers (de Jong *et al.*, 2003; Meulenbroek & de Jong, 2010; Van Wijck-Warnaar *et al.*, 2010), and others have explored the coping styles of specific voice disorder groups and populations across different countries (Epstein *et al.*, 2009; Oliveira, Hirani, Epstein, Yazigi, & Belhau, 2012). Overall, the findings suggest that the more healthy or *adaptive coping styles* reflect attitudes and behaviours where the person actively seeks information, attempts different solutions, and reaches out for emotion-focused social support. The more *maladapative coping styles* reflect a passive approach to coping characterised by different forms of avoidance such as denial, withdrawal from social interactions, and a reticence to seek social support. Across these studies it is evident that those participants with the more severe voice disorders, or those rating themselves as having a high Voice Handicap Index, were inclined to use more passive and avoidant coping strategies. For instance, in the study where Epstein *et al.* (2009) sought to validate their *Voice Disability Coping Questionnaire (VDCQ)*, comparisons between two different voice disorder groups showed that patients with muscle tension dysphonia were more likely to use active, problem-solving approaches while those with spasmodic dysphonia were more likely to use avoidant and passive coping styles.

The findings from these different studies highlight the fact that different approaches to coping may well represent different stages in the process of individuals coming to terms with a diagnosis, understanding the essential nature of their voice disorder, and preparing themselves for the prognosis after intervention. They suggest too that inevitably, individuals may resort to more passive or *avoidant coping styles* if there seems little hope of recovery, or if a person realises that further deterioration is pending (McLeod & Clarke, 2007). The authors cited above all stress that it is important for practitioners to be aware of the different coping styles or strategies that patients may adopt during the different phases of dealing with their vocal impairment, and as suggested by de Jong *et al.* (2003), efforts need to be made to ensure that individuals do not become stuck or 'deadlocked' with coping patterns that remain inflexible, that foster further denial, or that may lead the person to longer-term grieving and withdrawal.

Sense of loss and grief in relation to vocal impairment

The evidence suggests that vocal impairment may impact upon individuals and those close to them across a number of psychosocial domains. Clearly, the consequences of voice disorder can be significant, with implications for the ways in which practitioners might approach clinical management. The sense-of-loss associated with vocal impairment is not necessarily commensurate with the severity of the dysphonia, and many patients experience grief following changes to their voice. As a consequence, the counselling role of the speech pathologist is crucial in helping patients with vocal impairment to deal with their sense-of-loss and *altered sense-of-self*, whatever the aetiology of their dysphonia. The impact of vocal impairment may lead to a very normal grief reaction which should not be construed as a mental illness, as argued so movingly by Kleinman (2012), and it is my opinion that assisting patients to come to terms with their sense-of-loss is as important as the direct voice work focused upon restoring vocal function. In some groups of patients such as professional singers, where their identity is often inextricably tied to the voice, or for individuals suffering progressive neurological disorders, the grief can be profound. In some cases, with examples to be discussed in later chapters, more specialised grief counselling may be required (Miller, 2008; D. C. Rosen & Sataloff, 1997).

In the next chapter, I review several theoretical models that seek to explain how a range of psychosocial factors, both as unique influences and as they interact, may contribute to the onset and clinical presentations of voice disorders. Many of these factors have been shown to be causally related, especially in the FVD groups, but those related to the impact of both FVD and OVD on individuals tend to influence the maintenance, aggravation, and longer-term resolution of these disorders. I propose that the psychosocial factors related to the impacts of a given voice disorder deserve to be included in future theoretical models that seek to explain these complex processes.

References

Aronson, A. E. (1979). *Spastic dysphonia: Retrospective study of one hundred patients.* Unpublished manuscript.

Aronson, A. E., & Bless, D. M. (2009). *Clinical voice disorders* (4th ed.). New York: Thieme.

Aronson, A. E., Brown, J. R., Litin, E. M., & Pearson, J. S. (1968). Spastic dysphonia I. Voice, neurologic, and psychiatric aspects. *Journal of Speech and Hearing Disorders, 33,* 203–218.

Baker, J. (1981). *Your voice looks impotent: A transactional analysis perspective on voice therapy.* Paper presented at the Inaugural Transactional Analysis Conference, Australia, Adelaide.

Baker, J. (1998). Psychogenic dysphonia: Peeling back the layers. *Journal of Voice, 12*(4), 527–535.

Baker, J. (1999). Changes to women's voices following hormonal therapy. A report on alterations to the speaking and singing voices of four women. *Journal of Voice, 13*(4), 496–507.

Baker, J. (2002). Persistent dysphonia in two performers affecting the singing and projected speaking voice: A report on a collaborative approach to management. *Logopedics Phoniatrics Vocology, 27,* 179–187.

Baker, J. (2010). Women's voices: Lost or mislaid, stolen or strayed? *International Journal of Speech-Language Pathology, 12*(2), 94–106.

Baker, J., Oates, J., Leeson, E., Woodford, H., & Bond, M. J. (2014). Patterns of emotional expression and responses to health and illness in women with functional voice disorders (MTVD) and a comparison group. *Journal of Voice.* doi: http://dx.doi.org/10.1016/j.jvoic.2014.03.005

Baylor, C. R., Yorkston, K. M., & Eadie, T. L. (2005). The consequences of spasmodic dysphonia on communication-related quality of life: A qualitative study of the insider's experience. *Journal of Communication Disorders, 38,* 395–419.

Baylor, C. R., Yorkston, K. M., Eadie, T. L., Miller, R. M., & Amtmann, D. (2009). Developing the communicative participation item bank: Rasch analysis results from a spasmodic dysphonia sample. *Journal of Speech Language and Hearing Research, 52,* 1302–1320.

Benninger, M. S., Ahuja, A. S., Gardner, G., & Grywalski, C. (1998). Assessing outcomes for dysphonic patients. *Journal of Voice, 12*(4), 540–550.

Benninger, M. S., Gardner, G., & Grywalski, C. (2001). Outcomes of botulinum toxin treatment for patients with spasmodic dysphonia. *Archives of Otolaryngology Head and Neck Surgery, 127,* 1083–1085.

Bickford, J., Coveney, J., Baker, J., & Hersh, D. (2013). Living with the altered self. *International Journal of Speech-Language Pathology, 15*(3), 324–333.

Blumer, H. (1969). *Symbolic interactionism: Perspective and method.* Englewood Cliffs: Prentice-Hall.

Branski, R. C., Cukier-Blaj, S., Pusic, A., Cano, S. J., Klassen, A., Mener, D., Patel, S., & Kraus, D. H. (2010). Measuring quality of life in dysphonic patients: A sytematic review of content development in patient-reported outcomes measures. *Journal of Voice, 24*(2), 193–198.

Byrne, L. A. (2007). *My life as a woman: Placing communication within the social context of life for the transsexual woman.* (Doctoral Thesis), La Trobe University, Melbourne, Australia.

Cannito, M. P. (1991). Emotional considerations in spasmodic dysphonia: Psychometric quantification. *Journal of Communication Disorders, 24,* 313–329.

Charmaz, K. (1983). Loss of self: A fundamental form of suffering in the chronically ill. *Sociology of Health and Illness, 5*(2), 168–195.

Charmaz, K. (1990). 'Discovering' chronic illness: Using grounded theory. *Social Science and Medicine, 30,* 1161–1172.

Charmaz, K. (2003). Grounded theory: Objectivist and constructivist methods. In N. K. Denzin & Y. S. Lincoln (Eds.), *Strategies of qualitative inquiry* (2nd ed.). Thousand Oaks: Sage Publications.

Charmaz, K., & Belgrave, L. L. (2012). Qualitative interviewing and grounded theory analysis. In J. F. Gubrium, J. A. Holstein, A. B. Marvasti, & K. D. McKinney (Eds.), *The SAGE handbook of interview research: The complexity of the craft* (2nd ed.). London: Sage Publications.

Chomsky, N. (2006). *Language and mind.* Cambridge: Cambridge University Press.

Cohen, S. M., Jacobson, B. H., Garrett, C. G., Noordzij, J. P., Stewart, M. G., Attia, A., Ossoff, R. H.,& Cleveland, T. F. (2007). Creation and validation of the singing voice handicap index. *Annals of Otology, Rhinology & Laryngology, 116,* 402–406.

Colton, R. H., Casper, J., & Leonard, R. (2006). *Understanding voice problems: A physiological perspective for diagnosis and treatment.* Philadelphia: Lippincott, Williams & Wilkins.

Colton, R. H., & Casper, J. K. (1990). *Understanding voice problems. A physiological perspective for diagnosis and treatment.* London: Williams and Wilkins.

Connor, N. P., Cohen, S. B., Theis, S. M., Thibeault, S. L., Heatley, D. G., & Bless, D. M. (2008). Attitudes of children with dysphonia. *Journal of Voice, 22*(2), 197–209.

Courey, M. S., Garrett, C. G., Billante, C. B., Stone, C. R., Portell, M. D., Smith, T. L., & Netterville, J. L. (2000). Outcome assessment following treatment of spasmodic dysphonia with botulinum toxin. *Annals of Otology, Rhinology & Laryngology, 109*(9), 819–822.

Dacakis, G., Davies, S., Oates, J. M., Douglas, J. M., & Johnston, J. R. (2013). Development and preliminary evaluation of the transsexual voice questionnaire for male to female transsexuals. *Journal of Voice, 27*(3), 312–320.

de Jong, F. I. C. R. S., Cornelius, B. E., Wuyts, F. L., Kooijman, P. G. C., Schutte, H. K., Oudes, M. J., & Graamans, K. (2003). A psychological cascade model for persisting voice problems in teachers. *Folia Phoniatrica et Logopaedia, 55*(2).

Deary, I. J., Wilson, J., Carding, P., MacKenzie, K., & Watson, R. (2010). From dysphonia to dysphoria: Mokken scaling shows a strong, reliable hierarchy of voice symptoms in the Voice Symptom Scale. *Journal of Psychosomatic Research, 68,* 76–71.

Deary, I. J., Wilson, J. A., Carding, P. N., & MacKenzie, K. (2003). VoiSS: A patient-derived Voice Symptom Scale. *Journal of Psychosomatic Research, 68,* 67–71.

Eadie, T. L. (2003). The ICF: A proposed framework for comprehensive rehabilitation of individuals who use alaryngeal speech. *American Journal of Speech-Language Pathology, 12*(2), 189–197.

Eadie, T. L. (2007). Application of the ICF in communication after total laryngectomy. *Seminars in Speech and Language, 28*, 291–300.

Eadie, T. L., & Bowker, B. (2012). Coping and quality of life after total laryngectomy. *Otolaryngology Head and Neck Surgery, 146*(6), 959–965.

Eadie, T. L., Yorkston, K. M., Klasner, E. R., Dudgeon, B., Deitz, J. C., Baylor, C. R., Miller, R. M., & Amtmann, D. (2006). Measuring communicative participation: A review of self-report instruments in speech-language pathology. *American Journal of Speech-Language Pathology, 15*, 307–320.

Elliott, A. (2008). *Concepts of the self* (2nd ed.). Cambridge: Polity Press.

Epstein, R., Hirani, S. P., Stygall, J., & Newman, S. P. (2009). How do individuals cope with voice disorders? Introducing the Voice Disability Coping Questionnaire. *Journal of Voice, 23*(2), 209–217.

Etter, N. M., Stemple, J. C., & Howell, D. (2013). Defining the lived experience of older adults with voice disorders. *Journal of Voice, 27*(1), 61–67.

Franic, D. M., Bramlett, R. E., & Cordes Bothe, A. (2005). Pychometric evaluation of disease specific quality of life instruments in voice disorders. *Journal of Voice, 19*, 300–315.

Glaser, B. G., & Strauss, A. L. (1967). *The discovery of grounded theory*. Chicago: Aldine.

Gliklich, R., Glovsky, R. M., & Montgomery, W. M. (1999). Validation of a voice outcome survey for unilateral vocal cord paralysis. *Otolaryngology – Head and Neck Surgery, 120*, 153–158.

Hancock, A. B., Krissinger, J., & Owen, K. (2011). Voice perceptions and quality of life of transgender people. *Journal of Voice, 25*(5), 553–558.

Haselden, K., Powell, T., Drinnan, M., & Carding, P. (2009). Comparing health locus of control in patients with spasmodic dysphonia, functional dysphonia and nonlaryngeal dystonia. *Journal of Voice, 23*(6), 699–706.

Heidegger, M. (1962). *Being and time* (J. Macquarrie & E. Robinson, Trans.). New York: Harper & Row.

Hogikyan, N. D., & Sethuraman, G. (1999). Validation of an instrument to measure voice related quality of life (V-RQOL). *Journal of Voice, 13*(4), 557–569.

Husserl, E. (1970). *Logical investigations* (J. N. Findlay, Trans.). New York: Humanities Press.

Jacobs, M. (2011). *Psychogenic voice disorder and a compromised sense of self.* (Master of Science in Medicine (Psychotherapy)), University of Sydney.

Jacobson, B. H., Johnson, A., Grywalski, C., Silbergleit, A., Jacobson, G., Benninger, M. S., & Newman, C. W. (1997). The Voice Handicap Index (VHI): Development and validation. *American Journal of Speech-Language Pathology, 6*(3), 66–70.

Kaptein, A. A., Hughes, B. M., Scharloo, M., Hondebrink, M., & Langeveld, T. P. M. (2010). Psychological aspects of adductor spasmodic dysphonia: A prospective population controlled questionnaire study. *Clinical Otolaryngology, 35*, 31–38.

Kazi, R., De Cordova, J., Singh, A., Venkitaraman, R., Nutting, C. M., Clarke, P., . . . Harrington, K. J. (2006). Voice-related quality of life in laryngectomees: Assessment using the VHI and V-RQOL symptom scales. *Journal of Voice, 21*(6), 728–734.

Kleinman, A. (2012). The art of medicine: Culture, bereavement, and psychiatry. *The Lancet, 379*, 608–609.

Krischke, S., Weigelt, S., Hoppe, H., Kollner, V., Klotz, M., & Eysholdt, U. (2005). Quality of life in dysphonic patients. *Journal of Voice, 19*(1), 132–137.

Lauriello, M., Cozza, K., Rossi, A., DiRienzo, L., & Tirelli, G. C. (2003). Psychological profile of dysfunctional dysphonia. *ACTA Otorhinolaryngologica Italica, 23*, 467–473.

Laver, J. (1980). *The phonetic description of voice quality.* Cambridge: Cambridge University Press.

Lee, M. T. (2011). Head and neck cancer. In K. Hilari & N. Botting (Eds.), *The impact of communication disability across the lifespan* (pp. 263–277). Guildford: J&R Press Ltd.

Ma, E. P.-M., & Yiu, E. M.-L. (2001). Voice Activity and Participation Profile: Assessing the impact of voice disorders on daily activities. *Journal of Speech Language and Hearing Research, 44*(3), 511–524.

Ma, E. P.-M., Yiu, E. M.-L., & Verdolini Abbott, K. (2007). Application of the ICF in voice disorders. *Seminars in Speech and Language, 28*, 343–350.

Malchiodi, C. A. (2012). *Handbook of art therapy* (2nd ed.). New York: Guilford Press.

Mathieson, L. (2001). *Greene and Mathieson's: The voice and its disorders.* (6th ed.). London: Whurr.

McLeod, J. E., & Clarke, D. M. (2007). A review of psychosocial aspects of motor neurone disease. *Journal of Neurological Sciences, 258*, 4–10.

Mead, G. H. (1962). *Mind, self and society.* Chicago: Charles W Morris.

Meulenbroek, L. F. P., & de Jong, F. I. C. R. S. (2010). Trainee experience in relation to voice handicap, general coping and psychosomatic well-being in female student teachers: A descriptive study. *Folia Phoniatrica et Logopaedica, 62*, 47–54.

Miller, J. (2008). *The creative feminine and her discontents. Psychotherapy, art, and destruction.* London: Karnac Books.

Mirza, N., Ruiz, C., Baum, E. D., & Staab, J. P. (2003). The prevalence of major psychiatric pathologies in patients with voice disorders. *Ear Nose and Throat Journal, 82*(10), 808–812.

Murry, T., Cannito, M., & Woodson, G. E. (1994). Spasmodic dysphonia: Emotional status and botulinum toxin treatment *Archives of Otolaryngology Head and Neck Surgery, 120*, 310–316.

Murry, T., & Rosen, C. A. (2000). Outcome measures and quality of life in voice disorders. *Otolaryngologic Clinics of North America, 33*(4), 905–916.

Oates, J. (2011). Voice impairment. In K. Hilari & N. Botting (Eds.), *The impact of communication disability across the lifespan.* Guildford: J & R Press.

Oates, J., & Dacakis, G. (2014). *Voice and communication in the lives of male-to-female transsexual people.* Paper presented at the The Third Hong Kong Speech and Hearing Symposium, Hong Kong.

Oliveira, G., Hirani, S. P., Epstein, R., Yazigi, L., & Belhau, M. (2012). Coping strategies in voice disorders of a Brazilian population. *Journal of Voice, 26*, 205–213.

Pasricha, N., Dacakis, G., & Oates, J. (2008). Communicative satisfaction of male-to female transexuals. *Logopedics Phoniatrics Vocology, 33*(1), 25–34.

Pemberton, C. (2010). Voice injury in teachers: Voice care prevention programs to minimise occupational risk. Available at http://www.voicecareaustralia.com.au/Voice%20Injury%20in%20Teachers.pdf [Accessed October 2016]

Ramig, L. O., & Verdolini, K. (1998). Treatment efficacy: Voice disorders. *Journal of Speech, Language, and Hearing Research, 41*, s101.

Rammage, L., Morrison, M., & Nichol, H. (2001). *Management of the voice and its disorders.* San Diego: Singular Publishing Group.

Rosen, C. A., Lee, A. S., Osborne, J., Zullo, T., & Murry, T. (2004). Development and validation of the voice handicap index-10. *Laryngoscope, 114*, 1549–1556.

Rosen, D. C., & Sataloff, R. T. (1997). *Psychology of voice disorders.* San Diego: Singular Publishing Group.

Rough, J., & Brake, H. (2013). *Current issues for speech pathologists managing patients with spasmodic dysphonia.* Paper presented at the 4th Sydney Laryngology Course, St Vincent's Hospital, Sydney, Australia.

Roy, N., Merrill, R., Gray, S. D., & Smith, E. M. (2005). Voice disorders in the general population: Prevalence, risk factors, and occupational impact. *The Laryngoscope, 115*(11), 1988–1995.

Roy, N., Merrill, R. M., Thibeault, S., Parsa, R. A., Gray, S. D., & Smith, E. M. (2004). Prevalence of voice disorders in teachers and the general population. *Journal of Speech Language Hearing Research, 47*, 281–293.

Roy, N., Stemple, J., Merrill, R. M., & Thomas, L. (2007). Epidemiology of voice disorders in the elderly: Preliminary findings. *The Laryngoscope, 117*, 628–633.

Royal College of Speech and Language Therapists. (2009). *RCSLT Resource Manual for Commissioning and Planning Services for SLCN-Voice.* London: Royal College of Speech and Language Therapists.

Rubin, A. D., Wodchis, W. P., Spak, C., Kileny, P. R., & Hogikyan, N. D. (2004). Longitudinal effects of botox injections on voice-related quality of life (V-RQOL) for patients with adductory spasmodic dysphonia. *Archives of Otolaryngology Head and Neck Surgery, 130*, 145–420.

Russell, A., Oates, J., & Greenwood, K. (2005). Prevalence of self-reported voice problems in the general population in South Australia. *Advances in Speech-Language Pathology, 7*(1), 24–30.

Sataloff, R. T. (1991). *Professional voice. The science and art of clinical care.* New York: Raven Press.

Scott, S., Robinson, K., Wilson, J. A., & MacKenzie, K. (1997). Patient-reported problems associated with dysphonia. *Clinical Otolaryngology, 22*, 37–40.

Siupsinskiene, N., Razbadauskas, A., & Dubosas, L. (2011). Psychological distress in patients with benign voice disorders. *Folia Phoniatrica et Logopaedia, 63*, 281–288.

Smith, E., Verdolini, K., Gray, S. D., Nichols, S., Lemke, J., Barkmeier, J., Dove, H., & Hoffman, H. (1996). Effect of voice disorders on quality of life. *Journal of Medical Speech-Language Pathology, 4*(4), 223–244.

Smits, R., Marres, H., & de Jong, F. (2012). The relation of vocal fold lesions and voice quality to voice handicap and psychosomatic well-being. *Journal of Voice, 26*(4), 466–470.

Titze, I. R., & Verdolini Abbott, K. (2012). *Vocology. The science and practice of voice habilitation.* Salt Lake City: National Center for Voice and Speech.

Van Wijck-Warnaar, A., Van Opstal, M. J. M. C., Exelmans, K., Schaekers, K., Thomas, G., & de Jong, F. I. C. R. S. (2010). Biopsychosocial impact of voicing and general coping style in teachers. *Folia Phoniatrica et Logopaedica, 62*, 40–46.

Vilkman, E. (2000). Voice problems at work: A challenge for occupational safety and health. *Folia Phoniatrica et Logopaedia, 52*, 120–125.

Weingarten, K. (2012). Sorrow: A therapist's reflection on the inevitable and the unknowable. *Family Process, 51*(4), 440–455.

Willinger, U., Volkl-Kernstock, S., & Aschauer, H. N. (2005). Marked depression and anxiety in patients with functional dysphonia. *Psychiatry Research, 134*(1), 85–91.

Wilson, J., Deary, I. J., Millar, A., & MacKenzie, K. (2002). The quality of life impact of dysphonia. *Clinical Otolaryngology and Allied Sciences, 27*(3), 179–182.

Wojnar, D., & Swanson, K. M. (2007). Phenomenology: An exploration. *Journal of Holistic Nursing, 25*, 172–180.

World Health Organization. (2001). *International Classification of Functioning, Disability, and Health (ICF).* Geneva: World Health Organization.

Yiu, E. M.-L. (2002). Impact and prevention of voice problems in the teaching profession: Embracing the consumers' view. *Journal of Voice, 16*(2), 215– 228.

Zraick, R. I., & Risner, B. Y. (2008). Assessment of quality of life in persons with voice disorders. *Current Opinion in Otolaryngology and Head and Neck Surgery, 16*, 188–193.

8

Theoretical models for functional voice disorders

'Whether these vocal conditions simply represent quantitative differences along a single continuous dimension, for example laryngeal and extralaryngeal muscle tension, or are categorically and etiologically unique, is open for debate' (Roy & Bless, 2000a) (p. 462).

Introduction

Several theoretical models have now been developed to explain how various psychosocial factors may interact and operate as risk factors for the development of a range of voice disorders, and in particular, for the functional voice disorder (FVD) group. This includes the muscle tension voice disorder (MTVD) and psychogenic voice disorder (PVD) sub-groups. While poorly regulated extrinsic and intrinsic laryngeal muscle activity patterns are often observed, and issues related to heavy vocal demands across different occupational, social or performance settings are also key factors for many, the primary focus of the theoretical models discussed in this chapter will be on the *predisposing* or *precipitating psychosocial factors.* Reference will also be made to those psychosocial factors now shown to *aggravate, perpetuate* or *influence outcomes* in association with both FVD and organic voice disorder (OVD) groups. In some theoretical models these factors may be implicit but in others, such as personality traits or coping styles, they are represented as explicit feedback loops that not only contribute to onset but may also facilitate successful resolution of a vocal impairment, or operate to predict risk for the exacerbation, maintenance, or deterioration of the voice disorder.

In this chapter I present an overview of several *theoretical models for FVD* that delineate the complex interactions between a range of cognitive, affective, behavioural, and neurophysiological factors as these may contribute to the onset of FVD, and that may distinguish between the MTVD and PVD sub-groups. The models seek to integrate evidence from both clinical and empirical studies with the *neurophysiological correlates of emotion and stress*, and as these phenomena have been shown to influence voice production. Essentially, each model promotes a *bio-psychosocial perspective* reflecting global trends in medicine, neurology, and psychiatry. I highlight some of the key tenets underpinning each model, then comment on some of the similarities or different emphases given to specific factors, and how these distinctions may have implications for clinical management. I then raise a number of issues that remain somewhat controversial or warrant further clarification or exploration.

In concluding Part I of this book, I propose that the inclusion of psychosocial factors in theoretical models for FVD or OVD will have implications for the way in which students, generalist speech-language pathologists (SLP), and practitioners specialising in voice disorders may embrace a more holistic approach to clinical management. I also suggest that if practitioners felt both comfortable and competent in embracing a more comprehensive approach to intervention, this would enhance the long-term efficacy of treatment outcomes, and would reduce the *risk of recurrence* or relapse. Of equal importance, it would influence the way in which people with voice problems and those close to them might think about their voices, their vocal rehabilitation, and their overall well-being.[1]

Predominant themes regarding the aetiology of functional voice disorders

Across the published literature there has been a pervasive notion that functional voice disorders (FVD) may develop in association with *a range of psychosocial factors*, and that these may operate as predisposing, precipitating, exacerbating, or perpetuating influences (Aronson & Bless, 2009; Baker, 2008; Butcher *et al.*, 2007; O'Hara *et al.*, 2011; Oates & Winkworth, 2008; L. Rammage, Morrison, & Nichol, 2001; Roy & Bless, 2000b).

---

1 Please note that while I am maintaining the same terminology and acronyms that I have used throughout this text for FVD, which both includes and differentiates between MTVD and PVD sub-groups, when describing the different studies and theoretical models in this chapter, I refer to the diagnostic terminology and acronyms that have been nominated by the respective authors.

One predominant theme relates to *poor general health* and in particular, *upper respiratory tract infection* (URTI) (MacKenzie, Millar, Wilson, Sellars, & Deary, 2001). The self-reporting of an URTI might not normally be construed as a strictly psychosocial issue, but it is mentioned in this context because it is the most commonly cited 'stressful' incident reported by patients prior to onset, and is generally considered by patients to be causally related. Moreover, as shown in a recent study, the experience of three or more URTIs in any one year significantly increases the *life-time prevalence* of dysphonia (S. M. Cohen, 2010). However, as pointed out by House *et al.* (1987), it is difficult to verify viral URTI retrospectively. Furthermore, since general practitioners rarely carry out laryngoscopy, a diagnosis of URTI and treatment with antibiotics is often given even if there are no symptoms of infection. Therefore, Schalén and Andersson (1992) have suggested that a more accurate diagnosis in such cases might be PVD. However, these authors also caution that for those patients with a true URTI, persisting symptoms of cough, hypersensitivity of the vocal tract or vulnerability to asthma or bronchitis, these problems may lead to an ongoing preoccupation with symptoms in the laryngeal area that contributes to perpetuation of laryngeal symptoms.

Another pervasive theme relates to findings for palpable and observable *intrinsic and extrinsic laryngeal muscle tension patterns* in patients presenting across the full range of FVD, and the proposition that the misuse of the voluntary muscles associated with phonation is *the final common pathway* in all FVD (M. Morrison & Rammage, 1993; L. Rammage, 2011; L. Rammage *et al.*, 2001). However, as discussed in a previous paper in relation to diagnostic classification (Baker, Ben-Tovim, Butcher, Esterman, & McLaughlin, 2007), there is some controversy as to whether or not patterns of muscle tension are necessarily indicative of vocal dysfunction, or whether they categorically represent specific diagnostic categories of voice disorder (Behrman, Dahl, Abramson, & Schutte, 2003; Sama, Carding, Price, Kelly, & Wilson, 2001). Rather, these muscle tension patterns may merely be a symptom frequently observed with a range of FVD, or compensatory behaviours in association with organic voice disorders (OVD) such as those following laryngeal trauma, vocal fold paresis or laryngeal surgery (Koufman & Blalock, 1991; M. D. Morrison, Nichol, & Rammage, 1986). In patients where patterns of muscle tension and misuse are clearly observed, this generally arises from over-activity of the autonomic and voluntary nervous systems. These individuals seem to be unduly aroused and anxious, and often in association with stressful psychosocial factors (Demmink-Geertman & Dejonckere, 2002; Rammage, Nichol, & Morrison, 1987; Seifert & Kollbrunner, 2006). It has been emphasised that an awareness and thorough understanding of these associations is important for all practitioners (Colton, Casper, & Leonard, 2006; Rammage, 2011; Rammage *et al.*, 2001).

For instance, *stressful life events and difficulties* and *conflict over speaking out* (COSO) incidents are frequently reported in association with the onset of FVD (Andersson & Schalen, 1998; Aronson, 1990b; Baker *et al.*, 2013; Butcher *et al.*, 2007; House & Andrews, 1988), and predisposing factors such as *personality traits* and *coping styles* have been shown to influence ways in which individuals process their emotions and respond to stress (Epstein, Hirani, Stygall, & Newman, 2009; Gerritsma, 1991; Roy & Bless, 2000b; Roy *et al.*, 1997). Furthermore, patients with FVD often present with a dispositional profile typical of patients with somatoform and other *medically-unexplained conditions (MUS)*. These profiles may include an *elevated health concern* in association with *abnormal illness behaviours* (Baker, Oates, Leeson, Woodford, & Bond, 2014), or include personality traits of *perfectionism* in association with *fatigue* and a chronic sense of low energy as a person strives to meet responsibilities (Deary *et al.*, 2007; Deary & Miller, 2011; O'Hara *et al.*, 2011). This pattern of poor general health and fatigue, particularly in association with *elevated levels of anxiety* and *depression*, has led these authors to suggest that FVD might be construed as one of many 'common distress disorders' (O'Hara *et al.*, 2011, p.924).

Inherent in these psychosocial factors is the controversial notion that the *suppression* or *repression of negative emotion* may be used as a way of coping with threat or stress, and that this has aetiological significance for the onset and different clinical presentations of FVD (Andersson & Schalen, 1998; Aronson & Bless, 2009; Baker, 1998, 2003; Butcher *et al.*, 2007; House & Andrews, 1988). As highlighted in Chapter 6, the operational definitions of suppression and/or repression suggest that where there is a discrepancy between low levels of self-reported anxiety and a person's physiological and behavioural responses indicative of anxiety, this may have consequences for health (Myers & Derakshan, 2004; van Mersbergen, Patrick, & Glaze, 2008; Vingerhoets, Nyklicek, & Denollet, 2008). These constructs have led to the development of theoretical models proposing that individuals may suppress or even repress negative emotions in order to cope in response to stressful life events (Butcher, 1995; Butcher *et al.*, 2007), or may manifest different levels of emotional awareness (Baker *et al.*, 2013; Baker & Lane, 2009). In both cases, it is thought these psychological mechanisms may shape the different clinical presentations of FVD, such as MTVD and PVD.

Finally, in drawing upon some of the key elements highlighted in the models above, Dietrich *et al.* (2008, 2014; 2008) have sought to explain the *psychobiological correlates of stress* and how these processes may impact upon phonation. I will now present an overview of the major theoretical models that seek to explain the development and perpetuation of FVD, and as each may differentiate between PVD and MTVD (Box 8.1).

> ### Box 8.1 Theoretical Models for FVD including those with MTVD & PVD
>
> - Psychodynamic model for Conversion Reaction and PVD
>   - (Aronson & Bless, 2009; Aronson, Peterson, & Litin, 1964, 1966; Baker, 1998, 2003; Breuer & Freud, 1955/1893-1895; Sapir, 1995)
> - The Reformulated Psychoanalytic and Psychosocial model
>   - (Butcher, 1995; Butcher, Elias, & Cavalli, 2007)
> - The Bio-psychosocial model of Medically-Unexplained Symptoms and FVD
>   - (Chaturvedi & Bhandari, 1989; Deary, Chalder, & Sharpe, 2007; O'Hara, Miller, Carding, Wilson, & Deary, 2011)
> - The Dispositional Trait Theory model
>   - (Roy & Bless, 2000a, 2000b; Roy, Bless, & Heisey, 2000a, 2000b):
> - The Emotion Processing Deficits model
>   - (Baker, Ben-Tovim, Butcher, Esterman, & McLaughlin, 2013; Baker & Lane, 2009)
> - The Psychobiological Framework of Voice Disorders
>   - (Dietrich, Andreatta, Jiang, Joshi, & Stemple, 2012; Dietrich & Verdolini Abbott, 2008, 2012; Dietrich, Verdolini Abbott, Gartner-Schmidt, & Rosen, 2008 and Helou, 2014).

Psychodynamic model for conversion reaction and psychogenic voice disorder

As outlined in a previous overview of the literature (Baker, 2008), the predominant psychological explanation for psychogenic or functional voice loss was originally understood against a background of Freud's *psychodynamic theory*. Here, the emphasis was on the repression of feelings related to unconscious conflicts, which led to the notion of *hysterical conversion reaction* symptoms. Originally conceived by Janet (1920) and later developed by Freud (1955/1920), a conversion reaction was thought to result from the repression of *vehement emotions* related to internal conflicts or unbearable situations, and that these were then transformed into some form of bodily expression. Freud supported Janet's concept of *vehement emotions* as being at the root of traumatic neuroses and that the symptoms, whether affecting voluntary movement or sensation, could simulate a neurological or medical disorder. The unconscious intent was thought to prevent conscious awareness of emotionally charged thoughts or emotions, such as anger, sadness or anxiety, and to interrupt the normal functioning of the sensorimotor pathways. At one level the conversion symptom offered the *primary gain* of assisting the person to extricate him/herself from a difficult situation. Alternatively, where symptoms persisted, the illness behaviours and subsequent increase in attention were thought to provide *secondary gains*, serving to maintain or reinforce the conversion reaction.

In the field of speech pathology, Arnold Aronson has been one of the most prolific and influential authors on the subject of conversion reaction a/dysphonia and PVD. His work has been influenced by the psychodynamic model in combination with findings from more recent behavioural and neurophysiological perspectives (Aronson, 1969, 1978, 1985, 1990b; Aronson & Bless, 2009). He argues strongly that PVDs are broadly synonymous with those referred to as *functional*, although the diagnostic term 'psychogenic'

'has the advantage of stating positively, based on an exploration of its causes, that the voice disorder is a manifestation of one of more types of psychologic disequilibrium, such as anxiety, depression conversion reaction or personality disorder, that interfere with normal volitional control over phonation' (Aronson & Bless, 2009) (p.171).

Typically, patients with a PVD demonstrate: a *loss of voluntary control over the initiation and maintenance of phonation*; *incongruity of symptoms* in relation to the normal structure and neurological function of the laryngeal mechanism; and evidence of *reversibility of symptoms* during vegetative vocal activities such as coughing, laughing, or crying (Aronson, 1978; Sapir, 1995). The aphonia or dysphonia is thought to represent a symbolic expression of an internal conflict or threatening idea, invariably related to interpersonal conflicts within family or work settings where there is a dilemma over the expression of negative emotions, such as anger, anxiety, or sadness.

Aronson has emphasised that the extrinsic and intrinsic laryngeal muscles are highly responsive to emotional stress, and that 'their hyper-contraction is the common denominator behind the a/dysphonia in virtually all psychogenic voice disorders' (Aronson & Bless, 2009) (p.172). However, he has also argued that the fundamental aetiologic foundations lie not just in *patterns of muscle tension* that may manifest in a number of different ways, but rather, in response to a combination of *psychological processes* and *behavioural factors* that influence the different clinical profiles.

Interestingly, in his diagnostic classification for PVD, Aronson *et al.* (2009) include patients who fulfil the diagnostic criteria for *conversion reaction voice disorder* and those inclined to *vocal abuse* who may go on to develop behaviourally-related lesions such as vocal nodules or contact ulcers. Such patients would generally be diagnosed with a *hyperfunctional dysphonia*, or MTVD in other classification systems. These authors maintain that where individuals exhibit a proneness to entrenched patterns of vocal hyperfunction, such behaviours are often related to emotional or dispositional factors. They suggest that stable personality traits may influence a person's habitual patterns of responsiveness to illness or environmental stresses, or that other emotional factors may incline these individuals towards vocalising aggressively and perpetuating vocally abusive behaviours. Therefore, while patterns of muscle tension can be observed in patients with different clinical presentations of FVD, the fundamental aetiologic factors are embedded in *different psychological processes*. It is these processes that influence an individual's neurophysiological responsiveness to vocal demands, external stresses, or interpersonal relationships. In the theoretical models developed subsequently and as discussed below, it is interesting to note how efforts have been made to tease out what these specific psychological processes and their associated neural correlates might be, and how their interactions might explain the different clinical profiles of PVD and MTVD sub-groups.

Reformulated psychoanalytic and psychosocial model for PVD

Butcher, Elias and Cavalli (1995; 2007) prefer the diagnostic term psychogenic voice disorders (PVD) when referring to the broad non-organic or FVD group, and propose three alternative psychological models to account for the different PVD sub-types. These include: *a reformulated psychoanalytic model* for the classical Freudian conversion reaction voice disorders; *a psychosocial conversion model* that incorporates cognitive behaviour principles; and *a habituated conversion model* that accounts for those situations where symptoms persist after resolution of the original internal or external psychosocial stresses. In each PVD type, emphasis is given to the inhibitory effects of laryngeal musculoskeletal tension on voice production but again, it is the different psychological processes that are thought to be aetiologically significant in determining the different clinical sub-types. Key features for their three PVD models are shown in Box 8.2.

Box 8.2 Reformulated psychoanalytic and psychosocial model for PVD

Type 1: Reformulated classical hysterical conversion reaction a/ dysphonia

- Fulfils DSM-IV criteria for conversion of psychological stress into a physical symptom via *process of repression*
- Bland denial or indifference, evidence of primary and secondary gain
- Occurs rarely, estimated to be approximately 5% of all PVD
- Predisposed by personality, early or current life experiences, interpersonal difficulties, conflict over expression of sexual or aggressive feelings
- Unconscious conflict channelled into musculoskeletal tension and inhibited voice production symbolic of the nature of the conflict
- Resistant to resolution due to repression, denial, and lower motivation in response to primary and secondary gains

Type 2: Psychosocial cognitive-behavioural conversion

- Fulfils DSM-IV criteria for conversion of psychological stress into a physical symptom via a process of *conscious suppression*
- Concerns expressed regarding symptoms, evidence of some primary gains
- Occurs in 95% of all PVD cases
- Predisposed by personality, life experiences, anxiety, and ambivalence around assertiveness, emotional expressiveness, sense of powerlessness
- Conflict over speaking out leads to muscle tension & inhibition of phonation
- Resolution successful due to accessibility of suppressed emotions and amenability to psychotherapeutic approaches that help the patient to make sense of their conflicted feelings and to consider alternative ways of coping

Type 3: Habituated conversion

- Prior stressors have resolved but muscle tension patterns have persisted

(Extrapolated from Butcher, 1995; Butcher *et al.*, 2007)

Type 1 – Reformulated psychoanalytic conversion reaction voice disorder

In developing their reformulated psychoanalytic model, the authors have argued against Freud's earlier notion of the conversion of *intra-psychic conflicts over unacceptable libidinal impulses* as accounting for psychological processes that may be operating in functional voice symptoms. They suggest instead that although very rare, there are clear examples of conversion reaction a/dysphonia resulting from the unconscious repression of sexuality, bland denial of emotional distress in relation to significant recent or past trauma, and that these processes may be coupled with behaviours that suggest explicit primary and secondary gains in maintaining symptoms.

Butcher *et al.* (2007) have found that the psychological processes of repression or dissociation often render the more intense and conflicted emotions to be less accessible to either the patient or the therapist, accounting for those cases where conversion reaction symptoms remain intractable. They suggest that these *conversion reaction dysphonias* are not so readily resolved by traditional approaches to voice therapy, even when SLPs integrate psychotherapeutic approaches such as *cognitive behaviour therapy (CBT)*. Here, referral to a clinical psychologist or psychiatrist is considered more appropriate.

These authors refer to a number of published case reports describing severe and persistent PVD in association with prior traumatic situations, where individuals may have used *dissociation* as an unconscious means of repressing the traumatic event from conscious memory (Baker, 1998, 2003; Baker & Lane, 2009). In these reports, memories of traumatic events that had occurred months and even years prior to the onset of the current aphonia were triggered by recent events that were qualitatively similar, and that also focused on the throat and the voice. According to Butcher *et al.* (2007), these cases did not meet the criteria for their Type 1 reformulated classical Freudian conversion, or their Type 2 cognitive-behavioural classification of PVD as outlined below, because the traumatic events were not recent, and the patients expressed grave concern about their long-term aphonia and demonstrated high levels of motivation to resolve the issue. However, the authors suggest that these unusual cases were similar to those in their Type 1 model:

> *'and through the action of the unconscious process of repression and dissociation they have found a way of avoiding being conscious of an unacceptable experience, and as a result, have been unable to either assimilate or accommodate the experience into their view of themselves, their world and the behaviour of others'* (p. 20).

188

A more detailed discussion in relation to the clinical features and approaches to intervention with cases like these is presented in Chapter 12.

Type 2 – Psychosocial cognitive-behavioural conversion

The *psychosocial cognitive-behavioural conversion model* accounts for approximately 95% of the more common clinical presentations of PVD seen by Butcher *et al.* (2007), and draws upon constructs from the classical CBT model as originally proposed by Aaron Beck (1979). The CBT model recognises developmental experiences, predisposing vulnerability factors, and precipitating incidents that may contribute to the onset of a range of physical and mental health conditions. It also differentiates between the cognitive, behavioural, affective, and neurophysiological factors that may serve to exacerbate or perpetuate a given condition. Interactions between these features are evident in mental health disorders such as anxiety and depression, and several medically-unexplained disorders such as irritable bowel syndrome or chronic fatigue syndrome (Deary *et al.*, 2007).

In accounting for their *psychosocial cognitive-behavioural conversion model*, Butcher *et al.* emphasise the psychological processes of consciously *suppressed* emotional responses in association with threatening or stressful situations, many of which are recognised as being conflict over speaking out (COSO) dilemmas, which may then lead to tensional symptoms affecting vocal function. The authors suggest that through this process of suppressing negative emotions, and through dysfunctional beliefs or attitudes that may be reflected in 'rules for living, underlying assumptions, or automatic thoughts' (p. 12), individuals shape their emotions and subsequent behaviours.

Furthermore, drawing upon the earlier observations of other practitioners (Aronson & Bless, 2009; Brodnitz, 1969; House & Andrews, 1987), and from their own clinical experiences, they note that not only does this condition occur much more commonly in women but also, the social context of women may be formative in this process. Across their many publications Butcher and colleagues provide a rich foundation of qualitative data with respect to the socio-cultural context of so many patients who develop PVD. For instance, women with PVD frequently report undertaking an unrealistically *high burden of responsibility*, often complain of being overly committed and yet *also* admit that they feel *powerless to speak out* or to make the appropriate personal changes in order to cope.

These authors argue that we should not underestimate the fact that our Western society is still an essentially male-dominated culture, where social forces have continued to inhibit female self-esteem, assertiveness, confidence in self-expression, and feelings of personal efficacy. They propose that against such a sociocultural background there might be an interaction between life experiences and degrees of psychological vulnerability, rather than serious psychological disturbance or pathology, to explain why voice loss is more common in women. Their psychosocial model with emphasis on recent events and conflicts over expressing feelings is proposed accordingly:

> 'If predisposed by social and cultural bias as well as early learning experiences, and then if exposed to interpersonal difficulties that stimulate internal conflicts, particularly in situations involving conflict over self-expression or voicing feelings, intra-psychic conflict or stress becomes channeled into musculoskeletal tension which physically inhibits voice production' (Butcher, 1995) (p. 472).

These factors might well be recognised as *feminist issues* from a socio-political perspective, and it is somewhat ironic that they have only rarely been raised as a possible explanation for the very high prevalence of PVD in women (Baker, 2002). As PVD is so much more common amongst women in Western society, estimated to be at a ratio of at least 8:1 females to males (Aronson *et al.*, 1964; Baker, 2002; White, Deary, & Wilson, 1997; Wilson, Deary, & MacKenzie, 1995), and if sociocultural factors are thought to be formative in the process, I suggest that issues related to gender warrant further exploration. We might also consider what the situation might be in other cultures where women are so much more explicitly marginalised, or seem to be rendered invisible or silenced. The implications of these factors across different cultures clearly require additional sensitivities that would need to shape every clinician's approach to clinical management.

Type 3 – Habituated conversion

In this third model the authors propose that the PVD symptoms may persist long after the initial stressful situations that prompted onset have resolved, and that the ongoing a/dysphonia is due to *habituated muscle tension patterns*. This distinction makes good clinical sense when we consider how often patients report stressful circumstances in the weeks or months prior to onset of the voice disorder, but by the time they present for assessment, the circumstances may no longer seem relevant. In such cases, facilitation of normal phonation can be readily achieved, and there does not appear to be evidence of ongoing psychosocial distress. As emphasised by Morrison *et al.* (1986), the important clinical implication of this common occurrence is that it would be preferable if people could be seen as soon as possible after the onset of their symptoms, so that the psychological issues could be dealt with appropriately.

Muscle misuse sub-group

As clearly distinct from their three main PVD types, Butcher *et al.* (2007) refer to a further *muscle misuse sub-group* who typically come from occupations with heavy vocal demands, often producing their voices with excessive effort and without due attention to good voice care. Again, I would suggest that this sub-group would be classified as a *hyperfunctional dysphonia* or MTVD in other classification systems (Baker *et al.*, 2007; Mathieson, 2001).

Butcher and colleagues acknowledge that although there are some apparent similarities with respect to patterns of muscle tension also seen in patients with PVD, there are a number of physiological, perceptual, and aetiological factors that differentiate positively between those with PVD and the *muscle misuse* sub-group. PVD is more likely to develop for example: suddenly, or with episodic voice loss following stressful life events; normal phonation may inadvertently 'leak' during laughing, crying, coughing, or spontaneous moments in conversation; and generally, normal phonation can be elicited by the SLP with specific pre-verbal activities. In contrast, while many patients with *muscle misuse dysphonia* may be over-committed, with stressful situations occurring naturally in their lives, these individuals typically cope effectively. Butcher and colleagues argue that the *functional use of the voice* is the primary aetiological factor within this group.

Comments and implications of this model for clinical practice

Underpinning these theoretical models, we can recognise a more definite distinction between the possible *aetiologic pathways* for individuals a) broadly classified as having a functional voice disorder (FVD) but who may be further classified into the clinical sub-groups with a clinical profile typical of PVD and b) those presenting as a *muscle misuse* or MTVD. Essentially, there is a clear emphasis on psychological and emotional conflicts underlying the development of PVD, and more behavioural factors associated with the onset of MTVD. Similar distinctions were initially drawn by Aronson and colleagues *et al.* (1964)

and have been used subsequently by others (Baker *et al.*, 2007; Mathieson, 2001; M. Morrison & Rammage, 2001; Stemple, Roy, & Klaben, 2014).

The key tenets of the models proposed by Butcher *et al.* reflect both psychodynamic and cognitive-behavioural constructs related to emotional distress, and this team has led the field in recommending an integrated approach to clinical management incorporating *CBT with traditional voice therapy* (Butcher & Cavalli, 1998; Butcher & Elias, 1983; Butcher *et al.*, 2007; Butcher *et al.*, 1987). CBT is a well-evidenced therapy for a number of mental health disorders, such as depression anxiety (Clark, 2011), and is recognised as the preferred treatment of choice for *medically-unexplained syndromes* such as irritable bowel syndrome and chronic fatigue syndrome (Deary *et al.*, 2007; Miller *et al.*, 2014). It is the only psychotherapeutic model used in combination with direct voice therapy that has been subjected to scrutiny in treatment trials for FVD (Daniilidou *et al.*, 2007).

The theoretical formulations of Butcher *et al.* have led this team to encourage clinicians to feel comfortable in enquiring about the occurrence and possible impact of recent *stressful life events* prior to onset of voice disorders. They urge practitioners to be alert to patient reports of stressful life events that may be symbolically relevant, such as those imbued with COSO, or to dispositional traits that reflect a sense of vulnerability and powerlessness in effecting change. They also emphasise the importance of considering how the *suppression of negative emotions* in response to threat may influence a person's coping style, how this may contribute to muscle tension patterns and *dysregulated vocal function*, and how all of the above may influence ways in which individuals come to terms with their life situations and their altered vocal function.

Inherent in their model is the recognition that patients with different presentations of PVD may reflect *different levels of psychological distress* and *coping*. For instance, where individuals adapt and cope in a reasonably healthy way, traditional voice therapy approaches that include supportive counselling are likely to lead to straightforward resolution of the dysphonia. Others may benefit from a more psychodynamic approach carried out by a psychiatrist or clinical psychologist, with emphasis on the exploration of suppressed emotions in relation to previous traumas or inner conflicts that perpetuate feelings of low self-esteem, powerlessness, and difficulties with assertiveness.

Alternatively, where cognitive and behavioural strategies have led to *maladaptive ways of coping* that serve to perpetuate or exacerbate symptom severity, clinical intervention may involve direct voice therapy with CBT. The authors suggest that this could be carried out by the SLP with dual credentials in CBT, or in collaboration with a certified CBT practitioner (Butcher & Cavalli,

1998; Butcher *et al.*, 2007; Elias, Raven, Butcher, & Littlejohns, 1989). The CBT approach places emphasis on exploring beliefs and attitudes about the self, the world, or other people that may be limiting a person's choices for dealing with stressful issues. It also includes strategies to help patients address *stress management*, deal with their anxiety, or improve their *interpersonal communication* and resilience. In this sense, there is no undue emphasis on psychopathology but rather, on the development of an awareness of the nature and *meaning of their vocal symptoms* in the context of their daily life, and ways to modify beliefs and attitudes, feelings and behaviour that may lead to sustained and healthy changes. These authors provide excellent examples of how CBT may be used in conjunction with traditional voice therapy in realising these important objectives.

Bio-psychosocial model of medically-unexplained symptoms and functional dysphonia

Another research team has proposed a *bio-psychosocial model* that seeks to account for a range of factors that may contribute to the onset and maintenance of functional voice disorders (Deary, 2011; Deary & Miller, 2011; Miller *et al.*, 2014; O'Hara *et al.*, 2011). In this theoretical model, the authors use the term functional dysphonia (FD), which is defined as a voice disorder where there is no detectable organic pathology, or if there is, it is not commensurate with the degree of vocal dysfunction (O'Hara *et al.*, 2011). This model does not make a distinction between those that may present with MTVD or PVD, as proposed in other classification systems for FVD (Baker *et al.*, 2007; Mathieson, 2001), or as mapped out in some of the other theoretical models discussed previously in this chapter.

Following on from the ground-breaking work by Butcher and colleagues with respect to CBT and the clinical management of FVD, the *bio-psychosocial model* also draws upon the classical CBT framework of emotional distress, linking this to the extensive literature relating to a number of *medically-unexplained symptoms (MUS)*. These include disorders such as *chronic pain, fibromyalgia, chronic fatigue syndrome*, and *irritable bowel syndrome*. Deary and colleagues (2007) suggest that the predisposing, precipitating, and perpetuating factors typically associated with MUS are similar to those identified in patients presenting with FD. Reference is made to a number of key constructs underpinning the CBT model for MUS (see Box 8.3).

Box 8.3 Constructs from the CBT model and Medically-Unexplained Symptoms

Predisposing factors

- Genetics
  - Inheritable predisposition to general distress
  - Unexplained fatigue and somatisation
  - Vicariously learned illness behaviours, distress proneness
- Early experience of adversity including physical and sexual abuse
- Personality
  - Neuroticism, stress reactivity, emotional inhibition, perfectionism
- Anxiety/depressive mood

Precipitating factors

- Stressful life events
- Dilemmas with forced choices leading to negative consequences
- Acute and prolonged stress leading to 'perseverative cognition'

Perpetuating factors

- Hypothalamic pituitary adrenal axis (HPA-axis) and sensitisation
- Heightened attention and 'faulty filtering system'
  - Cognitive unconscious and 'embodied cognition' (Gallagher, 2005)
  - Cognitive bias and Cognitive Activation System (CAS) (Ursin, 2005)
  - Behavioural Inhibition System (BIS) (Gray, 1991)
- Attribution and illness beliefs
  - Activity avoidance, symptom maintenance
- Response to illness and coping in general
  - 'All or nothing coping' and avoidance, perpetuates symptoms

(Extrapolated from Deary *et al.*, 2007)

In the sections below I comment upon aspects of this CBT model for MUS that may contribute new perspectives on the nature and development of FD and the implications this may have for clinical management (Fig. 8.1).

PREDISPOSING AND PRECIPITATING FACTORS

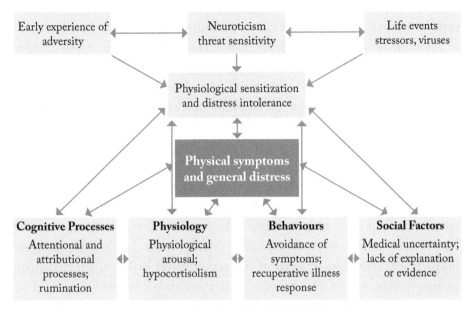

PERPETUATING FACTORS

Fig. 8.1 Expanded CBT model of MUS (Deary et al., 2007) and as proposed in relation to FVD (O'Hara et al., 2011)

Reproduced with permission Deary et al., (2007)

Key constructs of a bio-psychosocial model for medically-unexplained symptoms

In their expanded CBT model for MUS, Deary *et al.* (2007) highlight a number of *dispositional factors* that render some individuals vulnerable to the development of these disorders, and those stressful life situations that may precipitate the onset of the various physical symptoms. They note similarities in many of those factors underpinning a range of MUS, suggesting that it might be more realistic to construe the different syndromes along with anxiety and depression as *common distress disorders*.

For instance, individuals presenting with different MUS frequently manifest generic *somatopsychic distress*, with concomitant symptoms of poor *general health* and high levels of *fatigue*, and these symptoms often occur in association with stable dispositional traits of *perfectionism* (Deary & Chalder, 2010). While *healthy perfectionism* is recognised as reflecting high standards, attitudes of conscientiousness, and a desire to do things as well as possible, *unhealthy perfectionism* is characterised by efforts to do things very well but often against a background of self-doubt and misgivings about personal performance, and a determination to persevere in the face of considerable adversity.

Symptom development and perpetuation is thought to occur in two different stages. The first stage reflects a hypersensitivity to arousal, chronic stress, and mediation from the HPA axis that may lead to fatigue and poor general health, and eventually to the development of symptoms, even *physiological burnout*. The second stage develops in response to a *cognitive bias* that essentially selects or filters symptoms for conscious attention, and in a manner that enables a degree of recuperation.

As emphasised by these authors, much of our bodily activity and function is 'monitored and orchestrated unconsciously by more or less automatic mechanisms' (p.785) and as such, fails to draw our conscious attention. However, in some individuals, especially those prone to MUS, a cognitive bias for particular symptoms at times of vulnerability may lead to a hypersensitivity to proprioceptive and kinaesthetic sensations, and a lowered threshold for responding to anxiety-provoking situations. This in turn facilitates behavioural responses of avoidance that may include reduced activity or social withdrawal. Here, the authors refer to constructs derived from Ursin's (2005) model of the *Cognitive Activation System (CAS)*, which is thought to remain in a state of arousal until some particular action is taken to eliminate or reduce the stress. This is similar to the *Behavioural Inhibition System (BIS)* as proposed by Gray (1991), who has suggested that more anxious individuals respond with heightened arousal and selective attention in the face of threatening stimuli, followed by reduced activity or behavioural inhibition. Interestingly, both of these constructs give implicit support to the *dispositional trait theoretical model for FD* as proposed by Roy and Bless (2000a), and constructs related to *different levels of emotional awareness* as suggested by Baker and Lane (2009).

Another key tenet of their model is the notion that symptoms are maintained through recursive and autopoietic interactions between physical, cognitive, behavioural, and social factors. Through this process of *autopoiesis*, a concept taken from living systems theory (Maturana & Varela, 1980), these interactions generate the same network of processes that produced them. The authors emphasise that it is this vicious cycle of self-perpetuating interactions between domains that serves to maintain symptoms, distress, or disability, and that this supports a bio-psychosocial theoretical model for MUS. This research team makes a strong case for parallels between MUS and FD. They also propose that the CBT model for MUS, as shown in Fig.8.1, provides a useful theoretical framework to explain those factors that may contribute to the onset and perpetuation of these functional voice symptoms, and how principles of CBT may be effectively integrated into traditional voice therapy (Deary & Miller, 2011; Miller *et al.*, 2014; O'Hara *et al.*, 2011).

Parallels between the bio-psychosocial model for MUS and FD

Predisposing and precipitating factors

In proposing a CBT bio-psychosocial model for FD, O'Hara *et al.* (2011) offer a 'narrative summary' of the literature in relation to predisposing and precipitating factors, which suggests that individuals are predisposed to FD by:

'neurotic and introvert/repressive personality, coping style, and early experience of adversity; that individuals are precipitated into FD by life events and dilemmas, particularly those in which action or expression is difficult; and that once established, FD is maintained by an interplay of physiological and ongoing psychosocial difficulties' (p. 922).

They also refer to findings from semi-structured interviews conducted by Daniilidou *et al.* (2007) showing that individuals with FVD are prone to worry and distress, and that they have often gone through major life transitions prior to onset of their voice disorders. These findings reflect a similar pattern of dispositional features and stressful life events occurring in association with MUS, such as irritable bowel syndrome and chronic pain, and they are similar to those highlighted in an extensive overview of the empirical evidence for psychosocial factors associated with FVD (Baker, 2008).

O'Hara *et al.* (2011) also found that patients with FD, in comparison to their control groups, report two other related but independent factors. One is a description of themselves as being *'conscientious/perfectionist* individuals who persist in trying to deal with life difficulties, and perhaps to their detriment' (O'Hara *et al.*, 2011) (p. 922). The other is related to symptoms of low energy, a *marked susceptibility to fatigue* and a lack of mental and physical stamina. Similar findings have also been noted in patients presenting with MUS such as chronic pain and chronic fatigue syndrome.

In seeking to account for the development of functional vocal symptoms, these authors propose that unhealthy perfectionism, coupled with 'soldiering on' to meet vocal demands in the face of ongoing stress and anxiety, may lead to a lowering of the immune system and to frequent reports of poor general health and marked fatigue. This in turn may facilitate behaviours such as 'avoidance of anxiety-provoking situations, time off work, reduced activity and social withdrawal, all of which could cause or perpetuate anxiety, low mood, fatigue and reduced vocal use' (p. 924). The hypothesised interactions between *unhealthy perfectionism* and *physical and mental fatigue* strengthens the *bio-psychosocial* foundations of their theoretical model, and contributes a helpful perspective on the general health and personality traits of individuals with FD. This pattern also mirrors the two stage processes for the development and perpetuation of MUS outlined above.

These dispositional findings reflect some of the characteristics of individuals with FVD noted in the other theoretical models discussed in this chapter (Aronson & Bless, 2009; Baker *et al.*, 2013; Baker & Lane, 2009; Butcher *et al.*, 2007; House & Andrews, 1988; Roy & Bless, 2000b). As observed by these different research teams, women with FVD often experienced *stressful life events* preceding onset, many of which were imbued with *conflict over speaking out (COSO)*, or pressures to persevere, regardless of the chronic stress and detriment to themselves. A high percentage of the women in the respective cohorts were teachers or professional voice users working in occupations with a *heavy vocal load* and high levels of *emotional labour*. Qualitative data revealed that these individuals often reported fears of buckling under the burdens of *high levels of responsibility* while also sustaining efforts to meet professional expectations and standards. Although these factors were not necessarily framed in terms of 'unhealthy perfectionism' in these other theoretical models, many of the women with FVD, especially those within the psychogenic voice disorder (PVD) sub-groups, were also shown to be *introverted*. As previously highlighted, introversion is a personality trait commonly associated with perfectionistic attitudes and behaviours (Eysenck, 1967; Newman & Wallace, 1993a, 1993b). These findings for raised levels of perfectionism in association with fatigue support a recurring theme across all the theoretical models for FVD, which suggests that *persevering under stressful situations for sustained periods of time* inevitably impacts upon a person's overall physical and psychological well-being, and on their vocal function.

Comments on and implications of this model for clinical practice

Challenge to notions related to the suppression or repression of negative emotions

In proposing a bio-psychosocial CBT model for FD, Deary and colleagues strongly challenge the notion that the suppression or repression of negative emotions in response to psychological conflicts or stressful life events contributes to the development or the perpetuation of FD (Deary, 2011; Deary & Miller, 2011; Miller *et al.*, 2014; O'Hara *et al.*, 2011). This challenge is based partly upon the equivocal empirical evidence for *repressive coping* as highlighted in a previous review of the literature by Baker (2008). It is also supported by their own clinical experience and that of others, where patients with FD may acknowledge their concerns about stress in their lives, often reporting elevated health concerns with respect to their voice as a natural consequence of its pivotal role in their work.

These authors argue that loss of voice and other functional voice symptoms do not necessarily represent difficulties in the expression of negative emotion and psychological conflicts with symbolic meaning, or that vocal symptoms represent a dilemma over speaking out. They therefore challenge those theoretical models that encourage the exploration of suppressed or repressed emotions, or that advocate helping patients to make explicit those emotional responses that remain implicit (Aronson & Bless, 2009; Baker *et al.*, 2013; Baker & Lane, 2009; Butcher *et al.*, 2007).

Occupations with vulnerability to particular symptoms

This research team also emphasises that a high proportion of patients who present with FD are occupied in jobs or professions where the voice is the primary tool of trade, and that given the circumstances outlined above, it is not surprising that they are likely to be vulnerable to symptoms affecting the voice (O'Hara *et al.*, 2011). They therefore propose that while psychosocial issues need to be acknowledged and possible co-morbidities with anxiety and depression noted, it is equally important, if not more so, to recognise factors, such as *occupational voice use* with high vocal demands, life situations contributing to lowered immune system function, and poor overall general health with elevated levels of fatigue. They suggest that although vocal symptoms may bring these individuals to the clinic, FD may represent a more general impairment and that FD is merely another MUS or example of a *'common distress disorder'*.

Integration of CBT with traditional voice therapy

Taking all of these issues into account, O'Hara and co-workers have proposed that an expanded bio-psychosocial CBT model for MUS, with its emphasis on *autopoietic interactions* between biological and psychosocial factors, is a more relevant theoretical model to explain both the development and course of FD. As a corollary to this, they recommend that the principles of CBT might be successfully integrated into traditional voice therapy by speech-language therapists (SLT) who have undertaken formal CBT training, or SLT working in collaboration with mental health professionals with formal credentials in CBT (Daniilidou *et al.*, 2007; Deary & Miller, 2011; Miller *et al.*, 2014; O'Hara *et al.*, 2011).

As nicely summarised by Miller *et al.* (2014), the primary aim of CBT is to help clients understand how a vicious cycle of current life circumstances, thoughts, emotions, and behaviours might contribute to symptom development across a range of conditions, including MUS and voice disorders. A second aim is to appreciate how previous life experiences, beliefs, and attitudes may influence the way an individual responds to current life stressors. A third aim is to identify those responses that may operate to reinforce negative coping strategies, to maintain symptoms, or to perpetuate the cycle once again. The role of the therapist then, is to help the patient challenge and re-evaluate unhelpful thoughts, to facilitate more healthy behaviours and activities, and to regain a sense of mastery over their life circumstances.

In some cases, this CBT-enhanced voice therapy may target behavioural strategies to improve work-life balance or fatigue. In others, it may include emphasis on anxiety, depression, and stress-related difficulties. This reflects the recommendations of Butcher and colleagues (1995; 1983; 2007; 1993) who have also advocated that the different levels of input from a CBT framework may be determined by the nature and severity of the functional voice symptoms, and by the overall physical and mental health of the patient. As stressed by both of these research teams, in all circumstances the importance of the patient's overall well-being is considered paramount, with active participation and collaboration between patient and therapist as key components of CBT. Some of the steps that might be taken with a CBT-enhanced approach to voice therapy for FD as advocated by Deary and colleagues are shown in point form in Box 8.4.

Box 8.4 CBT enhanced voice therapy for Functional Dysphonia

Developing a formulation that accounts for the patient's dysphonia

- Socratic questioning to exploring predisposing and precipitating factors
- Guided discovery to explore assumption, contradictions, perpetuating factors
- Co-created formulations to help patients develop their own hypotheses

Specific techniques aimed at changing perpetuating factors

- Behavioural interventions
  - Related to rest, sleep management and levels of activity
  - Challenge avoidance and gradual exposure to anxiety-provoking situations
- Cognitive interventions
  - Identify negative thinking patterns
  - Challenge catastrophic beliefs around voice symptoms
  - Reshape thinking around the effects of voice use, misuse
  - Prevention of relapse
  - Identify future stressors
  - Identify coping strategies that may involve reduced levels of activity
  - Be alert to inappropriate reduction in voice use, social isolation

(Extrapolated from Daniilidou, Carding, Wilson, Drinnan, & Deary, 2007; Deary & Miller, 2011; Miller, Deary, & Patterson, 2014; O'Hara *et al.*, 2011).

Dispositional trait theory

Roy and Bless (2000a, 2000b) have developed a *dispositional trait theory model* to explain possible causal pathways to account for two different sub-groups within the functional voice disorder classification referred to as functional dysphonia (FD) and vocal nodules (VN). In this model, FD is defined as a voice disorder in the absence of visible structural or neurological pathology, with elevated scores on measures of anxiety, somatic complaints, and introversion. The *dispositional trait theory* model acknowledges many foundation concepts raised by previous researchers (Aronson, 1990b; Butcher, 1995; House & Andrews, 1988; M. Morrison & Rammage, 1993), and proposes a conflict between laryngeal inhibition and activation reflecting different personality types, cognitive processing, and behavioural patterns, all of which will be reflected in nervous system functioning. The theory draws upon the model developed by Newman and Wallace (1993a, 1993b); this reflects a synthesis of the biological theory of personality by Eysenck *et al.* (1967; 1985) and a neuropsychological model of the conceptual nervous system by Gray (1975, 1982). As expressed by Roy and Bless (2000a):

> *'Based upon differences in personality this theory predicts unique and contrasting signal sensitivities and behavioural response biases for individuals with functional dysphonia and vocal nodules. It is proposed that specific personality traits predispose one to develop these disorders, and to moderate the symptomatology and course of the voice pathology'* (p. 472).

The theoretic model developed by Roy and Bless (2000a, 2000b) is best appreciated by reading their two excellent seminal papers and the subsequent studies designed to test out the theory (Roy *et al.*, 2000a, 2000b). However, for the purposes of this chapter, I offer a brief overview of the key constructs with reference to their schematic diagram that shows how these processes may contribute to the different profiles for FD and VN (Fig 8.2). I then discuss several features identified in the model that may predispose individuals to recurrence of their vocal problem, and the implications of this for clinical management.

As shown above, the model proposes associations between the neural correlates of the *Behavioural Activation System (BAS)*, the *Behavioural Inhibition System (BIS)*, and the *Nonspecific Arousal System (NAS)* (Gray, 1975, 1982, 1985, 1987; Gray & McNaughton, 2000), and as these may interact with Eysenck's (1967; 1985) *'big three' superfactors* to contribute to the development of FD and VN.

The BIS/BAS as originally proposed by Gray (1975) is a neurophysiological framework for understanding how mechanisms for behavioural regulation relate to motivation and personality in normal and abnormal human behaviours. These same constructs have been explored in relation to a broader range of cognitive and self-regulatory processes that may account for disturbances in affect leading to psychological dysfunction and psychiatric disorders (Amodio, Master, Yee, & Taylor, 2007; Kasch, Rottenberg, Arnow, & Gotlib, 2002).

In essence, the construct of the BAS corresponds to 'going' once a plan of action is devised, and the BIS corresponds to 'stopping' in the face of threat. As proposed by Gray (1975), there is a reciprocal interaction between the BAS and BIS so that increased activity in one leads to decreased activity in the other, any increase in either the BAS or BIS system augments the activity in the NAS, and when the NAS activity increases, this in turn influences the intensity of

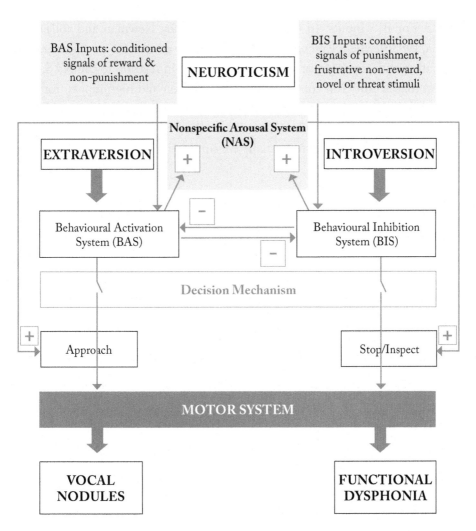

Fig. 8.2 A theory of the dispositional bases of vocal nodules and functional dysphonia

Adapted from Newman and colleagues synthesis of Eysenck's (1967) and Gray's (1975) biological theories of personality. Extraversion and Neuroticism are mapped onto the three systems within Gray's conceptual nervous system model. FD and VN are seen as behavioural consequences of the signal sensitivities and response biases of BIS dominant neurotic introverts, and BAS dominant neurotic extraverts respectively.

With kind permission Roy & Bless, (2000a, p.474)

the BAS or BIS inputs. In the model developed by Newman and colleagues (1993a, 1993b), where Eysenck's (1967) personality constructs are considered in association with inputs from the BAS or BIS, and in relation to the NAS, they suggest that neuroticism combined with extraversion and high inputs from the BAS leads to *impulsivity*. In contrast, neuroticism with introversion and high input from the BIS leads to *anxiety and inhibition*. Some of the key differences between these two interacting systems are summarised in point form in Table 8.1.

Table 8.1 Key constructs related to the NAS, BAS & BIS and links to 'Big-Three' Personality Superfactors

NAS
Responsive to changes in the autonomic nervous system such as flight/flight reactions, and coupled with higher levels of Neuroticism, prepares the organism for the different motivational or emotional inputs from the BAS and BIS

BAS/Extraversion	BIS/Introversion
Motivational system for coordinating goal driven approach/avoidance associated with positive affective states	Motivational system for inhibitory behaviours associated with negative affective states such as anxiety
Sensitive to signals related to reward and non-punishment	**Hyper-vigilance** and anxiety in response to threat
Focus of attention on action, engagement and approach toward a rewarding system, or direct action away from threat/punishment	Focus of attention to novelty, uncertainty, or anticipation of non-reward or punishment leading to passive avoidance
Approach, escape or active avoidance behaviours to attain goals	Reflection, interruption, inhibition or stopping behaviours
Frustrative non-reward or punishment leads to active avoidance	**Frustrative non-reward/punishment leads to passive avoidance**
Extraversion (optimism/joy/aggression) + Neuroticism links to impulsivity & perseveration of action despite negative outcome	Introversion (tension/anxiety/depression/low self-esteem) + Neuroticism links to inhibition & suppression/extinction of action
Neural correlates-mesolimbic dopaminergic system & PFC* *prefrontal cortex	Neural correlates-amygdala & septohippocampal system & ACC* *anterior cingulate cortex

Extrapolated from (Amodio, Master, Yee, & Taylor, 2007; Eysenck, 1967; Eysenck & Eysenck, 1985; Gray, 1975; Gray & McNaughton, 2000; Kasch, Rottenberg, Arnow, & Gotlib, 2002; Newman & Wallace, 1993a, 1993b; Roy & Bless, 2000a, 2000b; Xu et al., 2012)

Functional dysphonia (FD)

In their theoretical model, Roy and Bless (2000a, 2000b) speculate that the patterns of laryngeal tension underpinning FD are directly influenced by enduring personality and dispositional traits in association with nervous system functioning, and in particular, the BIS. The authors propose that the combined effects of personality traits, such as introversion and neuroticism (as reflected in trait anxiety), contribute to predictable and conditioned *laryngeal inhibitory responses* to certain environmental signals, and that this in turn leads to 'muscularly inhibited voice production'. The mechanisms by which this may occur are related to the ways in which BIS and NAS-dominant individuals may respond with ongoing *hyper-vigilance to threat*, or to experiences of *frustrative non-reward or punishment.*

Hyper-vigilance to threat in the forms of novel, uncertain, or conflicting messages from the external environment, or from changes in internal bodily states, is typically noted in individuals who are BIS dominant (Fig. 8.2). As applied to people with FD, Roy and Bless (2000a) suggest that hyper-vigilance to ambiguous stimuli, such as those associated with URTI, oedema, reflux laryngitis, or emotional states, may lead to increased focus of attention and sensitivity to these conflicting stimuli, with elevated levels of arousal and muscle tone, and when sustained, to inhibition of phonation. In linking these processes to possible neural correlates, the authors propose that while the phylogenetically newer neocortical control of speech remains unaffected, thus enabling the communication of whispered or articulated spoken language, the sustained inhibitory control by the more primitive *septohippocampal system* facilitates increased motor inhibition of phonation, resulting in aphonia or dysphonia. In other studies using self-report questionnaires and EEG recordings designed to identify the neural correlates of BIS functioning, these processes have been referred to as a *'bottom up' process of inhibition* associated with conflict monitoring and the slowing or stopping of an ongoing action, and notably raised levels of activity in the *anterior cingulate cortex (ACC)* (Amodio *et al.*, 2007) .

Frustrative non-reward or *anticipation of punishment* has also been noted in BIS-dominant individuals, and when coupled with dispositional features of introversion in association with anxiety, may lead to more passive forms of avoidance, suppression, or even extinction of a particular action (see Table 8.1). As applied to individuals with FD, Roy and Bless (2000a) have integrated these constructs into their model (Fig. 8.2) with those previously articulated in relation to conflict over speaking out (COSO) (Aronson, 1990b; Butcher, 1995; House & Andrews, 1988). They propose that when threatening situations or frustrating outcomes have been paired with previous attempts to speak out, the BIS is activated in the *anticipation of non-reward*, just as it might be in the face of actual punishment. Here, the conflict between inhibition and activation is thought to precipitate *laryngeal freezing*, which may take the form of passive avoidance of a situation through failing to perform a given action. Clinically, this may present as a complete aphonia or strained dysphonia and again, despite normal structure and neurological innervation of the larynx.

Vocal Nodules

Alternatively, BAS-dominant individuals are generally motivated to undertake goal-driven activities where the rewards of attention and interaction are high, or to actively take the necessary steps to avoid threat and punishment. When coupled with the combined personality traits of extraversion and neuroticism, BAS-dominant individuals are likely to be optimistic, joyful, and even aggressive. At the more extreme end of the continuum, they may be highly impulsive, and may fail to modulate behaviours that may be harmful. In other studies using self-report questionnaires and EEG recordings designed to identify the neural correlates of BAS functioning, these processes have been referred to as an intentional *'top down' form of inhibition* or avoidance of an activity, with raised levels of neuronal activity in the *left prefrontal cortex (PFC)* (Amodio *et al.*, 2007).

In exploring these parallel constructs in relation to individuals with vocal nodules (VN), Roy and Bless propose that here, the extraverted personality traits, coupled with BAS dominance and levels of anxiety and NAS sensitivity, may contribute to patterns of excessive voice use and engagement in vocally damaging behaviours. The model proposes that BAS-dominant and extraverted individuals are inclined to persist in the misuse of the voice in the face of advice to the contrary, or despite the obvious harmful effects, and that this may be due to a raised level of impulsivity and lack of constraint. These interacting factors have implications for the aggravation of entrenched patterns of vocal hyperfunction, and inevitably too for the risk of recurrence of lesions such as vocal nodules, whether after medical, surgical, or voice therapy.

Comments and implications of this model for clinical practice

This model makes a most valuable contribution towards our understanding of the actual processes that might contribute to the different clinical profiles of individuals within the FVD classification. As operationally defined in Chapter 1, the broad heterogeneous FVD group includes the psychogenic voice disorder (PVD) and muscle tension voice disorders (MTVD) sub-groups (Baker *et al.*, 2007). I would respectfully suggest that those in the functional dysphonia (FD) group as defined by Roy and Bless (2000a) are similar to patients referred to as PVD in the classification system cited above, and that those in the VN group are typical of patients diagnosed with muscle tension voice disorder MTVD, which may include those with minor pathologies such as nodules (MTVD, Type 2a).

Their model draws upon data from both early and recent empirical studies, and successfully incorporates what we intuitively know from clinical experience. In this sense it is both theoretically sound and clinically useful. One of the major strengths of their model is the way in which it proposes strong hypotheses about the interactions between the various cognitive, affective, and behavioural factors that may then be understood within a meaningful neuropsychological framework. This has subsequently generated excellent efforts to reconcile neurophysiological aspects of voice production with psychological correlates, such as anxiety and stress, and personality traits discussed later in this chapter (Dietrich *et al.*, 2012; Dietrich & Verdolini Abbott, 2008, 2012, 2014; Dietrich *et al.*, 2008; van Mersbergen *et al.*, 2008).

This model provides a useful way to conceive laryngeal constriction and total loss of voice in the BIS-dominant and introverted individuals who may respond with elevated levels of emotional sensitivity in the face of interpersonal conflict, traumatic, and stressful circumstances. Alternatively, some individuals may be inclined to respond with heightened neurophysiological reactivity to sensory changes in the larynx following upper respiratory tract infection. While the sensitivity to stressful interpersonal situations makes good sense, the emphasis on responsiveness to 'ambiguous sensory changes' is perhaps less obvious but also fascinating.

This construct might help to explain those cases diagnosed with PVD or 'functional dysphonia' where neither the patient nor the therapist is able to identify any emotionally stressful situations associated with the onset of voice loss. I am not suggesting that if stressful incidents are not readily identified or recalled that they did not occur. On the contrary, it often takes time and considerable skill to elicit recall of such incidents (Baker, 1998, 2003). However, as this theoretical model suggests, individuals who are BIS dominant may be more generally prone to motor inhibition in response to ambiguous physiological sensory signals. When this occurs in the laryngeal and associated areas, it may well translate to persistent motor inhibition that over time becomes habituated, even long after the resolution of the original sensory changes that occurred in association with infection, reflux, or other biochemical changes.

The model also offers a most plausible explanation for the way in which interactions between dispositional features of extraversion and anxiety, coupled with high levels in the BAS, can predispose individuals to lifestyle choices and vocal behaviours that lead to hyperfunctional vocal misuse, and even to the development of vocal nodules. Of equal significance is the proposal that where individuals are predisposed to extreme levels of BAS involvement they are also inclined to perpetuate poorly regulated impulsive behaviors, despite the adverse consequences. Here, it is implied that these individuals may fail to modify their lifestyle or vocal behaviours in a judicious manner that would enable healing after acute phonotrauma or long-term patterns of vocal misuse, with the inevitable aggravation of their vocal impairment or recurrence of the dysphonia.

In this sense the model provides a most helpful new perspective for clinicians who may be concerned about a patient's apparent *non-compliance* with treatment recommendations so commonly seen in individuals with vocal nodules. Therefore, rather than viewing this in a somewhat pejorative light as 'highly defended', 'resistant to change', or 'failing to adhere to recommendations', it might be construed as an individual genuinely *restrained from changing* (to use a construct from systems theory), and that these *restraints to change* are represented in the stable and somewhat entrenched dispositional, emotional, and neurophysiological processes. This may help to obviate a practitioner's feelings of frustration, or inclination to blame, with implications for clinical intervention. However, the tantalising question remains as to how we as clinicians might use this knowledge and understanding to modify approaches to clinical management. Such issues will be addressed in Part II.

The emotion processing deficits model for functional voice disorders

A new causal model of *emotion processing deficits* in women presenting with FVD has been proposed by Baker and Lane (2009). The development of this theoretical model arose directly from the empirical findings of my doctoral project entitled '*An Investigation into Life Events and Difficulties and Patterns of Emotional Expression in women with Functional Voice Disorders'*. This was inspired by the original and ongoing writings of Arnold Aronson, my own clinical practice, and the significant contributions of the many researchers whose work has culminated in the theoretical models discussed throughout this chapter. Some of the key trends in the findings for stressful life events preceding onset and other psychological correlates were reviewed in Chapters 5 and 6, respectively. Aspects of these findings are highlighted below in order to show how they prompted the formulation of our proposed *Emotion Processing Deficits model for FVD*.

Life events and difficulties

Key statistically significant findings show that women with FVD, in comparison to OVD and non-voice disordered controls, experience more *severe events* and *major difficulties* and more *Conflict over Speaking Out (COSO)* events and difficulties, including those characterised by *Powerlessness in the System (PITS)* in the 12 months prior to onset and or interview. Many events were related to health and employment, disintegration of significant relationships through infidelity or divorce, sudden estrangement from children, and sudden loss of close confidantes and support figures. Others were traumatic, such as strangulation and violent sexual assault, serious illness, or loss of close ties through death.

The COSO events and difficulties occurred primarily across the domains of work, other relationships including children, and marital and partner relationships. These incidents involved interpersonal conflicts where women with FVD felt unable to speak out, seek assistance, or to protest against the status quo for fear of grave consequences. Significantly more FVD group women were likely to report COSO difficulties with PITS occurring in relationships at work, with partners, and with close family members. This was notable in women in close relationships with violent partners who threatened them with assault if they asserted themselves It was commonly reported by women in occupations with high levels of contact and service to the public, and particularly amongst school teachers who comprised 32% (23/73) of the FVD cohort. These women often reported frustration over the management of student behaviours and a sense of futility in seeking support, despite efforts to communicate reasonably with senior personnel. They reported being ignored or threatened with loss of employment if they persisted in being assertive, or if their behaviour implied that they could not cope.

Based upon these data it was proposed that the impact of severe events and major difficulties and COSO situations with PITS, viewed against a background of occupations with *high levels of emotional labour* and *low job control*, may be a helpful way of thinking about the context in which FVD develops. The results suggested that many women with FVD were both vocally and emotionally burnt out, having lost not only their physiological voice but also, 'their voice' in the larger systems to which they belonged (Baker *et al.*, 2013).

Psychological traits and emotional expression

In addition, across a range of standardised self-report questionnaires related to personality traits, dispositions, and *patterns of emotional expressiveness* and *attachment in adult relationships*, the FVD group women were more likely to report the following: a vulnerability to anxiety, anger, and depression with lower levels of optimism; at least one previous experience of sexual or physical abuse in their lifetime; an insecure attachment style in current adult relationships as reflected in attitudes and behaviours indicating a fearful attachment profile, and fewer social supports (See Chapter 6).

More FVD group women reported coming from families with less emotional expressiveness, an ambivalence over the expression of negative emotions, and a preference for suppressing feelings in the face of threat. This was echoed in reports of a *high-anxious coping style*, which is operationally defined as a tendency to interpret one's own behaviour as being more anxious than it really is, a capacity to identify one's own distress, and an emotional rather than rational approach to solving problems (Derakshan & Eysenck, 2001). Overall, the high scores on anxiety indicated that many women with FVD could admit to being anxious generally, and in relation to their voice disorder.

The high levels of anxiety and *high-anxious coping style* amongst FVD group women suggested a pattern of emotional expressiveness more consistent with the conscious or even sub-conscious suppression of emotion. Contrary to predictions, there was little evidence of *la belle indifférence* and ironically, FVD group women were the least likely to report a *repressive coping style*. This was reserved for the 'healthy' controls!

Interestingly, statistical models representing *interactions* between *stressful situations* preceding onset and *psychological traits* showed that the LEDS and COSO situations were the strongest risk factors for the onset of FVD, and that psychological traits were not. As highlighted in Chapter 6, this was an unexpected finding and we concluded that traits such as anxiety, ambivalence over emotional expression, and insecure attachment may have influenced the ways in which some individuals reacted to stressful life events and difficulties, especially those qualitatively imbued with COSO.

Comparisons between MTVD and PVD sub-groups

The secondary focus of this study was to explore how the same psychosocial dimensions may have interacted to create risk for the development of the FVD sub-groups, PVD (n = 37) and MTVD (n = 36). Key features of the PVD group were sudden onset, difficulty in the voluntary initiation of phonation, symptom incongruity, and symptom reversibility. Other differences revealed that those with PVD presented with total loss of voice and symptoms of globus, with intrinsic muscle tension patterns characterised by more marked involvement of the false vocal folds and anterior-posterior constriction of the aryepiglottic sphincter than in MTVD group women. These findings led the specialists to judge individuals with PVD as suffering from a 'more severe voice disorder' at the point of diagnosis.

The above observations prompted us to hypothesise that the PVD group women may have experienced a greater number of severe events and difficulties and more potent COSO situations characterised by PITS, than the MTVD sub-group. This was not so. Although women in both PVD and MTVD groups experienced a high number of severely stressful events and major difficulties, including many with COSO and PITS, neither the events data nor the psychological traits data clearly predicted voice disorder group membership. Furthermore, statistical models reflecting the *interactions* between the same psychosocial measures failed to differentiate significantly between the PVD and MTVD sub-groups.

Questions arising from these findings

These findings prompted us to consider a number of questions. First, does sudden and/or total loss of voice, as seen with PVD, necessarily mean that the condition has arisen in response to more severely threatening events or COSO difficulties than those incidents that precede MTVD? It was not the case in this study.

Secondly, given that the LEDS and COSO events were the highest risk factors for the onset of FVD, and equally high between the PVD and MTVD sub-groups, would their different clinical presentations have been better explained by dispositional factors that we had not explored? For instance, would we have seen more differences between FVD sub-groups if we had used traditional personality measures that highlighted different degrees of neuroticism in association with extraversion and introversion as so strongly demonstrated by Roy *et al.* (2000b)? I suspect we would have done.

Thirdly, was repression of negative emotion in response to the many stressful LEDs and COSO situations the primary psychological process operating? Clearly, a pervading theme in our findings was that FVDs are associated with a greater amount of emotional distress and negative affect. Another theme suggested some kind of inhibition or alteration in the ability to process emotional distress that included both recent and more remote *developmental factors*. This was evidenced by self-reports of growing up in a family with less emotional expressiveness, and insecure and anxious attachments in current relationships. However, was this psychological process repression?

In seeking to answer that question, it was notable that very few women with FVD, and even those in the PVD sub-group, manifested *la belle indifference*. On the contrary, they expressed deep concerns about their voice disorders and obvious relief when the symptoms resolved. Furthermore, those with FVD were least likely to report a repressive coping style in comparison to the other groups. For example, one woman who was raped chose not to tell her parents about it or press charges against her assailant, but she told a friend and her local doctor about it shortly after the incident. In another case, a woman who was struggling to cope in her workplace was aware of having violent fantasies towards clients at the time but had never discussed these fantasies with anyone.

These were not examples of repression that would have been followed by catharsis during therapy. Rather, they were examples of women with a recollection of such incidents at some level, but the conscious processing of the emotions associated with the traumatic events was somehow limited. So is there another way to account for this? Was there a different way of understanding the traditional Freudian construct related to unconscious repression of emotion leading to different forms of bodily expression?

Some modern interpretations of the Freudian notion of repression challenge the notion conversion reaction symptoms representing 'a transmutation of repressed emotions into some form of bodily expression', and propose an updating of psychoanalytic concepts with constructs drawn from a Piagetian conceptualisation of emotion (Baker & Lane, 2009). For instance, rather than mental contents lying in the unconscious fully formed waiting to be unveiled at the point when the forces of repression are overcome, it has been shown that these are undifferentiated sensorimotor schemas that are not yet represented symbolically (Schimek, 1975). Donnel Stern (1983) has also observed that when individuals experience trauma, they often have difficulty in describing what happened and what they felt at the time. Contrary to classic Freudian theory, he suggests that their emotions are not fully formed and differentiated lying in the unconscious waiting to be uncovered by overcoming defenses.

Rather, it is more a matter of these negative emotions and memories remaining 'undifferentiated' until they can be brought to the light of conscious scrutiny. Therefore, severely stressful events or difficulties might remain associated with a relatively undifferentiated negative affect that remains persistent until the emotions can be discussed and formulated with another person. Only then can the traumatic experience be processed and experienced fully as feelings for the first time.

More recently, differences in *emotional awareness*, and the processing of negative emotions such as those described above, have been shown to determine different degrees of physiological arousal in wider populations, such as eating disorders, psoriasis, and depression (Bydlowski *et al.*, 2005; Consoli *et al.*, 2006; Donges *et al.*, 2005). Deficits in emotional awareness also manifest in individuals with *alexithymia*, which is a profound difficulty in finding and using words to describe emotions in relation to the self and others (Subic-Wrana, Bruder, Thomas, Lane, & Kohle, 2005; Waller & Scheidt, 2004).

Emotional processing deficits model

Overall, the findings from the study by Baker *et al.* (2013) provided a solid foundation for considering how the differences in processing of negative emotions might help to explain the development and perpetuation of FVD, and in collaboration with Richard Lane, we proposed a new theoretical model of *Emotional Processing Deficits in FVD* (Baker & Lane, 2009). This model offers a possible explanation for the development and exacerbation of the broad group of FVD, and may help to account for the different clinical presentations and profiles of patients in the PVD and MTVD sub-groups. In the sections below I highlight key aspects of the model and implications for clinical practice.

Levels of Emotional Awareness

The model draws directly upon concepts from the *Levels of Emotional Awareness Scales (LEAS)* as originally developed by Lane and Schwartz (1987). The LEAS model holds that an individual's ability to recognise and describe emotion in self and others is a cognitive skill that undergoes a developmental process similar to that which Piaget described for cognition in general (Piaget, 1952). A fundamental tenet of this model is that individual differences in emotional awareness reflect variation in the degree of differentiation and integration of the schemata used to process emotional information, whether the information comes from the external world or from the internal world through introspection. The five levels of emotional awareness in ascending order are: 1) Physical sensations; 2) Action tendencies; 3) Single Emotions; 4) Blends of Emotions; 5) Blends of emotional experience (the capacity to appreciate the complexity in the experience of self and others) (R. D. Lane & Schwartz, 1987).These authors have proposed possible neural correlates in relation to both *implicit and explicit emotional experience*. This has led to the development of 'a unifying framework that will potentially contribute to a theory of emotion that includes both unconscious emotional processes and conscious emotional experience' (R.D. Lane, 2000) (p. 346). A rudimentary neuroanatomical model of emotional awareness that distinguishes between these implicit and explicit processes as formulated by Lane is shown in Fig. 8.3.

NEUROANATOMICAL   **PSYCHOLOGICAL**

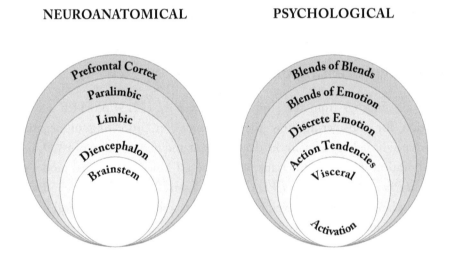

Fig. 8.3 Parallels in the hierarchical organisation of emotional experience and its neural substrates

The shell structure is intended to convey that each succeeding level adds to and modulates lower levels but does not replace them. Although each model contains five levels, a one to one correspondence between each level in the psychological and neuroanatomical models is not intended. Lower levels with white backgrounds correspond to implicit processes. Higher levels with grey background correspond to explicit processes.

From "Emotional Processing Deficits in Functional Voice Disorders by J. Baker and R.D. Lane in *Emotions in the Human Voice, Volume III* (p.128–129) by K. Izdebski (Ed.). Copyright © 2009 Plural Publishing, Inc. All rights reserved. Used with permission.

The five levels of emotional awareness can be mapped onto the distinctions between implicit and explicit processes. Therefore, individuals operating at the lower end of the developmental continuum may experience emotions in an undifferentiated somatic way. Their awareness of emotion under these circumstances may only be *implicit*, experienced at the sensorimotor level, consisting of peripheral and physiological arousal or action tendencies that occur in the absence of the feeling that is characteristic of a given emotion. These emotions are *implicit* in the sense that they occur automatically and do not require conscious processing in order to be executed efficiently. Therefore, when a traumatised individual develops particular medically-unexplained or functional symptoms, this model proposes that the emotions associated with the trauma are unformulated and undifferentiated, and are primarily expressed in the physiological domain (Level 1).

Alternatively, as elaborated further by Lane (2000), individuals who are able to process emotions at the higher end of the continuum experience their emotions consciously through the use of language in a more differentiated way. In being able to process emotions at this more *explicit level*, such individuals can then make sense of their emotional response as feelings, not only to themselves but also in relation to others. When emotions are conscious, an individual can draw upon understandings of past and present interactions with his or her environment 'to think ahead, avoid, plan and generalise to similar but unfamiliar situations' (p. 346). This enables more flexibility in responses, including the potential for greater emotional control.

In order to understand how this may occur, Lane (2000) has postulated cortical and sub-cortical neural substrates thought to be activated in response to the different levels of explicit emotional experience such as *'background feelings'*, *'attention to feelings'*, and *'reflective awareness of feelings'* in relation to the self and others. These are summarised in Table 8.2.

In explaining further the implications of the levels of emotional awareness model with its integrated neuroanatomical and psychological constructs, Lane *et al.* (2001) referred to recent imaging studies of emotional arousal. These studies have shown how particular structures on the medial surface of the frontal lobe may be differentially involved in the processing of background feelings, attention to feelings, and reflective awareness of feelings, as shown in Fig. 8.4.

Table 8.2 Possible neural correlates of different levels of emotional awareness

Cortical and sub-cortical neural substrates	Psychological model
L1 – Thalamus & hypothalamus & brainstem L2 – Amygdala for aversive stimuli-essential for implicit processing L2 – Ventral striatum & nucleus accumbens for reward stimuli	Level 1 – implicit processes that are automatic, modular & cognitively impenetrable- unconscious processing Level 2 – sensorimotor enactive level where distinctions between globally positive or negative states can be made
Paralimbic structures including anterior cingulate cortex (ACC), insula, temporal pole & orbitofrontal cortex (L3–4) Area 1 – Prefrontal cortex + ventromedial frontal cortex (Fig. 8.4) Area 2 – Dorsal anterior cingulate cortex (Fig. 8.4) Area 3 – Rostral anterior cingulate prefrontal cortex (Fig. 8.4)	Levels 3–5 explicit processes influenced by higher cognitive processes including prior explicit knowledge a) **Background feelings**-conscious emotional experience not associated with attention to it or reflection upon it b) **Attention to feelings** c) **Reflective awareness of feelings** in relation to self/others, control over emotional behaviour, future planning etc

Extrapolated from (Baker & Lane, 2009; R.D. Lane, 2000; R. D. Lane, Reiman, Ahern, & Thayer, 2001; R. D. Lane & Schwartz, 1987)

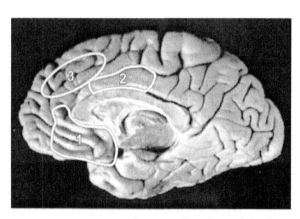

Fig. 8.4 Structures on the medial surface of the frontal lobe that participate in: (1) background feelings, (2) attention to feelings and (3) reflective awareness of feelings

These studies also revealed that as activity in the *anterior cingulate cortex (ACC)* increases, *cardiac vagal tone*, as measured by the high frequency component of *heart rate variability (HRV)*, also increases (Baker & Lane, 2009; R.D. Lane, 2000). The correlation between HRV and ACC therefore supports the hypothesis that routing emotional information from sub-cortical structures to these phylogenetically more advanced cortical areas has the effect of modulating the visceral expression of emotion. Furthermore, as summarised by the *neurovisceral integration model* (Thayer & Lane, 2000), becoming consciously aware of emotions involves a *bottom-up* transfer of information from subcortical to cortical structures. If an individual has an accepting attitude and experiences the feelings, this is associated with cortical and paralimbic processing that in turn leads to a *top-down* inhibition or modulation of subcortical activation modulated by vagal activation. Therefore, conscious processing has a dampening effect on emotional arousal associated with increased cardiac vagal tone. If the emotions are not consciously processed, or are only consciously processed in a limited way, vagal tone will be lower and the dampening effect will occur to a lesser extent.

Applications to FVD

On the basis of the data from our study (Baker *et al.*, 2013), the *Levels of Emotional Awareness* model as described by Lane and colleagues provides a way of understanding how both a strong negative affect and some interference with the conscious processing of it could lead to physiological changes that could contribute to the emergence of FVD. The developmental model is consistent with data suggesting that the problem experienced by patients with FVD in emotion processing arose earlier in life. It is also consistent with the observations that patients with FVD struggle with unacceptable or painful emotions, such as those that may be difficult to accept and process at a conscious level in association with life stress or trauma.

The *Emotion Processing Deficits model* as proposed by Baker and Lane (2009), suggests that FVD may reflect a difficulty in the processing of negative emotions in response to stressful life events or COSO situations, leading to different degrees of subcortical arousal. It is further proposed that an individual's unique emotional and neurophysiological responses to these stressful situations against a background of their early psychosocial development, personality traits, and emotional expressiveness may influence the severity or perpetuation of a FVD, and may shape the different clinical presentations of FVD as represented in the MTVD and PVD sub-groups.

As has been previously shown, patients with FVD frequently exhibit constriction of the extrinsic and intrinsic laryngeal muscles induced by heightened sympathetic arousal, attenuated vagal stimulation, and interactions between these complex processes (Demmink-Geertman & Dejonckere, 2002; Rosen & Sataloff, 1997). The neurovisceral integration model, as cited above, can account for the chain of events that appears to lead to the onset of FVD. Stressful life experiences under certain circumstances induce emotions that are difficult or impossible to consciously process, and that in turn leads to deficit in cardiac vagal tone. This *lowering in vagal tone* contributes to an increase in the constriction of the extrinsic and intrinsic laryngeal muscles, and then to excessive vocal fold tension and FVD.

Our model proposes that some individuals with FVD who may be functioning at the lower end of the developmental continuum are more likely to be struggling with emotions that are essentially implicit, and situated at the more undifferentiated somatic levels of expression. These individuals may be inclined to respond in a more basic manner, reverting to a more primitive physiological reaction as reflected in a readiness for 'fight or flight'. As emphasised by Aronson (1990b), this appears to be an unconscious reaction, and is thought to prepare the organism for increased physical work 'by fixing the upper extremities to the thoracic cage for combat requiring firm adduction of the vocal folds, and wide abduction to facilitate an increased volume and flow of oxygen in order to meet the body's increased metabolic demands' (p. 119). In some cases, this may manifest in the form of a complete closing down of the laryngeal sphincter with total loss of voice, or as a generalised tension leading to hyperfunctional patterns of vocalisation and dysphonia in others. In both cases, awareness of emotions may only be implicit and without 'the feelings' that are generally associated with a particular emotion. For those patients who continue to operate at the lowest levels of emotional awareness, symptoms may persist for weeks and months, and in rare cases, for years.

Alternatively, other individuals with FVD who function with a higher level of emotional awareness are more likely to be sensitive to physical sensations associated with visceral arousal, and will be able to consciously process their emotions by thinking and talking about them more explicitly. Through the use of language, they will be able to make sense of the feelings arising from stressful events and COSO difficulties in their lives, not only to themselves but also, in relation to others. For these individuals, vocal symptoms are more likely to be transient and FVD more readily resolved.

In seeking to offer a theoretical explanation for the differences between the FVD sub-groups, it is my hypothesis that patients diagnosed with PVD may be functioning at a *lower level of emotional awareness*. It is suggested that these individuals are more likely to be struggling with emotions that are essentially implicit, undifferentiated, and situated at a more primitive somatic level of expression. This may be reflected in a readiness for fight or flight, and in their unique clinical profile of difficulties in the voluntary initiation of phonation, symptom variability and incongruity, and demonstrable symptom reversibility.

In contrast, I suggest that patients diagnosed with MTVD, including those with vocal nodules and other small lesions associated with vocal hyperfunction, are likely to be operating at a relatively *higher level of emotional awareness* than those with PVD. These patients generally seem to be more 'in tune' with physical sensations associated with visceral arousal, and are able to process their emotions more readily by consciously thinking about them and discussing them explicitly with another. The apparently higher levels of emotional awareness in which these patients are operating seems to enable them to integrate the voluntary and involuntary aspects of voice production more effectively, and to be more proactive in doing something to relieve their anxiety.

Comments and implications of this model for clinical practice

Our model draws together those emotional, cognitive, behavioural, and neuro-physiological components in relation to stress that seem to be operating across a heterogeneous group of FVD, and may also help to explain differences between the PVD and MTVD sub-groups.

Essentially, our new model offers a *bio-psychosocial perspective* to the under-standing of FVD, not unlike the other theoretical models discussed throughout this chapter, and as so ardently pursued in other aspects of health (O'Dea & Daniel, 2001).

The implications for clinical practice suggest that if negative emotions in response to stressful events and/or traumatic experiences could be identified and formulated with another person, they could then be assimilated and experienced as feelings for the first time. The role of therapeutic intervention would be to help patients shift from an undifferentiated and *implicit level of emotional awareness* (involving a 'bottom-up' transfer of information from sub-cortical to cortical structures), to a more *explicit level of emotional awareness* as mediated by language (leading to a 'top-down' inhibition or modulation of subcortical activation). Patients would then be in a position to identify and differentiate between their emotions in a more formulated manner. In so doing, they would be in a position to gain greater regulatory control over these lower level processes.

This would not be an aimless and interminable foray into the inner emotional life of the patient by an overly curious therapist resembling Eric Berne's 'phallus in wonderland'. It would, however, require that clinicians have the emotional awareness and skills themselves to join with patients at their particular level of emotional functioning, beginning with the diagnostic psychosocial interview and then throughout the therapeutic process. Here, the aim would be to help patients to progress gradually to the higher levels of emotional awareness and integrate the voluntary and involuntary aspects of their voice production, enabling a greater sense of mastery and control over their vocal function.

Significantly too, being able to talk about their feelings within the context of situations that had preceded the voice disorder, such as health issues, stressful events, longer-term difficulties, and COSO incidents would help patients to understand the *meaning of their vocal symptoms*, and to appreciate how their voice problem might 'make sense'. This would enable individuals to consider a broader range of coping responses to stressful life situations in the future, and to be empowered to do something about it.

The model offers a theoretical framework that encourages patients and clinicians alike to think beyond the *physical voice* and to consider the *metaphorical voice* in the context of family, work, and extended social networks. In this sense the model offers further support for those advocating integration of traditional voice therapy strategies with principles of CBT, or other models of counselling and psychotherapy as may be deemed appropriate, such as family therapy. The ways in which these different psychotherapeutic approaches may be integrated into clinical practice are discussed in Part II.

Future directions for research on the basis of this model

The general framework of our model generates new hypotheses to be tested, and offers a way forward to investigate the neural substrates of FVD. For instance, it would be important to examine whether there is evidence of a deficit in emotional awareness in women with FVD and if as predicted, that there is a difference in the levels of emotional awareness between individuals with MTVD or PVD.

Furthermore, since low cardiac vagal tone as measured by low resting HRV is typically observed in patients with generalised anxiety disorder and depression, and in others suffering a range of health problems such as hypertension (Park &

Thayer, 2014), one would predict that vagal tone as indexed by respiratory sinus arrhythmia would be diminished in patients with FVD and would therefore increase with successful treatment.

In a *functional imaging* context, we might anticipate that recall of traumatic experiences would be associated with deficits in *anterior cingulate cortex (ACC)* functioning during the symptomatic phase of FVD, especially those with PVD, and that with recovery of vocal function there would be a reversal of this deficit accompanied by an increase in vagal tone. These processes have been demonstrated in an imaging study with male and female Vietnam war veterans, where changes to regional blood flow in the amygdala and medial prefrontal cortex were observed during traumatic imagery (Shin *et al.*, 2004).

Following on from these precepts, one would also predict that with successful treatment of the voice disorder, the ability to describe the emotions associated with the stressful life experiences would improve as explanations become more complex and differentiated. If the different hypotheses generated by our new model could be confirmed, such findings would be useful in making the diagnosis of FVD and tracking the recovery process during treatment.

Psychobiological framework for voice disorders

Underpinning each of the theoretical models discussed in the sections above has been the notion that *acute* or *chronic stress* may contribute in different ways to both FVD and OVD. As a result, more concerted efforts have recently been made to study the specific role of *stress* on normal vocal function in general, and on extrinsic and/or intrinsic laryngeal muscle groups in particular, with implications for the development and aggravation of a range of voice disorders.

Dietrich and Verdolini Abbott (2008) have drawn upon the clinical and empirical evidence from the professional literature suggesting possible links between stress and vocal function, and integrated these with findings from the extant literature reporting on the effects of *acute* and *chronic stress* on various aspects of physical and mental health (see my overview of these issues in Chapter 3). This has led to the formulation of the *Psychobiological Framework for Voice Disorders* (Dietrich & Verdolini Abbott, 2008), which seeks to explain the effects of stress on laryngeal behaviour as determined by interactions between the somatic and autonomic nervous systems, and as mediated by the limbic system. This framework has generated a number of hypotheses and new empirical data to support the model (Dietrich *et al.*, 2012; Dietrich & Verdolini Abbott, 2012, 2014; Dietrich *et al.*, 2008), with a recent project leading to the proposal of a

Revised Psychobiological Framework for Voice Disorders (Helou, 2014). I will now highlight some of the key elements of the original model with reference to their schematic diagram as shown in Figure 8.5.

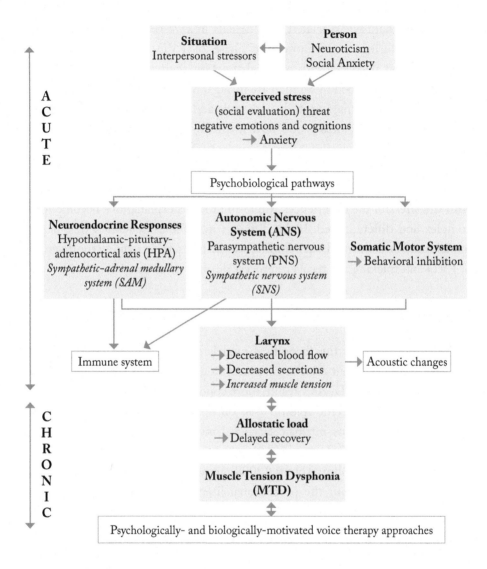

Fig. 8.5 Psychobiological framework of voice disorders

From "Psychobiological Framework of Stress and Voice" by M. Dietrich and K. Verdolini Abbott in *Emotions in the Human Voice, Volume II*, (p.161) by K. Izbedski (Ed.). Copyright © 2008 Plural Publishing, Inc. All rights reserved. Used with permission.

Definition of terms

As reflected in the title, the *Psychobiological Framework for Voice Disorders* does not limit itself solely to FVD. Rather, the model seeks to explain how psychological stress in association with a range of psychosocial factors may impact upon different neurobiological systems, with implications for both normal and abnormal vocal function across a range of voice disorders. The authors have chosen Primary Muscle Tension Dysphonia (MTD-Primary) as defined in the *Classification Manual of Voice Disorders-1* (Verdolini, Rosen, & Branski, 2006) in order to illustrate how constructs from the stress/health research may be applied. MTD-Primary in this classification system refers to a hyper or hypo adducted hyperfunctional voice disorder, where the essential features of the dysphonia occur 'in the absence of current organic vocal fold pathology, without obvious psychogenic or neurological aetiology, and in association with excessive, atypical or abnormal laryngeal movements during phonation' (p. 249). As the empirical evidence for abnormal muscle tension patterns is scarce, MTD-Primary is more economically defined in this system as 'a persistent unexplained dysphonia that is behaviourally modifiable' (p. 249). It is also suggested that precipitating factors may include: events 'possibly unrecognised and/or previously resolved' (p. 250); that 'introverted personality may be a contributing factor' (p.250); and that 'persistent primary MTD may lead in the longer term to the development of *phonotraumatic lesions* as one potential sequela to these disorders' (p. 250).

Dietrich *et al.* (2008) define stress according to Cohen *et al.* (1995) as 'a process in which environmental demands tax or exceed the adaptive capacity of an organism, resulting in psychological and biological changes that may place persons at risk for disease' (p.3). Some of the key constructs in relation to *stress* and *perceived stress* that have informed their theoretical framework are summarised in Box 8.5.

Box 8.5 Key psychological and physiological issues in relation to stress

- Different types of stressors are perceived as being more or less stressful
  - *Challenging* situations shown to be perceived as less stressful
    - Leading to increased cardiac performance
  - *Threatening* situations characterised by social evaluative threat and little control over outcome perceived as markedly more stressful-*shame stress*
    - Leading to increased blood pressure
- Stress responses may be specific with felt distress related to particular emotions
  - Fight–flight stress response associated with anxiety, fear, anger
  - Possible differences between stress associated with anger, fear, or shame
  - Ongoing debate over links between stress, emotion, and cognition
- Acute stress – responses initially adaptive, even life saving
  - normal allostatic response for appropriate time, then turned off
- Chronic stress – overload of adaptations or under-activity of biological systems
  - Abnormal allostatic load increasing with different kinds of responses
    - Repeated hits, lack of adaption, prolonged response with delayed shutdown and recovery, hyperactivity and compensatory response
- Individual differences in ways of responding to stress moderated by
  - Personality traits e.g. introversion, negative affect, neuroticism
  - Stress reactivity e.g. social anxiety, somatic complaints
  - Coping styles e.g. emotion oriented coping, denial, suppression, repression
- Implications of chronic stress for physical and mental health
  - Behaviours, illness perceptions, compliance
  - Vulnerability to infection, immune function, wound healing

(Extrapolated from Dietrich & Verdolini Abbott, 2008)

Descriptive overview of this model

The authors propose that interactions between environmental situations and dispositional factors shape the way in which individuals appraise and respond to these scenarios. If perceived as being stressful, this leads to negative thoughts and emotions, prompting concurrent and interactive involvement of the *neuroendocrine, autonomic nervous system (ANS),* and *somatic motor system,* with potential impacts on the *immune system.* These changes then stimulate alterations to the physiology of the larynx as reflected in decreased blood flow and decreased upper airway secretions, with concomitant increase in muscle tone and tension in the extrinsic and intrinsic laryngeal musculature. In essence, these authors suggest that increased laryngeal tension is one aspect of an overall bodily response to stress as mediated by the ANS, and that stress invokes 'an intertwined psychological, emotional, cognitive, physiological, immunological and behavioural cascade of events that may affect the larynx' (Dietrich & Verdolini Abbott, 2008) (p.160).

The model offers a framework for addressing hypotheses designed to assess 'potential psychobiological pathways linking stress to vocal functioning' (p. 174). One hypothesis suggests that under circumstances where acute stress becomes chronic, this may contribute to stress-induced changes in the larynx and over time, to the development of a voice disorder. Here, the authors postulate a central mechanism such as *delayed recovery* that may account for differences between an acute rather than chronic laryngeal disturbance. They suggest further that dispositional factors such as *personality traits* and *stress reactivity* may influence individual responses to stress. For some, this may facilitate the *behavioural inhibition* and laryngeal muscle tension often seen in MTD-Primary, or as *behavioural activation* and laryngeal muscle tension that may be observed in others, leading to phonotrauma and tissue changes such as vocal nodules. Findings from several studies undertaken by this research team, as outlined below, have generated further empirical data to support these proposed links between stress, personality, and vocal function.

Empirical evidence to support aspects of the psychobiological framework

Perceived stress

In a preliminary study, Dietrich *et al.* (2008) explored the frequency of *perceived stress, anxiety*, and *depression* as measured by standardised questionnaires in a heterogeneous group of patients diagnosed with different voice disorders. These groups included patients with MTD, benign vocal fold lesions (VN), *paradoxical vocal fold movement disorder (PVFMD)*, and *glottal insufficiency*. The primary aim of the study was to explore the relationship between stress, anxiety, and depression across a group of patients with common pathologies, and then more specifically in relation to laryngeal diagnosis.

For the pooled group data, perceived stress, anxiety, and depression scores were within the range typically found in a healthy population. However, 25% of patients reported scores above the healthy norm for *stress*, 36.9% with elevated scores for *anxiety* and 31.2% for *depression*. The authors emphasised that while these figures suggest that between 25 and 37% of the whole patient group displayed elevated scores on stress, anxiety, or depression, the remainder did not. Therefore, 'caution should be exercised in making *a priori* assumptions about the presence of psychological conditions in patients with voice disorders in general' (p.483).

The results in relation to the specific diagnostic groups revealed that PVFMD showed the more elevated scores across all three dimensions, and that patients with glottal insufficiency had lower scores for stress and anxiety. Interestingly, although patients with MTD and benign lesions had similar profiles, with approximately 50% reporting abnormal state anxiety and 25% reporting elevated stress and depression, they did not have higher scores on either of these measures than those with PVFMD or glottal insufficiency. In addition, analysis of sub-groups within the MTD cohort failed to show differences in scores for stress, anxiety, or depression between those with functional dysphonia, functional aphonia, or primary MTD. These findings led the authors to suggest that MTD may be construed as 'a wide spectrum of conditions ranging from psychogenic aphonia, to little or no psychological involvement as may occur in "musculogenic" MTD' (p.484). Once again they warned against overestimating psychological factors as being necessarily causal in the average individual with MTD.

Personality, stress reactivity, and extrinsic laryngeal muscle tension

In subsequent studies, Dietrich *et al.* (2012, 2014) explored further the possible links between personality and stress reactivity, and the frequently held assumptions that increased levels of laryngeal muscle tension will reflect these links. More specifically, their studies investigated *Trait Theory*, whereby Roy *et al.* (2000a) have proposed that introversion and extraversion may influence individual responses to stress, which in turn will be reflected in differentiated vocal behaviours and laryngeal muscle tension patterns in the functional voice disorder sub-groups (i.e., those with MTD primary and those with vocal nodules).

In these studies, the authors investigated the proposal that *introversion* would predictably influence vocal behaviour and *extra-laryngeal muscle function* in vocally healthy individuals compared with those with *extraversion*. They suggested that if this were so, thee differences might support a risk-hypothesis for MTD (Primary). The authors sought to determine whether exposure to an *acute social evaluative stressor* such as public speaking would influence extra-laryngeal muscle activity differently in introverted versus extraverted vocally healthy individuals and secondly, whether stressor-induced changes in extra-laryngeal behaviours were associated with an *increased perception of vocal effort*.

Participants were vocally healthy females divided equally into an introversion and extraversion group. The primary measures were surface electromyography (sEMG) of the submental (SM) and infrahyoid (IH) extralaryngeal sites, including sEMG of the anterior tibialis of the leg as a control site. These measures were taken before, during, and after exposure to the psychological stressor task. These extralaryngeal muscle groups have been shown to indicate elevation and depression of the larynx. Other measures included self-reported vocal effort, Voice Handicap Index (VHI) for voice-related to quality of life, and acoustic measures of voice during overt speech. Key findings revealed:

- Greater *IH muscle activity* in the *introversion group* in comparison to extraverts during all stages of the protocol and particularly in the stressor task
- Greater *IH muscle activity* and *introversion* were significantly correlated with VHI
- Differences in extra-laryngeal muscle activity were sufficient to support a risk hypothesis for voice problems (taking into account self-reports of vocal fatigue)
- Interactions between *IH muscle activity* and *introversion* coupled with *neuroticism* were not as significant as introversion on its own.

227

These data gave further support to a key construct of the Trait Theory, which proposes that under stressful conditions introverted individuals are more likely to respond with *behavioural inhibition*. Since behavioural inhibition has been shown to involve slowing, halting, or abrogation of an ongoing behaviour in the face of challenge or perceived threat (Amodio *et al.*, 2007), it would be anticipated that this behavioural inhibition would be reflected in suppressed laryngeal behavior in association with muscle tension of some kind. Dietrich *et al.* (2012) proposed 'that a pattern of *increased IH muscle activity* may be one manifestation of behavioural inhibition or response suppression' (p. 984).

These authors concluded that while their study clearly showed greater *IH muscle activity* in response to a stressor task amongst vocally healthy introverted individuals in comparison to extraverts, the findings did not allow generalisations to patients with MTD. Furthermore, it was equally important to view interactions between an individual's personality and stress reactivity in the context of his or her professional and social life. Here, they were referring to additional risk factors such as vocal demands at work, interpersonal stresses, or poor physical well-being, all of which need to be elucidated in each person's unique 'situation–person' interactions located at the top of their *Psychobiological Framework*, as shown earlier in Fig. 8.5.

In the second part of this study, Dietrich *et al.* (2014) sought to determine whether groups of vocally healthy individuals who responded with High extralaryngeal muscle activity as determined by *surface EMG (sEMG)* during a stressor task would differ from those with Low extralaryngeal muscle activity on *personality* and other measures related to *emotional reactivity* and *autonomic cardiovascular reactivity*. Their predictions were that those with High sEMG in comparison with those with Low sEMG (for both the submental (SM) and infrahypoid (IH) muscle sites) would score lower on Extraversion and social potency, higher on general social anxiety, and with greater fear and rumination during the stressor task of public speaking. On measures of autonomic cardiovascular arousal as measured by systolic blood pressure (SBP) they did not anticipate a significant difference between groups. The key findings for this second stage of the study showed:

- High sEMG groups for both the SM and IH muscle sites were associated with significantly lower scores on Extraversion and Social Potency
- High sEMG for the IH muscle site was associated with significantly *greater basic perceived fear* across all phases of the protocol than in the Low sEMG group
- There were no significant differences between groups for SBP

These findings strengthened their proposed Psychobiological Framework and lent further support to Trait Theory, since low-Extraversion was once again shown to be associated with heightened extra-laryngeal behaviour under stressful conditions, and where fear had contributed to this process.

Stress reactivity, limbic system, and central neural control of vocalisation

Dietrich Andreatta, Jiang, Joshi and Stemple (2012) subsequently extended this line of enquiry to investigate the relationship between *trait stress reactivity* and the possible role of the *limbic system* in the *central neural control of vocalisation*. As background to this study, they undertook a comprehensive overview of the literature in relation to the central neural correlates of stress, emotions in humans, and emotional vocalisation, with additional reference to studies investigating motor conversion disorders. They then proposed 'that the limbic vocal control pathway overlaps with neural networks that process emotion and stress in humans, and thus may modulate input to motor cortical networks' (p.380). These proposed interactions in relation to voice are shown in Fig. 8.6.

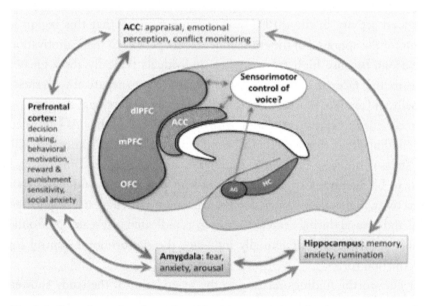

Fig. 8.6 Overview of prefrontal and limbic regions involved in processing of emotion and stress and their potential influence on the sensorimotor cortical control of voice (the periaqueductal gray is not pictured). The dashed arrows do not imply direct functional connectivity (Dietrich et al., 2012)

Reproduced with kind permission Maria Dietrich et al., and reprinted by permission of Taylor & Francis Ltd., Publisher of International Journal of Speech-Language Pathology.

The primary aims of their study were to ascertain 'whether trait stress reactivity influences activity in the prefrontal and limbic areas during an overt sentence reading task' (p. 385), and 'whether stress reactivity and associated individual differences in prefrontal and limbic activations correlate with sensorimotor cortical activity during overt sentence reading' (p.386). The study was undertaken using a *functional Magnetic Resonance Imaging (fMRI)* paradigm. Participants included a group of vocally healthy adults, divided into *high stress reactivity* and *low stress reactivity* sub-groups, who then carried out a series of overt (with voice and articulation), whispered (articulation but without voice), and covert (in their head) sentence reading tasks. The key findings revealed:

- The *high stress reactive* group demonstrated elevated *prefrontal* and *limbic* activity during the overt sentence reading task versus low stress reactive group
  - Dorsolateral prefrontal cortex (dlPFC) and periaqueductal gray (PAG)
- The *high stress reactive* group showed elevated *primary somatosensory cortex* (S1), *motor cortex* (M1), and *premotor* activity during sentence reading.

The authors have highlighted several aspects of the findings that are significant and that further support their Psychobiological Framework. For instance, the increased activity in the dlPFC was of interest, given that this region is important for the appraisal of the environment and operates to shape motivation and behaviour, because high stress reactive individuals typically show greater vigilance in the face of change, judge situations more negatively, overreact emotionally, and tend to recover more slowly from emotionally charged situations. Furthermore, the associated correlation with elevated levels in the PAG affirmed previous findings that this region is a neural correlate of physiological arousal, such as stressor-induced autonomic cardiovascular reactivity, and in this case appeared to be facilitated by the reading task in participants with high trait stress reactivity. The authors concluded that this new data suggests 'heightened appraisal and arousal during sentence reading, as indicated by greater prefrontal and limbic activity, may differentially influence the sensorimotor control for voice production' (p. 387).

Other noteworthy findings relating to the second aim of the study showed correlations between high stress reactive individuals and increases in the somatosensory motor and premotor cortex during the reading tasks. More specifically, heightened activity in the motor cortex was negatively correlated with the personality trait of *social potency*. This showed that individuals with low social potency, who would, by definition, be low in social dominance and persuasiveness and prefer to remain in the background, were more likely to show increased activity in the motor cortex. The authors suggested that this further supported aspects of Trait Theory (Roy & Bless 2000), which proposes that introversion, including low social potency, influences behavioural inhibition in association with patterns of increased laryngeal muscle tension.

Revised psychobiological framework for voice disorders

As pointed out by Helou and colleagues (2014; 2013), the literature regarding processes underpinning the development and aggravation of FVD frequently refers to interactions between the somatic and autonomic nervous systems (ANS), and how these processes may contribute to muscle tension. With respect to the ANS and vocal function in general, stage fright has been shown to facilitate a 'fight-or-flight' response through activation of the sympathetic nervous system, with observable changes in vocal pitch and quality, and concomitant autonomic physiological changes such as sweaty palms and dizziness. Furthermore, clinical populations with 'non-organic dysphonia' have reported significantly more *neurovegetative symptoms* than vocally normal individuals (Demmink-Geertman & Dejonckere, 2002, 2008), and data from the studies cited in the sections above show clear links between *high stress reactivity* as mediated by the ANS and elevated levels of *extrinsic laryngeal muscle activity*.

However, as also emphasised by Helou *et al.*, less is known about how *stress reactivity* as mediated by the ANS (e.g., cardiac vagal control via the parasympathetic nervous system) may impact upon the function of the *intrinsic laryngeal muscles*. Moreover, if there is a functional response in the larynx, how might this response influence the *duration* of the increased muscle activity, and would such effects be selective to either the *adductory* or the *abductory* muscles? Further, how might these processes have implications for the development of an FVD? In order to answer these questions, and with a view to investigating some of the key tenets of the *Psychobiological Framework* further, the research team undertook two further studies.

Initially, Helou *et al.* (2013) used an experimental laboratory cold-pressor task (CP) to stimulate a whole body ANS response in vocally healthy adult females. Measures included: *cardiovascular readings* of heart rate, systolic and diastolic blood pressure; *surface electromyographic (sEMG)* response of the *trapezius muscle*; and *fine wire EMG* of the *intrinsic laryngeal muscles* – all at rest and after exposure to the stressor task.

The key findings revealed concurrent increases in cardiovascular readings with increases in muscle activity generally. Co-activation of both the laryngeal abductors and adductors was noted, and statistically significant increases were evident in the right posterior cricoarytenoid (PCA), bilateral thyroarytenoid/ lateral cricoarytenoid (TA/LCA) muscle complex, and bilateral cricothyoid (CT) muscles during the CP task. This elevated muscle activity persisted well after cessation of the task, and after cardiovascular recovery from the task as well. The authors suggested that these unique findings lent further support to possible associations between stress, anxiety, and patterns of increased laryngeal muscle tension, and that this may have implications for our understanding of processes in the FVD group of disorders. They also suggested that the data with respect to duration after cessation of the stressor might support traditional notions of muscle tension dysphonia (MTD), being characterised by 'chronic, tonic levels of increased muscle tension in the larynx, including the intrinsic laryngeal muscles' (p. 2763).

In the second study, which formed the basis of a doctoral project, Helou (2014) investigated whether an intrinsic laryngeal muscle response in vocally healthy females occurs in the face of a psychological stressor, such as a speech preparation task, a known socially evaluative task, and if so, the specific features of that muscular response. A further aim of the project was to ascertain whether either a psychological variable such as trait *stress reactivity* or a physiological variable such as *cardiac vagal control* was operating as a mediator in this process, and if so, how might the mediating mechanisms be interrelated. Measures included: a standardised personality questionnaire to establish trait stress reactivity; heart rate, blood pressure, and respiratory sinus arrhythmia (RSA) as extracted from the ECG signal for cardiac vagal control; sEMG in the trapezius muscle as a positive control site and in the anterior tibialis as a negative control site; fine wire electromyography (EMG) of the intrinsic laryngeal muscles, namely the posterior cricoarytenoid (PCA), thyroarytenoid/lateral cricoarytenoid (TA/ LCA), and the cricothyroid (CT). Key statistically significant findings revealed:

- Elevated levels of activity in the trapezius and tibialis (which was unexpected)
- Increases in the activity of the PCA, TA/LCA muscle complex, but not the CT
- The magnitude of the stress response in the intrinsic laryngeal muscles was greater than in the trapezius and tibialis and accompanied by a clear respiratory response
- High stress reactivity predicted higher trapezius, tibialis, and attenuated TA activity
- Low levels of RSA values as an indicator of low cardiac vagal tone that also predicted increased activity of the all the muscles under investigation.

The study clearly showed both heightened overall somatic muscle activity and increased intrinsic laryngeal muscle responses to a psychological stress condition, and that the psychological variable of stress reactivity and the physiological variable of autonomic function played a mediating role in this process. In view of these significant findings, Helou suggested that the original *Psychobiological Framework* (Dietrich & Verdolini Abbott, 2008) might be expanded in several ways. These are mentioned briefly and are shown in the *Revised Psychobiological Framework of Voice Disorders* (Fig. 8.7).

Suggested changes incorporated in the revised Psychobiological Framework (Helou, 2014)

1. The framework 'should explicitly include the trachea and conducting airways as an effector organ of stress' (p. 152). This would support the concomitant respiratory response that was observed during the stressor task, and the close structural and functional association of the larynx to the lower airways.
2. More concerted research efforts are warranted to explore the roles of both the parasympathetic and sympathetic nervous systems under conditions of stress, and as their interactions upon laryngeal and respiratory function. A greater emphasis on the parasympathetic nervous system enables further investigation of the links between the low cardiac vocal tone with its concomitant increases in intrinsic laryngeal muscle activity as frequently found in individuals with anxiety and related physical and mental health disorders, including medically-unexplained conditions.
3. The links between the different stress systems (i.e., neuroendocrine, autonomic, and somatic systems), and the effector organs (i.e., larynx, lower airways, and skeletal muscles) should be *bi-directional*. Given that alterations within these different stress systems are likely to have an impact on a person's perception of stress, these interactions should be represented bi-directionally as well.
4. The notion of 'chronic stress' would be more appropriately subsumed under the more comprehensive construct of 'allostatic load', which refers to the cumulative effects of the autonomic nervous system, the HPA-axis, and the immune systems on an individual, and allostatic load increases with 'repeated hits', 'lack of adaption', 'prolonged response with delayed shutdown and recovery', and 'hyperactivity and compensatory response'(McEwen, 1998) (See Box 8.5). Helou suggests that 'The Allostatic Load Model' complements 'The Cinderella Hypothesis' (Hagg, 1991), both of which offer explanations for the persisting effects of lack of rest and recovery on voluntary muscle

behaviours, and the implications for the development of musculoskeletal disorders.

5. One final proposition that might further enrich the psychobiological framework is to incorporate 'Risk Factors for Laryngeal Reaction to Stress' at the top of the model alongside the Person-by-Situation interaction. The role of environment and behavioural risk factors in the pathogenesis of hyperfunctional voice disorders is explicit in current patient care models, as evidenced by standard application of indirect therapy techniques early in the course of voice therapy. This may include reducing the amount of talking, reducing vocal loudness, identifying and minimising vocal use, and manipulating the environment. The developers of the Psychobiological Framework of Voice Disorders have noted this issue but to date, the framework has not been adjusted to accommodate the change. Dietrich *et al.* (2012) write that 'introverted individuals appear to possess a unique vulnerability for laryngeal reactions in response to stress. However this vulnerability may contribute to a voice disorder only in interaction with other risk factors, such as occupational voice use, work stress, an overtaxing person situation or poor physical well-being' (p. 984). It follows therefore that a person's dispositional vocal behaviour must first become counterproductive or dysfunctional in social or professional contexts to manifest as a voice disorder. Since the goal of the psychobiological framework is to reflect the stress-related pathogenesis of voice impairment, it stands to reason that this *'make or break factor'* should be represented alongside the other top-level predisposing elements, Person-by-Situation interaction (Helou, 2014) (p. 158) (see Fig. 8.7.).

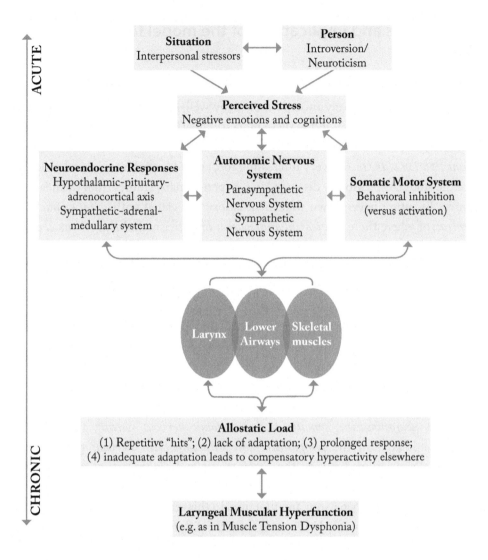

Fig. 8.7 Revised Psychobiological Framework of Voice Disorders (Doctoral Thesis, Helou, L. 2014, University of Pittsburgh)

Reproduced with kind permission Leah Helou.

Comments and implications of the model for clinical practice

One of the strengths of the Psychobiological Framework (original and revised) is that it most effectively incorporates many well-known constructs related to acute and chronic stress, and as these processes may be reflected in allostatic load. The choice to include socially evaluative tasks with some measures taken during *'anticipation of the task'* is very interesting too, and adds to the ecological validity of the study. As previously discussed in Chapter 3, many studies from the health/ stress literature have shown that in situations associated with *social evaluative threat*, or where there is a *fearful anticipation* of criticism and *lack of control over outcomes*, these chronic conditions are more likely to lead to higher levels of 'stress' (Dedovic, Duchesne, Andrews, Engert, & Pruessner, 2009; Dickerson & Kemeny, 2004; Fisher & Baum, 2010). The model then links these concepts in relation to acute and chronic stress in a meaningful way to the current evidence for stressful life events and personality traits that have been shown to contribute to onset or to influence outcomes for many individuals with voice disorders.

The model gives a comprehensive account of the way in which psychological stress may generate neurophysiological changes in the body overall. It highlights many interacting psychobiological processes: the effects of *psychological stress* on the *neuroendocrine, somatic,* and *autonomic nervous systems;* the relative contributions from the *sympathetic* and *parasympathetic nervous systems;* the possible associations between the *limbic system* and *higher cortical regions of the brain;* and then as interactions between these different systems may specifically influence laryngeal behaviour and function. In this sense, the model is meticulous in its attention to potential influences from the different neurobiological systems operating, and it has provided valuable empirical data that endorse aspects of earlier explanations on the effects of stress on vocal function (Aronson & Bless, 2009; M. Morrison & Rammage, 2001; Rosen & Sataloff, 1997). Significantly, the recent emphasis on parasympathetic nervous system responses, such as cardiac vagal tone, as these may relate to laryngeal and respiratory function, gives encouraging support to the hypotheses raised by Baker and Lane (2009) in their Emotion Processing Deficits Model for FVD as previously discussed.

The Psychobiological Framework has generated a number of studies showing that in vocally healthy speakers, personality traits such as *introversion* or *low social potency* may influence an individual's response to psychological stress as triggered by *social evaluative tasks*. Moreover, these differentiated responses will be directly associated with elevated levels of activation both centrally in the motor cortex, and peripherally, in specific extra-laryngeal muscles such as the infrahyoid and submental, and in the intrinsic laryngeal muscles such as the PCA and TA/LCA. It has long been a contention that the FVD group of disorders is characterised by patterns of muscle tension to various degrees, but it has not been entirely certain which laryngeal muscles may be implicated under conditions of psychological stress. These new findings contribute important missing pieces to the jigsaw puzzle, while also giving additional support to Trait Theory.

In the development of the Psychobiological Framework, Dietrich *et al.* (2008, 2012, 2014; 2008) have undertaken studies with both vocally healthy individuals and clinical populations. They have emphasised that while stress, anxiety, and depression may be reflected in the clinical profile of many patients with different voice disorders, particularly those with MTD, it is important *not to presume* that these issues are always present. However, they warn that where stress, anxiety, and/or depression are integral to the clinical picture, the long-term efficacy of treatment may be compromised, and the risk of relapse and recurrence of the voice disorder is likely to be high. The authors propose that it is important to find ways of interrupting the vicious cycle that often ensues if such issues are not recognised and resolved.

In view of their preliminary findings on the links between trait stress reactivity and the *central control of vocalisation*, Dietrich *et al.* (2012) suggest that if *limbic motor pathways underlying vocal control* could be directly linked with vocal dysfunction, then voice therapy could incorporate approaches 'that would capitalise on limbic system neuroplasticity to modulate sensorimotor control for voice production' (p. 387). Here, they suggest 'top-down' strategies that might include models of counselling, such as CBT or *mindfulness meditation*, in combination with direct voice therapy as a further approach to managing chronically stressful situations (McEwen & Gianaros, 2010). These recommendations closely reflect those advocated in all of the other theoretical models above, where more in-depth counselling or the integration of psychotherapeutic approaches with traditional voice therapy may be considered as an option. This will be the focus of Part II.

Conclusions

It can be seen that while there are different emphases in each of the theoretical models discussed in this chapter, it is also possible to recognise several recurring themes. The primary focus of most of the models has been on psychosocial factors contributing to the onset, aggravation, and outcomes of FVD, with efforts in several models to distinguish between the PVD and MTVD sub-groups. Some authors would suggest that all of these disorders lie somewhere on a continuum reflecting different degrees of laryngeal muscle tension; others would argue that there are different psychological processes operating that then shape the different clinical presentations of these disorders.

The psychosocial factors recognised in the models above relate to acute and chronically stressful life situations preceding onset, and to dispositional features and health-related issues that may influence how individuals respond to these challenges. Each model has attempted to explain how interactions between these factors may impact upon an individual's thoughts, emotions, and behaviours, and how these processes may contribute to the onset, aggravation, or perpetuation of the different voice disorders.

Reference is made in each model to the role of early life experiences in shaping individual vulnerabilities, and to other issues such as gender, family, social, and work-related demands that may contribute to a vulnerability for the development of one kind of voice disorder over another. Each model then postulates *neurophysiological correlates* that reflect the impact of the negative emotions arising in response to these complex psychosocial factors, with inferences about 'bottom-up' or 'top-down' regulation and how such processes may influence muscle tension patterns and vocal function.

Implicit in these models has also been the suggestion that FVD are not unlike other medically-unexplained symptom disorders, and that FVD might well be construed as a further example of a medically-unexplained 'distress condition'. This has strong merit, and certainly the role of acute and chronic stress in association with the many psychosocial factors that seem to contribute to these disorders, or that serve to exacerbate or maintain them, are very similar to those that we see with FVD.

It is also evident that FVD, and certainly the PVD sub-group, has striking similarities to the *Psychogenic Movement Disorders* described by Hallett and colleagues (2006; 2011), and as more recently encompassed under the broad classification of the *Functional Neurological Disorders* (Carson, Lehn, Ludwig, & Stone, 2016; Stone, 2016).These multidisciplinary clinical and research teams highlight the diverse nature of the functional symptoms, the impact of psychosocial factors contributing to their onset, and their clinical course, and offer more contemporary explanations to account for these disorders. In my opinion there is much that we can extrapolate for our understanding regarding the full range of FVD and the PVD and MTVD sub-groups from these explanations.

For example, a number of functional imaging studies are now generating further evidence for the neural correlates of the functional movement disorders.

Of particular interest are recent laboratory and functional magnetic resonance imaging (fMRI) studies, now confirming differentiated neural correlates during recall of traumatic life events in individuals with other conversion reaction symptoms, or functional neurological disorders (Aybek *et al.*, 2013). These findings are providing empirical evidence that may affirm the construct of repression, and support earlier hypotheses with respect to 'some form of blocking of the sensorimotor pathways' (Baker, 1991). They have fascinating implications for our understanding in relation to FVD where we continue to debate whether or not the processing of negative emotions, and their possible suppression or repression, may impact upon the initiation and control of voluntary phonation. They are also generating discussions about *willed movement* (Haggard, 2008), and whether or not functional symptoms and/or the frank conversion disorders represent 'excessive facilitation' or 'impaired inhibition'. These are important questions, with direct relevance to the field of FVD in general and as we may construe PVD and the more rare, but still omnipresent, conversion reaction voice disorders. Some of these issues will be discussed in more detail in Chapter 12 in relation to the clinical management of PVD.

While it is acknowledged that there are still questions to be answered about the exact mechanisms operating, the authors of all of these models conclude that the evidence points to strong interactions between psychosocial factors and laryngeal function. Significantly, most of the models propose that approaches to therapeutic intervention need to capitalise on our knowledge about these psychobiological 'bottom-up' and 'top-down' pathways.

The findings from each model would suggest that it is simply not enough, nor appropriate, to focus on vocal hygiene and behavioural voice therapy with symptom removal alone without due recognition of the underlying aetiology. As proposed recently by Stemple, Roy and Klaben (2014), *'If the situational, emotional and/or personality features that contributed to the development of the voice disorder remain unchanged following behavioural treatment, it would be logical to expect that such persistent factors would increase the probability/risk of future recurrences'* (p. 99).

The respective authors of each theoretical model have stressed that not all patients with voice disorders suffer from psychological distress. I would agree. However, I would argue that at all levels of the therapeutic intervention, beginning with the diagnostic interview, specialists involved should be aware of, and be prepared to address, psychosocial issues as they become evident (Baker, 2008). This would mean at the very least being able to join with the patients at different levels of emotional functioning, and to conduct a psychosocial interview. On a number of occasions Aronson had made a passionate plea for speech-language pathologists to become accomplished in conducting psychosocial interviews, not only with voice patients but with all patients with communication disorders (Aronson, 1973, 1990a). However, some clinicians continue to ask, all these years later, "But is this our role? Do we have a right to deal with these issues?" On the basis of all the theoretical models discussed in this chapter, and the considerable evidence for psychosocial factors in relation to voice disorders presented in Part 1 of this book, I would re-iterate once more: *'It is not a matter of having the right – it is our ethical and professional obligation to understand and deal with the psychosocial issues arising with patients with voice disorders'* (Baker, 2010) (p.103).

References

Amodio, D. M., Master, S. L., Yee, C. M., & Taylor, S. E. (2007). Neurocognitive components of the behavioural inhibition and activation systems: Implications for theories of self regulation. *Psychophysiology, 44,* 1–9. doi: 10.1111/j.1469-8986.2007.00609.x

Andersson, K., & Schalen, L. (1998). Etiology and treatment of psychogenic voice disorder: Results of a follow-up study of thirty patients. *Journal of Voice, 12*(1), 96–106.

Aronson, A. E. (1969). Speech pathology and symptom therapy in the interdisciplinary treatment of psychogenic aphonia. *Journal of Speech and Hearing Disorders, 34*(4), 321–341.

Aronson, A. E. (1973). *Psychogenic voice disorders.* Philadelphia: Saunders.

Aronson, A. E. (1978). Differential diagnosis of organic and psychogenic voice disorder. In F. Darley & R. Spriesterbach (Eds.), *Diagnostic methods in speech pathology.* New York: Harper and Row.

Aronson, A. E. (1985). *Clinical voice disorders.* New York: Thieme.

Aronson, A. E. (1990a). Importance of the psychosocial interview in the diagnosis and treatment of "functional" voice disorders. *Journal of Voice, 4*(4), 287–289.

Aronson, A. E. (1990b). Psychogenic voice disorders. *Clinical voice disorders: An interdisciplinary approach.* (3rd ed., pp. 116–159). New York: Thieme.

Aronson, A. E., & Bless, D. M. (2009). *Clinical voice disorders* (4th ed.). New York: Thieme.

Aronson, A. E., Peterson, H. W., & Litin, E. M. (1964). Voice symptomatology in functional dysphonia and aphonia. *Journal of Speech and Hearing Disorders, 28,* 367–380.

Aronson, A. E., Peterson, H. W., & Litin, E. M. (1966). Psychiatric symptomatology in functional dysphonia and aphonia. *Journal of Speech and Hearing Disorders, 31,* 115–127.

Aybek, S., Nicholson, T. R., Zelaya, F., O'Daly, O. G., Craig, T. K., David, A. S., & Kanaan, R. A. (2013). Neural correlates of recall of life events in conversion disorder. *JAMA Psychiatry.* doi: doi:10.1001/jamapsychiatry.2013.2842

Baker, J. (1991). *How much am I bid for this exquisite little dysphonia: The money or the witness box?* Paper presented at the Inaugural Voice Symposium of Australia, Adelaide.

Baker, J. (1998). Psychogenic dysphonia: Peeling back the layers. *Journal of Voice, 12*(4), 527–535.

Baker, J. (2002). Psychogenic voice disorders – heroes or hysterics? A brief overview with questions and discussion. *Logopedics Phoniatrics Vocology, 27,* 84–91.

Baker, J. (2003). Psychogenic voice disorders and traumatic stress experience: A discussion paper with two case reports. *Journal of Voice, 17*(3), 308–318.

Baker, J. (2008). The role of psychogenic and psychosocial factors in the development of functional voice disorders. *International Journal of Speech-Language Pathology, 10*(4), 210–230.

Baker, J. (2010). Women's voices: Lost or mislaid, stolen or strayed? *International Journal of Speech-Language Pathology, 12*(2), 94–106.

Baker, J., Ben-Tovim, D. I., Butcher, A., Esterman, A., & McLaughlin, K. (2007). Development of a modified diagnostic classification system for voice disorders with inter-rater reliability study. *Logopedics Phoniatrics Vocology, 32,* 99–112.

Baker, J., Ben-Tovim, D. I., Butcher, A., Esterman, A., & McLaughlin, K. (2013). Psychosocial risk factors which may differentiate between women with Functional Voice Disorder, Organic Voice Disorder, and Control group. *International Journal of Speech-Language Pathology, 15*(6), 547–563.

Baker, J., & Lane, R. D. (2009). Emotion processing deficits in functional voice disorders. In K. Izdebski (Ed.), *Emotions in the human voice* (Vol. 3, pp. 105–136). San Diego: Plural Publishing.

Baker, J., Oates, J., Leeson, E., Woodford, H., & Bond, M. J. (2014). Patterns of emotional expression and responses to health and illness in women with functional voice disorders (MTVD) and a comparison group. *Journal of Voice*. doi: http://dx.doi.org/10.1016/j.jvoic.2014.03.005

Beck, A. T. (1979). *Cognitive therapy and the emotional disorders.* Madison: Penguin.

Behrman, A., Dahl, L. D., Abramson, A. L., & Schutte, H. K. (2003). Anterior-posterior and medial compression of the supraglottis: Signs of nonorganic dysphonia or normal postures? *Journal of Voice, 17*(3), 403–410.

Breuer, J., & Freud, S. (1955/1893–1895). Studies on hysteria. In J. Strachey (Ed.), *The standard edition of the complete works of Sigmund Freud.* (Vol. 2, pp. 1–305). London: Hogarth Press.

Brodnitz, F. S. (1969). Functional aphonia. *Annals of Otolaryngology, (St Louis), 78,* 1244–1253.

Butcher, P. (1995). Psychological processes in psychogenic voice disorder. *European Journal of Disorders of Communication, 30,* 467–474.

Butcher, P., & Cavalli, L. (1998). Fran: Understanding and treating psychogenic dysphonia from a cognitive-behavioural perspective. In D. Syder (Ed.), *Wanting to talk.* London: Whurr.

Butcher, P., & Elias, A. (1983). Cognitive-behavioural therapy with dysphonic patients: An exploratory investigation. *The College of Speech Therapists Bulletin,* (377), 1–3.

Butcher, P., Elias, A., & Cavalli, L. (2007). *Understanding and treating psychogenic voice disorder: A CBT framework.* Chichester: Wiley.

Butcher, P., Elias, A., & Raven, R. (1993). *Psychogenic voice disorders and cognitive behaviour therapy.* San Diego: Singular Publishing Group.

Butcher, P., Elias, A., Raven, R., Yeatman, J., & Littlejohns, D. (1987). Psychogenic voice disorder unresponsive to speech therapy: Psychological characteristics and cognitive-behaviour therapy. *British Journal of Disorders of Communication, 22,* 81–92.

Bydlowski, S., Corcos, M., Jeammet, P., Paterniti, S., Berthoz, S., Laurier, Chamby, J., & Consoli, M. (2005). Emotion processing deficits in eating disorders. *International Journal of Eating Disorders, 37*(4), 321–329.

Carson, A., Lehn, A., Ludwig, L., & Stone, J. (2016). Explaining functional disorders in the neurology clinic: A photo story. *Practical Neurology, 16,* 56–61. doi: 10.1136/practneurol-2015-001242

Chaturvedi, S. K., & Bhandari, S. (1989). Somatisation and illness behaviour. *Journal of Psychosomatic Research, 33*(2), 147–153.

Clark, D. M. (2011). Implementing NICE guidelines for the psychological treatment of depression and anxiety disorders: The IAPT experience. *International Review of Psychiatry, 23,* 375–384.

Cohen, S., Kessler, R. C., & Gordon, L. U. (1995). Strategies for measuring stress in studies of psychiatric and physical disorders. In S. Cohen, R. C. Kessler & L. U. Gordon (Eds.), *Measuring stress. A guide for health and social scientists.* (pp. 3–26). Oxford: Oxford University Press.

Cohen, S. M. (2010). Self-reported impact of dysphonia in a primary care population: An epidemiological study. *Laryngoscope, 120,* 2022–2032.

Colton, R. H., Casper, J., & Leonard, R. (2006). *Understanding voice problems: A physiological perspective for diagnosis and treatment.* Philadelphia: Lippincott, Williams & Wilkins.

Consoli, M., Rolhion, S., Martin, C., Ruel, K., Cambazard, F., Pellet, J., & Misery, L. (2006). Low levels of emotional awareness predict a better response to dermatological treatment in patients with psoriasis. *Dermatology, 212,* 128–136.

Daniilidou, P., Carding, P., Wilson, J., Drinnan, M., & Deary, V. (2007). Cognitive behavioural therapy for functional dysphonia: A pilot study. *Annals of Otology, Rhinology & Laryngology, 116*(10), 717–722.

Deary, V. (2011). *Cognitive behaviour therapy for functional dysphonia: Development of a complex intervention.* Newcastle University ePrints.

Deary, V., & Chalder, T. (2010). Personality and perfectionism: A closer look. *Psychological Health, 25,* 465–475.

Deary, V., Chalder, T., & Sharpe, M. (2007). The cognitive behavioural model of medically unexplained symptoms: A theoretical and empirical review. *Clinical Psychology Review, 27,* 781–797.

Deary, V., & Miller, T. (2011). Reconsidering the role of psychosocial factors in functional dysphonia. *Current Opinion in Otolaryngology and Head and Neck Surgery, 19*(3), 150–154.

Dedovic, K., Duchesne, A., Andrews, J., Engert, V., & Pruessner, J. C. (2009). The brain and the stress axis: The neural correlates of cortisol regulation in response to stress. *NeuroImage, 47*, 864–871.

Demmink-Geertman, L., & Dejonckere, P. H. (2002). Non-habitual dysphonia and autonomic dysfunction. *Journal of Voice, 4*, 549–559.

Demmink-Geertman, L., & Dejonckere, P. H. (2008). Neurovegetative symptoms and complaints before and after voice therapy for nonorganic habitual dysphonia. *Journal of Voice, 22*(3), 315–325.

Derakshan, N., & Eysenck, M. W. (2001). Manipulation of focus of attention and its effects on anxiety in high-anxious individuals and repressors. *Anxiety, Stress and Coping., 14*, 177–191.

Dickerson, S. S., & Kemeny, M. E. (2004). Acute stressors and cortisol responses: A theoretical integration and synthesis of laboratory research. *Psychological Bulletin, 2004*(130), 355–391.

Dietrich, M., Andreatta, R. D., Jiang, Y., Joshi, A., & Stemple, J. C. (2012). Preliminary findings on the relation between the personality trait of stress reaction and the central neural control of vocalization. *International Journal of Speech-Language Pathology, 14*(4), 377–389.

Dietrich, M., & Verdolini Abbott, K. (2008). Psychobiological framework of stress and voice. In K. Izdebski (Ed.), *Emotions in the Human Voice: Volume 2* (pp. 159–178). San Diego: Plural Publishing.

Dietrich, M., & Verdolini Abbott, K. (2012). Vocal function in introverts and extraverts during a psychological stress reactivity protocol. *Journal of Speech, Language and Hearing Research, 55*, 973–987.

Dietrich, M., & Verdolini Abbott, K. (2014). Psychobiological stress reactivity and personality with high and low stressor-induced extralaryngeal reactivity. *Journal of Speech, Language and Hearing Research, 57*, 2076–2089.

Dietrich, M., Verdolini Abbott, K., Gartner-Schmidt, J., & Rosen, C. L. (2008). The frequency of perceived stress, anxiety, and depression in patients with common pathologies affecting voice. *Journal of Voice, 22*(4), 472–487.

Donges, U., Kersting, A., Dannlowski, U., Lalee-Mentzel, J., Arolt, V., & Thomas, S. (2005). Reduced awareness of others' emotions in unipolar depressed patients. *Journal of Nervous and Mental Diseases, 193*(5), 331–337.

Elias, A., Raven, R., Butcher, P., & Littlejohns, D. (1989). Speech therapy for psychogenic voice disorder: A survey of current practice and training. *British Journal of Disorders of Communication, 24*, 61–76.

Epstein, R., Hirani, S. P., Stygall, J., & Newman, S. P. (2009). How do individuals cope with voice disorders? Introducing the Voice Disability Coping Questionnaire. *Journal of Voice, 23*(2), 209–217.

Eysenck, H. J. (1967). *Biological basis of personality.* Springfield: Thomas.

Eysenck, H. J., & Eysenck, M. W. (1985). *Personality and individual differences.* New York: Plenum Press.

Fisher, M., & Baum, F. (2010). The social determinants of mental health: Implications for research and health promotion. *Australian and New Zealand Journal of Psychiatry, 44,* 1057–1063.

Freud, S. (1955/1920). Beyond the pleasure principle. In J. Strachey (Ed.), *The standard edition of the complete works of Sigmund Freud.* (Vol. 18, pp. 3–64). London: Hogarth Press.

Gallagher, S. (2005). *How the body shapes the mind.* Oxford: Oxford University Press.

Gerritsma, E. J. (1991). An investigation into some personality characteristics of patients with psychogenic aphonia and dysphonia. *Folia Phoniatrica, 43,* 13–20.

Gray, J. A. (1975). *Elements of a two process theory of learning.* London: Academic Press.

Gray, J. A. (1982). *The neuropsychology of anxiety: An enquiry into the functions of the septo-hippocampal system.* New York: Oxford University Press.

Gray, J. A. (1985). Issues in the neruo-psychology of anxiety. In A. H. Tuma & J. D. Maser (Eds.), *Anxiety and the anxiety disorders* (pp. 5–25). Hillsdale: Erlbaum.

Gray, J. A. (1987). *The psychology of fear and stress* (2nd ed.). London: Cambridge University Press.

Gray, J. A. (1991). Neural systems, emotion and personality. In J. Madden, IV (Ed.), *Neurobiology of learning, emotion and affect* (pp. 273–306). New York: Raven Press.

Gray, J. A., & McNaughton, N. (2000). *The neuropsychology of anxiety.* London: Oxford University Press.

Hagg, G. (1991). Static work loads and occupational myalgia – a new explanation model In P. A. Anderson, D. J. Hobart & J. V. Danhoff (Eds.), *Electromyographical Kinesiology* (pp. 141–144). Amsterdam: Excerpta MedicaBV/ Elsevier.

Haggard, P. (2008). Human volition: Towards a neuroscience of will. *Nature Reviews Neuroscience, 9,* 934–946.

Hallett, M., Fahn, S., Jankovic, J., Lang, A. E., Cloninger, C. R., & Yudofsky, S. C. (Eds.). (2006). *Psychogenic movement disorders: Neurology and neuropsychiatry.* Philadelphia: Lippincott Williams & Wilkins.

Hallett, M., Lang, A., Jankovic, J., Fahn, S., Halligan, P. W., Voon, V., & Cloninger, C. R. (Eds.). (2011). *Psychogenic movement disorders and other conversion disorders.* Cambridge: Cambridge University Press.

Helou, L. B. (2014). *Intrinsic laryngeal muscle response to a speech preparation stressor: Personality and autonomic predictors.* (Ph.D. Doctoral Dissertation), University of Pittsburgh.

Helou, L. B., Wang, W., Ashmore, R. C., Rosen, C. A., & Verdolini Abbott, K. (2013). Intrinsic laryngeal muscle activity in response to autonomic nervous system activation. *The Laryngoscope, 123,* 2756–2765.

House, A., & Andrews, H. B. (1987). The psychiatric and social characteristics of patients with functional dysphonia. *Journal of Psychosomatic Research, 31,* 483–490.

House, A., & Andrews, H. B. (1988). Life events and difficulties preceding the onset of functional dysphonia. *Journal of Psychosomatic Research, 32*(3), 311–319.

Janet, P. (1920). *The major symptoms of hysteria.* New York: Hafner.

Kasch, K. L., Rottenberg, J., Arnow, B. A., & Gotlib, I. H. (2002). Behavioural activation and inhibition systems and the severity and course of depression. *Journal of Abnormal Psychology, 111*(4), 589–597.

Koufman, J. A., & Blalock, P. D. (1991). Functional voice disorders. *Otolaryngologic Clinics of North America, 24*(5), 1059–1073.

Lane, R. D. (2000). Neural correlates of conscious emotional experience. In R. D. Lane & L. Nadel (Eds.), *Cognitive neuroscience of emotion.* (pp. 345–370). Oxford: Oxford University Press.

Lane, R. D., Reiman, E., Ahern, G., & Thayer, J. F. (2001). Activity in medial prefrontal cortex correlates with vagal component of heart rate variability during emotion. *Brain and Cognition, 47*, 97–100.

Lane, R. D., & Schwartz, G. E. (1987). Levels of emotional awareness: A cognitive-developmental theory and its application to psychopathology. *American Journal of Psychiatry, 144*, 133–143.

MacKenzie, K., Millar, A., Wilson, J. A., Sellars, C., & Deary, I. J. (2001). Is voice therapy an effective treatment for dysphonia? *British Medical Journal, 2001*(323), 658–661.

Mathieson, L. (2001). *Greene and Mathieson's: The voice and its disorders.* (6th ed.). London: Whurr.

Maturana, H., & Varela, F. J. (1980). Autopoiesis and cognition: The realization of the living. In R. S. Cohen & M. W. Wartofsky (Eds.), *Boston studies in the philosophy of science.* Dordrecht: D. Reidel.

McEwen, B. S. (1998). Stress adaptation and disease. Allostasis and allostatic load. *Annals of the New York Academy of Science,* (840), 33–44.

McEwen, B. S., & Gianaros, P. J. (2010). Central role of the brain in stress and adaptation: Links to socioeconomic status, health and disease. *Annals of the New York Academy of Science, 1186*, 190–222.

Miller, T., Deary, V., & Patterson, J. (2014). Improving asscess to psychological therapies in voice disorders: A cognitive behavioural therapy model. *Current Opinion in Otolaryngology and Head and Neck Surgery, 22*(3), 201–205.

Morrison, M., & Rammage, L. (1993). Muscle misuse voice disorders: Description and classification. *Acta Otolaryngologica, 113*(3), 428–434.

Morrison, M., & Rammage, L. (2001). *Management of the voice and its disorders* (2nd ed.). Clifton Park: Delmar/Cengage Learning.

Morrison, M. D., Nichol, H., & Rammage, L. (1986). Diagnostic criteria in functional dysphonia. *Laryngoscope, 94*, 1–8.

Myers, L. B., & Derakshan, N. (2004). The repressive coping style and avoidance of negative affect. In I. Nyklicek, L. Temoshok & A. Vingerhoets (Eds.), *Emotional expression and health* (pp. 169–184). Hove and New York: Brunner-Routledge.

Newman, J. P., & Wallace, J. F. (1993a). *Cognition and psychopathy in psychopathology and cognition.* New York: Academic Press.

Newman, J. P., & Wallace, J. F. (1993b). Diverse pathways to deficient self-regulation: Implications for disinhibitory psychopathology in children. *Clinical Psychology Review, 13*, 699–720.

O'Dea, K., & Daniel, M. (2001). How social factors affect health: Neuroendocrine interactions. In R. Eckersly, J. Dixon & B. Douglas (Eds.), *The social origins of health and well-being.* Cambridge: Cambridge University Press.

O'Hara, J., Miller, T., Carding, P., Wilson, J., & Deary, V. (2011). Relationship between fatigue, perfectionism, and functional dysphonia. *Otolaryngology-Head and Neck Surgery, 144*(6), 921–926.

Oates, J., & Winkworth, A. (2008). Current knowledge, controversies and future directions in hyperfunctional voice disorders. *International Journal of Speech-Language Pathology, 10*(4), 267–277.

Park, G., & Thayer, J. F. (2014). From the heart to the mind: Cardiac vagal tone modulates top-down and bottom-up visual perception and attention to emotional stimuli. *Frontiers in Psychology.* doi: 10.3389/fpsyg.2014.00278/full#B70

Piaget, J. (1952). *The origins of intelligence in children.* New York: International Universities Press.

Rammage, L. (2011). Emotional expression and voice dysfunction. *Perspectives on voice and voice disorders, 21*(3), 8–16. doi: 10.1044/vvd 21.1.8

Rammage, L., Morrison, M., & Nichol, H. (2001). *Management of the voice and its disorders.* San Diego: Singular Publishing Group.

Rammage, L., Nichol, H., & Morrison, M. D. (1987). The psychopathology of voice disorders. *Human Communication Canada/Communication Humaine Canada, 11*(4), 21–25.

Rosen, D. C., & Sataloff, R. T. (1997). *Psychology of voice disorders.* San Diego: Singular Publishing Group.

Roy, N., & Bless, D. M. (2000a). Toward a theory of the dispositional bases of functional dysphonia and vocal nodules: Exploring the role of personality and emotional adjustment. In R. D. Kent & M. J. Ball (Eds.), *The handbook of voice quality measurement.* (pp. 461–481). San Diego: Singular Publishing Group.

Roy, N., & Bless, D. M. (2000b). Personality traits and psychological factors in voice pathology: A foundation for future research. *Journal of Speech, Language, and Hearing Research, 43*, 737–748.

Roy, N., Bless, D. M., & Heisey, D. (2000a). Personality and voice disorders: A multitrait-multidisorder analysis. *Journal of Voice, 14*, 521–548.

Roy, N., Bless, D. M., & Heisey, D. (2000b). Personality and voice disorders: A superfactor trait analysis. *Journal of Speech, Language and Hearing Research, 43*, 749–768.

Roy, N., McGory, J. J., Tasko, S. M., Bless, D. M., Heisey, D., & Ford, C. (1997). Psychological correlates of functional dysphonia: An investigation using the Minnesota Multiphasic Personality Inventory. *Journal of Voice, 11*(4), 443–451.

Sama, A., Carding, P. N., Price, S., Kelly, P., & Wilson, J. A. (2001). The clinical features of functional dysphonia. *The Laryngoscope, 111*(3), 458–463.

Sapir, S. (1995). Psychogenic spasmodic dysphonia: A case study with expert opinions. *Journal of Voice, 9*(3), 270–281.

Schalen, L., & Andersson, K. (1992). Differential diagnosis and treatment of psychogenic voice disorder. *Clinical Otolaryngology, 17*, 225–230.

Schimek, J. G. (1975). A critical re-examination of Frued's concept of unconscious mental representation. *International Review of Psycho-Analysis, 2*, 1710187.

Seifert, E., & Kollbrunner, J. (2006). An update in thinking about nonorganic voice disorders. *Archives of Otolaryngology Head and Neck Surgery, 132*, 1128–1132.

Shin, L. M., Orr, S. P., Carson, M. A., Rauch, S. L., Macklin, M. L., & Lasko, N. B. (2004). Regional cerebral blood flow in the amygdala and medial prefrontal cortex during traumatic imagery in male and female Vietnam veterans with PTSD. *Archives of General Psychiatry, 61*(2), 168–176.

Stemple, J. C., Roy, N., & Klaben, B. K. (2014). *Clinical voice pathology* (Fifth ed.). San Diego: Plural Publishing.

Stern, D. (1983). Unformulated experience: From familiar chaos to creative disorder. *Contemporary Psychoanalysis, 19*(1), 71–99.

Stone, J. (2016). Functional neurological disorders: The neurological assessment as treatment. *Practical Neurology, 16*, 7–17. doi: 10.1136/practneurol-2015-001241

Subic-Wrana, C., Bruder, S., Thomas, W., Lane, R. D., & Kohle, K. (2005). Emotional awareness deficits in inpatients of a psychosomatic ward: A comparison of two different measures of alexithymia. *Psychosomatic Medicine, 67*, 483–489.

Thayer, J. F., & Lane, R. D. (2000). A model of neurovisceral integration in emotion regulation and dysregulation. *Journal of Affective Disorders, 61*, 201–216.

Ursin, H. (2005). Press stop to start: The role of inhibition for choice and health. *Psychoneuroendocrinology, 30*(1059–1065).

van Mersbergen, M., Patrick, C., & Glaze, L. (2008). Functional dysphonia during mental imagery: Testing the trait theory of voice disorders. *Journal of Speech, Language, and Hearing Research, 51*, 1405–1423.

Verdolini, K., Rosen, C. A., & Branski, R. C. (Eds.). (2006). *Classification Manual for Voice Disorders – I*. Mahwah: Laurence Erlbaum Associates.

Vingerhoets, A., Nyklicek, I., & Denollet, J. (Eds.). (2008). *Emotion regulation: Conceptual and clinical issues*. New York: Springer.

Waller, E., & Scheidt, C. E. (2004). Somatoform disorders as disorders of affect regulation: A study comparing the TAS-20 with non-self-report measures of alexithymia. *Journal of Psychosomatic Research, 57*, 239–247.

White, A., Deary, I. J., & Wilson, J. A. (1997). Psychiatric disturbance and personality traits in dysphonic patients. *European Journal of Disorders of Communication, 32*, 307–314.

Wilson, J. A., Deary, I. J., & MacKenzie, K. (1995). Functional dysphonia. Not 'hysterical' but seen mainly in women. *British Medical Journal, 311*, 1039–1040.

Part II

Addressing psychosocial factors throughout the therapeutic process

9

Therapeutic processes and different levels of counselling

Introduction

'It is often the case that therapy is what one needs, and treatment is what one gets, which may or may not be therapeutic' (Pieter Geerkens, 2013).

The clinical management of organic voice disorders (OVD) and functional voice disorders (FVD) is a complex process, and often involves different members of a multi-disciplinary team to various degrees, depending upon the nature of the voice disorder. The general practitioner and otolaryngologist co-ordinate the medical and surgical interventions, and the speech-language pathologist (SLP) undertakes the voice therapy. In those cases where a professional voice user requires more advanced development of the singing and speaking voice, the specialised knowledge and skills of vocal pedagogues are highly recommended. If a serious co-morbid psychiatric disorder is thought to be causally related, or where psychological issues arising in response to a particular voice disorder are thought to be aggravating or maintaining the vocal disorder, referral to a clinical psychologist or psychiatrist may be suggested. In such cases the mental health professional may be invited to offer a second opinion, supervise the therapist undertaking the voice therapy, work collaboratively with the SLP, and occasionally, take over the management of the case.

Generally, however, it is the SLP who is well placed to conduct a detailed case history and *psychosocial interview*, carry out assessment and diagnosis of the vocal problem, and facilitate aspects of treatment and voice therapy. Here, the primary aims are to assist patients in restoring their voice to as normal as possible and help them come to terms with any residual dysphonia. These objectives are achieved with a combination of *indirect approaches* that emphasise education about vocal health and hygiene, and with more *direct approaches* that draw upon principles of perceptual-motor learning and exercise physiology, designed to assist patients in modifying their vocal behaviours.

Different levels of counselling may be integrated throughout the phases of intervention to support these indirect and direct approaches. In some cases, counselling strategies may play a rather peripheral role and in others, a stronger psychotherapeutic emphasis may be required. To some extent, the priority given to counselling may be influenced by the nature of the voice disorder, but it will also be determined by the clinician's psychological mindedness, his or her attitudes and beliefs about the place of counselling within the scope of practice for SLPs, and the appropriate knowledge, skills, and training in relation to different models of counselling or psychotherapy.

Initially, strategies chosen to facilitate changes in vocal behaviors will be determined by any structural or neurophysiological limitations affecting the patient's respiratory and phonatory systems, their physical and mental health, habitual vocal patterns, and their vocal demands in relation to work, interpersonal and social settings. For professional voice users, particular attention will be given to the more stringent demands of vocal excellence required for maintaining standards in acting or singing performance.

At a deeper level, approaches to intervention will take into account the context of any external and internal psychosocial factors contributing to the onset, maintenance, or aggravation of a voice disorder. Other psychosocial issues may well compound the psychological impact that the voice disorder has been having on an individual. Practitioners from all disciplines have often observed that it is these psychosocial factors that interfere with a patient's motivation to adhere to the lifestyle changes necessary to ensure their vocal health. They may also limit a patient's capacity to engage fully in the behavioural strategies necessary to modify or improve vocal function, or may undermine an individual's resilience and longer-term ways of coping.

During the last decade when the drive for *evidence-based practice (EBP)* in SLP and otolaryngology has been such a strong imperative, there have been few methodologically sound randomised control outcome studies exploring different approaches to the treatment of voice disorders, especially in relation to the broad group of FVD which includes both the psychogenic voice disorder (PVD) and muscle tension voice disorder (MTVD) sub-groups. In the few studies that have compared outcomes between groups where indirect therapy alone, direct behavioural therapy alone, or a combination of these two approaches has been used, evidence suggests that direct approaches to voice therapy do offer patients some benefit. Several excellent systematic reviews evaluating the behavioural treatment of MTVD highlight the most effective studies to date (Eastwood, Madill, & McCabe, 2015; Ruotsalainen, Sellman, Lehto, & Verbeek, 2008; Speyer, 2006).

Somewhat ironically however, with all that we know about psychosocial factors in association with both FVD and OVD, little attention has been paid to interventions that have included different levels of counselling during stages of intervention, or specific *models of counselling* and/or *psychotherapy* that may have been used, either in combination with direct voice therapy, or as the primary intervention. Exceptions to this have been a number of single case reports or case series of patients with PVD (Aronson & Bless, 2009; Baker, 1998, 2003; Demmink-Geertman & Dejonckere, 2010; Hammarberg, 1987; Jacobs & van Biene, 2015; Kollbrunner, Menet, & Seifert, 2010; MacKenzie, Millar, Wilson, Sellars, & Deary, 2001; Sudhir, Chandra, Shivashankar, & Yamini, 2009). Other exceptions include several more rigorous *outcome studies* reporting on cognitive behavior therapy (CBT) in combination with direct voice therapy (Butcher & Elias, 1983; Butcher *et al.*, 2007; Carding, Deary, & Miller, 2013; Daniilidou, Carding, Wilson, Drinnan, & Deary, 2007).

Significantly, little emphasis has been placed upon the role, skills, and qualities of the clinician during the different approaches to intervention, and whether or not the quality of the *therapeutic relationship* may have contributed to, or detracted from, the more readily measured behavioural outcomes. All of these anomalies raise questions about what we mean by terms such as empirical evidence, whether all evidence is quantifiable and if it is not, whether this means that the role and skills of the clinician and/or the patient's qualitative experience of the therapeutic relationship are not relevant to outcomes.

This same drive for EBP has been an essential requirement across all domains of medicine and mental health in recent years, with many researchers and clinicians acknowledging that measurable outcomes of psychotherapy are much more difficult to validate than those involving surgery or medications. This has challenged mental health practitioners to clarify how *treatment* might be distinguished from *therapy*, what is meant by *counselling* or *psychotherapy*, and to explain how psychotherapy works. Although recent functional imaging studies are now providing neurophysiological evidence that psychotherapeutic processes *do* facilitate changes to the brain and behavior, further evidence is being demanded to show *how* psychotherapy works, and whether these changes may be reflected in measurable improvements in the physical and mental well-being of patients seeking help (Aybek *et al.*, 2013; Levy & Ablon, 2010).

Running parallel with this research agenda has been the prodigious production of well over 10,000 texts promoting various models of counselling and psychotherapy that attempt to compare and contrast the relative emphasis given by each model to facilitating changes in cognitive, emotional, or behavioural processes. While there are now several excellent texts for SLP and audiologists advocating counselling as a key component of the therapeutic process across many hearing and communication disorders, little emphasis has been given to disorders of the voice. These texts are listed later in this chapter.

Much of the counselling and psychotherapeutic literature highlights commonalities across the different approaches that include: the *different levels of counselling and psychotherapy* that may take place during the different phases of intervention; a range of essential *skills and strategies* to facilitate change; the *personal qualities* and *clinician behaviours* that can be typically observed in effective therapists; and in some cases, particular features that characterise *master clinicians*. These efforts have culminated in a number of master clinicians seeking to identify the essential *pragmatics of therapeutic practice* (Gibney, 2010). Here, the emphasis has been on teasing out the fundamental tenets underpinning what 'therapy' is all about, and the more elusive features that characterise the nature of the *therapeutic alliance*. It is interesting to note that recent empirical evidence across a range of studies now highlights *the significance of the therapeutic relationship* over and above any particular counselling or psychotherapeutic model being used in enabling individuals to achieve their desired changes. See Fig 9.1.

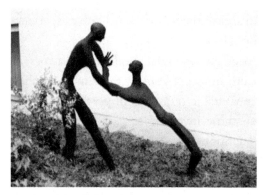

Fig. 9.1 Untitled sculpture outside Psychotherapy Clinic in Bungalor that suggests elements of the therapeutic relationship

With acknowledgment to psychotherapist, Veena Chakravarthy for efforts to find original source

In this and the following chapters I draw together many of these core concepts related to the pragmatics of therapeutic practice in counselling and psychotherapy, and suggest ways in which these may be extrapolated into the clinical management of voice disorders. These constructs are drawn from the counselling and psychotherapy literature in relation to the broad field of mental health, from recent texts and discussion papers mapping out ways for SLP to integrate counselling with disorder-specific interventions for a range of communication disorders, and from the approaches of a number of author/practitioners specialising in the clinical management of voice disorders.

I argue that counselling in relation to both OVD and FVD is not only within the scope of practice for SLPs, it is also our clinical responsibility to undertake the work. This entails counselling to the level of our knowledge, training, and competence whilst recognising too, when it is appropriate to seek supervision, to work in collaboration with others, or to refer on.

In concluding this chapter I propose that offering different levels of counselling, or even holding a *psychotherapeutic state of mind* during the different phases of intervention, may help to create a better psychological space for direct approaches to changing vocal behaviours to be learnt and assimilated. I suggest that in some cases, counselling in relation to the voice disorder will be just as important, if not more so, than the mastery of micro-skills in phonatory movements. In my experience as a clinician, clinical educator, and supervisor of qualified practitioners, I have often observed that the integration of counselling with the essential and necessary traditional voice work elevates the patient's clinical experience from one of *treatment* being administered by a *competent technician* to *therapy* as an interpersonal process in collaboration with a *healing therapist*.

What do we mean by the terms counselling and psychotherapy?

It is an important first step to consider what we mean by the terms counselling and psychotherapy, and what the implications of these differences might be for either SLP or other practitioners integrating the work with direct approaches to voice therapy.

Across some of the literature these terms are used interchangeably. This is notable in many texts introducing theoretical constructs related to different models, and where a range of generic skills and capacities underpinning the practice of counselling and psychotherapy are described. When used interchangeably, the two terms refer to professional activities that utilise an interpersonal relationship to enable people to develop understanding about themselves and to make changes in their lives (Psychotherapy and Counselling Federation of Australia, www.pacfa.org.au, accessed July 17, 2015).

In other settings, different meanings are attributed to the terms *counselling* and *psychotherapy*. To some extent this depends upon the clientele seeking help and the nature of their problems. It also depends upon the underlying theoretical perspectives, qualifications, and training of the professionals involved (Sullivan, 2008). It may be considered that making such distinctions between these terms is somewhat academic, but amongst professionals conducting this important work, the differences do matter. Furthermore, for SLPs considering issues related to scope of practice and the role of counselling in the management of voice disorders, such distinctions are relevant too.

Counselling

In one recent definition, counselling has been defined as *'a professional relationship that empowers diverse individuals, families, and groups to accomplish mental health, wellness, education, and career goals' (Kaplan, Tarvydas, & Gladding, 2014).* This definition was the outcome of a special meeting entitled *"20/20: A Vision for the Future of Counselling"* that was held in Pittsburgh in 2010. It was not intended that this definition would encroach upon the more formal scope of practice elements that would be included for the counselling profession or other professionals engaged in counselling. Rather, the aim of the meeting was to develop a new, concise definition by consensus that could be easily understood by those without a professional background in counselling.

In another definition, *professional counselling* has been defined as 'the application of mental health, psychological, and human development principles through cognitive, affective, behavioural, and systemic intervention strategies that address the wellness, personal growth and career development as well as pathology' (American Counselling Association, 2004). Although this definition refers only to 'counselling', it includes normal, developmental, and more disturbing psychological problems. This suggests that counselling may lie at one end of a continuum and psychotherapy at the other end. Hackney and Cormier (2013) propose that this definition is appropriate to professional counselling across many specific areas of health or education, but that in order to conduct counselling, practitioners would require unique knowledge and training, with advanced skills in communication, assessment, and intervention strategies within the context of the therapeutic relationship.

In a sense, this definition also implies *different forms of counselling* that may be determined by the nature of the service being offered by a particular institution. For instance, at one end of the continuum it may involve helping another by providing information, offering wise advice or guidance. In other situations, it may require practical suggestions about how best to manage a particular problem. Individuals offered these two forms of counselling are sometimes euphemistically referred to as 'the worried well'.

Further along the continuum, counselling may entail helping clients to explore concerns about their feelings, thoughts, and behaviours in response to specific life events and difficulties, and to offer strategies for optional ways of coping. These may be the typical problems of everyday living, troubling interpersonal conflicts, or issues arising in relation to particular medical or mental health conditions. Under these circumstances counsellors with specialist knowledge and expertise may be required to advise on best practice for clinical management, medical treatment, or other forms of intervention, and to help patients come to terms with a particular diagnosis or health condition. Counselling of this nature is likely to be *short-term* with *problem-focussed* or *solution-focussed interventions* directed specifically to the issues at hand. Crago and Gardner (2012) suggest that these models of counselling are more 'instrumental' and action-focussed, where change is expected to occur as a result of the direct interventions of the counsellor.

However, experience shows that some individuals who seek help for what seem to be everyday problems or specific health issues may also reveal marked emotional distress, or may develop psychological problems that interfere with the process of changes being undertaken. Under these circumstances they are more likely to benefit from deeper psychological work where it is more helpful to construe counselling as 'an interpersonal process in which clients can change, not as a result of the counsellor's direct interventions (doing) but as a result of the way the counsellor is with them (being)' (Crago & Gardner, 2012) (p. 10).

Psychotherapy

'But at heart, the personal exchange defines psychotherapy. All else flows from it'
(Marzillier, 2004) (p. 394).

As originally proposed by Freud and Jung, this deeper psychological work
with the primary aim of healing the psyche entails exploration, awareness, and
acceptance of the unconscious workings of the mind. As these processes become
more transparent and consciously acknowledged through the use of language,
healing and change can take place. This 'talking cure', or 'psychoanalysis'
as initially proposed by Freud and Jung, was undertaken in the context of a
significant, non-judgmental relationship where the dynamics of *transference* and
countertransference could be played out. This emphasis on helping the 'unconscious
to become conscious' with attention to the 'here and now' *psychodynamics of the
therapeutic relationship* has become the hallmark distinction made by mental
health professionals between counselling and psychotherapy (Crago, 2000).

The significance attributed to the nature and quality of the therapeutic
relationship has also been exemplified in the work of Carl Rogers (Rogers, 1951,
1961, 1980) and that of many counselling and psychotherapy practitioners who
have followed (Corey, 2012; Crago & Gardner, 2012; Egan, 2009; Geldard &
Geldard, 2009; Sullivan, 2008; I.D. Yalom, 2002). Rogers supported the original
premise of Freud and Jung that troubling behaviours and attitudes are often
symptomatic of deeper psychological conflicts, but in the development of his
person-centered models of counselling, he paid less attention to unconscious
mental processes. He also distanced himself from the medical model, and
maintained that many people seeking help with emotional and interpersonal
problems were not necessarily psychologically sick or suffering severe mental
illness.

At the same time he challenged the more didactic forms of counselling and
behaviourist approaches that advocated direct instrumental interventions from
therapists in the form of education, advice, or strategies, and argued it was not
the task of the therapist to change client behavior. Rather, it was the therapist's
job to create the psychological space for individuals to explore and discover what
needed to be changed. Carl Rogers proposed that this could take place within
the context of 'a significantly influential relationship', and that in this setting
clients would be capable of finding their own solutions. He believed that if the
therapist could offer this different type of relationship, the client would be able
'to discover within himself the capacity to use that relationship for growth and
change, and personal development will occur' (Rogers, 1961) (p.33).

This relationship was typically 'non-directive' and was characterised by 'non-possessive warmth', 'unconditional positive regard', and 'an accepting and non-judgmental stance'. While he and many others who followed acknowledged some differences between counselling and psychotherapy, they also observed that at advanced levels of training and practice there is considerable overlap, and that it is difficult to distinguish intensive and effective counselling from intensive and equally successful psychotherapy. The essence of this co-operative relationship and the duality of purpose and effort are captured most effectively in Robin Halliday's sculpture entitled *Dyad* as shown in Figure 9.2.

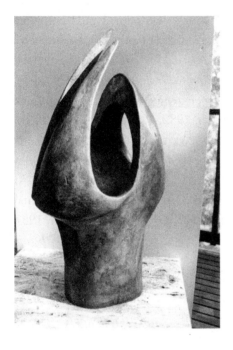

Fig. 9.2 "Diad" by Robin Holliday, PhD., FRS, FAA

"Diad represents two individuals maintaining a sociologically significant relationship, or two persons involved in an ongoing relationship or interaction".

Courtesy of Lily Huschtscha and Collection Galeria Aniela (art@galeriaaniela.com.au)

Are counselling and psychotherapy different and if so how?

In the interesting discussions devoted to the question of whether or not there is a difference between counselling and psychotherapy, Crago *et al.* (2000; 2012) have challenged a number of assumptions about some of the seemingly opposing factors that are often used to distinguish between these different ways of helping. These may include: the giving of advice, information, and education versus non-directive exploration; working with the 'worried well' rather than those with psychological adjustment problems or psychological illness; a focus on conscious psychological processes versus emphasis on subconscious or unconscious processes; coaching towards change versus the therapist-client relationship as a means to facilitate new awareness and behaviour; and judicious sharing of the self by the therapist versus total therapeutic neutrality, etc. Rather than denigrating one approach over another, these authors argue that there is a place for each of the constructs in the practice of both counselling and psychotherapy, albeit with different emphases for particular problems or at different stages within the helping process. These are important considerations for clinicians undertaking voice work.

Crago (2000) proposes a continuum along which the training and clinical practice of several different models of counselling and psychotherapy might be placed. He suggests that the following models of therapy would be placed towards the counselling end of the continuum: mainstream *behaviourist approaches, psycho-educational*, and *cognitive behaviour models of therapy* (Beck, 1979; Beck & Weishaar, 2014); *problem solving therapies* (Egan, 2009, 2014) (Geldard & Geldard, 2009); *motivational interviewing* (W. R. Miller & Rollnick, 2013); *brief solution-focused therapy* (de Shazer, 1982, 1985, 1988; Papp, 1983); *narrative therapy* (Freedman & Combs, 1996; White, 1995, 2011; White & Epston, 1990); and some *structural and strategic models of family therapy* (Hayley, 1971; Minuchin, 1974).

He suggests that the Bowenian and Milan schools of family therapy may occupy an intermediate position (Boscolo, Cecchin, Hoffman, & Penn, 1987; Winek, 2010), and that the *relational, humanistic*, and *existential models of therapy* would be placed at the psychotherapeutic end of the continuum. These would include the *psychoanalytic therapies* of Freud and Jung and neo Freudians such as Anna Freud (1954); the *humanistic models* of counselling as developed in the early work of Rogers (1951) and Egan (1997); the *existential psychotherapies* of practitioners such as Yalom (1970; 1989, 2002); and their own model of *relational psychotherapy* as described in *A Safe Place for Change* (Crago & Gardner, 2012).

In seeking to draw a line between the two different ways of helping, Crago (2000) suggests that *counselling* is more like a 'close-up' view of a particular image in a picture where prominence in the therapeutic work is given to *the problem*. From this perspective, facilitating changes in thoughts, feelings, and behaviours is likely to be achieved through *giving information*, psycho-educational insights, and *implementation of strategies*.

Alternatively, *psychotherapy* may be construed as a 'long-shot' view, with emphasis given to the wider context of which the problem is a part, such as the individual's gender, early family history, and social context. Crago suggests that in taking this wider view, *the therapeutic relationship* becomes more important as the vehicle of change, and that 'it is ultimately *the person of the therapist* which will be efficacious and internalised, regardless of the stance she takes, and/or the information she provides' (Crago, 2000; p. 78). It is within the context of this significant relationship that the therapist must be able to name the 'here-and-now' processes related to the psychodynamics of the therapeutic relationship, and help the client to understand this in the context of his or her unconscious processes related to earlier relationships. This skill of '*immediacy*' in relation to transference and counter-transference issues may only achieved with more advanced levels of training, and is the key distinguishing feature of psychotherapy (Crago & Gardner, 2012).

In a later discussion paper that expands upon differences between these *content and problem-based approaches of counselling* versus the *process and relationally-based psychotherapies*, Crago (2012) draws upon insights about the distinctive but inter-related functions of the left and right hemispheres of the brain as proposed by McGilchrist (2009).

In his text *The Master and his Emissary*, McGilchrist writes from the perspectives of recent brain imaging research, Western art and literature, philosophy, psychology, and psychiatry to show how the two hemispheres may process data and function differently.

Crago suggests that the neurophysiological distinctions between the two hemispheres may offer a helpful 'evidence-based explanation' that can account for the differences between the disciplines of *psychology* versus *counselling and psychotherapy*, and may give further support to his proposed distinctions between *counselling* and *psychotherapy*. Here, he suggests that the more scientific field of psychology that gives attention to particular parts, with an emphasis on the analysis, categorisation, and synthesis of these parts into a whole, derives more strongly from *left hemisphere dominance*. Models of counselling reflecting these psychological processes are more likely to be content-driven, problem- or solution-focussed, with therapist interventions emphasising strategies for action and behavioural change. Crago suggests that while these pragmatic approaches can be very effective, and that operationally defined outcomes are more amenable to measurement, some of the risks may be an undue adherence to diagnostic criteria, emphasis on symptoms and disorders rather than the person, and *recipe book approaches* to treatment that can seem rather prescriptive and depersonalised. For SLP in general and those working in the specialty of *Vocology*, these warnings are most apt.

In contrast, the more process-driven and relational models of psychotherapy tend to reflect phenomena related to the *right hemisphere*. Typically, functions of the right hemisphere enable an awareness of the whole, as well as individual parts, 'to perceive patterns and inter-relationships, to embrace apparent contradiction, to recognise metaphor and symbol, and to respond to them in kind' (Crago, 2012) (p.63). Extending these notions into the context of effective relational psychotherapy, he then proposes that it is essential for the two hemispheres to work together for the development of rational thought and understanding. 'In its true sense rationality is a product of *both* hemispheres operating together, and not something we arrive at by dismissing the evidence of our senses, emotions, and relationships, or isolating ourselves in a tight little world of logical propositions'. He argues that: 'It is not a question of rational reality-oriented left hemisphere (Freud's conscious) that 'tames' an irrational right hemisphere which thinks in pictorial terms (Freud's 'unconscious). Instead *both* hemispheres are conscious' (p. 62). From this perspective, details, symptoms, and pathologies certainly need to be named and recognised, but they are better understood in relation to the wider context.

In highlighting the relative strengths of the more pragmatic approaches to counselling for some clients, or the more relational approaches of psychotherapy for others, Crago (2012) stresses that the therapist's personality may be better suited to one way of helping as opposed to another, and that attention needs to be given to the matching of client and therapist accordingly. He concludes that regardless of any particular theoretical model, it will be the quality of the therapeutic relationship that is the 'primary vehicle of change', and that it is not so much the model, techniques or strategies used but 'what happens has more to do with the counsellor's *way of being with* the client' (p. 64).

When considering these notions in relation to the SLP working with voice, I suggest there is a place for both perspectives, with the 'close-up' view giving detailed focus to the problem and the 'long-shot' view giving primacy to wider contextual factors. This would apply at the very beginning when we draw upon information from laryngeal examination using the rigid endoscope for exquisite details related to the vocal fold structures, and then the flexible scope with stroboscopy for a more functional view during different phonatory activities. Similarly, in relation to intervention, approaches to direct voice therapy and counselling may well focus on the problem with emphasis on solutions, strategies for action, advice, and education. However, this would not preclude aspects of the 'long-shot' view as described by Crago that foster sensitivity to wider contextual factors relevant to the individual, or the therapist reflecting upon the effectiveness of the therapeutic alliance. As emphasised in the discussions about the different functions of the left and right hemispheres, and the potential for both 'close-up' and 'long-shot' views, what matters most is the capacity of therapists with their clients to integrate the two (Crago, 2012; McGilchrist, 2009).

Professional concerns about counselling in relation to communication disorders

In setting out to discuss ways in which counselling may enrich the therapeutic experience for individuals with voice disorders and contribute to more effective outcomes, it is relevant to mention several concerns that continue to plague our profession. These are inevitably raised by fledgling SLP students but just as often by experienced clinicians, academics, professional associations, and sometimes, by practitioners from other mental health disciplines. Authors have recently identified a number of limiting perspectives and barriers that may be contributing to some SLPs being reluctant to embrace counselling as a natural component of their professional responsibility (DiLollo & Neimeyer, 2014; Fourie, 2011b; Holland, 2007) (see Box 9.1).

Box 9.1 Myths, misconceptions & barriers in relation to counselling for SLP

- Counselling is only the province of mental health professionals
- Counselling infers psychopathology and this is not the SLP's domain
- Behavioural principles in facilitating change are sufficient
- Counselling is something done in addition to, or after 'proper therapy'
- Counselling is outside the job description and brief of the SLP
- Constraints of managed care limit the clinician's time for counselling
- Training in SLP is insufficient for competent practice in counselling
- Counselling is often only included at the end of disorder-specific topics
- Students are not taught *how* counselling is used to help resolve problems confronting people with communication disorders

(Extrapolated from Holland, 2007 and Di Lollo & Neimeyer, 2014)

Box 9.2 Questions about counselling raised by SLP

- Does counselling or psychotherapy fall within our scope of practice?
- Is the education & training in counselling sufficient in SLP programmes?
- Is counselling or psychotherapy an evidence-based intervention?
- What is the aim of counselling in relation to communication disorders?

These concerns have generated a number of questions related to *scope of practice* issues. They centre around the rights of the SLP to engage in counselling activities with patients or their families with communication disorders, including those with voice disorders. Some of these questions are shown in Box 9.2 and are discussed below.

Scope of practice

For some clinicians, this immediately raises questions previously mentioned at the beginning of this chapter with respect to professional boundaries, and whether or not it is appropriate for SLP to undertake counselling in conjunction with disorder-specific interventions across a range of communication disorders. These scope of practice issues have been thoroughly addressed by several author/practitioners (DiLollo & Neimeyer, 2014; Fourie, 2011b; Holland, 2007) with reference to mandates from professional association bodies such as the American Association of Speech-Language and Hearing Association (ASHA, 2007). For instance, in the current *Scope of Practice* document, counselling is recognised as an essential part of the SLP responsibilities, and is regarded as integral to the process of assisting families and children with speech, language, voice, and hearing disorders, and adults with similarly acquired disorders. The clinician's responsibilities include counselling individuals, families, co-workers, educators, and others in the community regarding acceptance, adaptation, and decision making about communication and swallowing disorders.

Furthermore, in the *Preferred Practice Patterns for the Profession of Speech-Language Pathology (ASHA 2004)* document it is emphasised that counselling should be conducted by appropriately credentialed and trained SLP 'providing timely information and guidance to patients/clients, families/caregivers, and other relevant persons about the nature of the communication or swallowing disorders, the course of interventions, ways to enhance outcomes, coping with disorders, and prognosis'.

Similarly, the Audiology *Scope of Practice* documents from ASHA recommend that counselling by audiologists should address the communicative and behavioural adjustment problems associated with auditory disorders, and the ways in which these difficulties may be impacting on the overall psychosocial well-being of the patients and their family members. These principles are reflected in the *Scope of Practice* documents from Speech Pathology Australia (2015), where counselling in relation to communication disorders, swallowing disorders, and therapy is integral to speech pathology practice, with emphasis on 'holistic patient care and management, considering all aspects of the individual's life and well-being' (p.8).

Limitations to scope of practice

In addition to clear statements about the counselling role and responsibilities of the SLP, it is implicit in these professional association documents that where *pre-existing psychopathology* appears to be having an adverse effect on a person, or where mental health issues have arisen in response to communication disorders, consulting with a *mental health professional* would be essential. In cases where an SLP might choose to undertake this deeper relational work, this would *only* be appropriate if he or she had an *advanced level training* and the recognised qualifications to practise psychotherapy. These stipulations and limitations to scope of practice are strongly set out in all texts in the field devoted to the application of counselling to communication disorders.

In multidisciplinary settings that foster a team approach, the SLP may seek *mentoring, co-therapy* or *supervision* from mental health colleagues, or may recommend referral for psychiatric evaluation and intervention (Nichol, Morrison, & Rammage, 1993). However, this also requires that practitioners have sufficient knowledge, skills, and experience to be sensitive to the emotional or psychological distress of their patients, to recognise how more serious mental health issues may be impacting on the individual with a communication or voice disorder, and to instigate timely referral for expert psychological or psychiatric opinion in these situations (DiLollo & Neimeyer, 2014; Holland, 2007).

Adequacy of education and training

Despite the strong mandates from professional bodies advocating different levels of counselling as integral to our professional role, there is also a general consensus that the *education and training in counselling* for SLP is inadequate (Phillips & Mendel, 2008). This mismatch between scope of policy statements and clinical training curricula may explain why some clinicians feel ill-equipped to draw upon skills in counselling, or may be reluctant to enter into a counselling relationship with their patients. This discrepancy is further exacerbated by some of the limiting attitudes and barriers, mentioned earlier in this chapter, that continue to constrain some therapists from engaging in this important work, or from undertaking further training to advance their skills in these areas (DiLollo & Neimeyer, 2014; Holland, 2007). These authors are adamant that education and training for SLP at both undergraduate and post-graduate levels needs to address such deficiencies more effectively. However, despite the ongoing barriers, the authors state very firmly that counselling in relation to communication disorders *is* the professional domain of the SLP and needs to be consciously integrated into all of our work.

This has led a number of practitioners to emphasise the need for academic curricula to provide designated coursework focussed upon different models of counselling and psychotherapy, with appropriate allocation of time and space for the development and clinical practice of generic counselling skills in relation to communication and related disorders (Geller & Foley, 2009; Iwarsson, 2015; Kaderavek, Laux, & Mills, 2004; Riley, 2002). In the field of medicine, similar calls for curricula to focus upon the importance of the physician-patient relationship and sensitivity to the role of emotions in relation to illness are also being made (Cohn, 2001; Schoenberg & Yakeley, 2014).

The firm distinctions continually being made between *counselling in relation to communication disorders* and *professional counselling* or p*sychotherapy* (Flasher & Fogle, 2012) have prompted many practitioners to seek advanced qualifications in these disciplines. This reflects the profession's increasing awareness of the highly sensitive nature of many psychosocial issues associated with many communication disorders, and the need for a more holistic approach to clinical management. While these calls for additional education and training have been for the profession as a whole, a number of practitioners specialising in voice disorders have been advocating for clinicians to avail themselves of more advanced training for many years (Aronson, 1990; Baker, 1998, 2008, 2010; Butcher *et al.*, 2007; Cavalli, 2009; Deary & Miller, 2011; Elias, Raven, Butcher, & Littlejohns, 1989; Parkinson & Rae, 1996; Rammage, 2011; Rammage, Morrison, & Nichol, 2001; Shewell, 1998, 2009).

In summarising these prevailing issues over scope of practice, professional territoriality, education, and training, I am once again drawn to the previously cited discussion paper by Hugh Crago (2000). In this challenging paper he reminds us that while psychiatrists and psychologists undertake the professional functions of counselling and psychotherapy, so too do practitioners from other professions such as nursing, teaching, and the ministry. He suggests that counselling and psychotherapy should be seen as 'a specific set of skills and understandings which may be practised across many different helping professions, rather than being 'owned by' any one of them' (p.74). Going one step further he writes: 'Despite its increasingly vocal insistence that it is the sole occupant of the territory, the discipline of psychology does not own counselling and psychotherapy, nor counselling and psychotherapy training' (p. 74). This point of view is both refreshing and affirming for our profession and for other practitioners specialising in voice. It strongly endorses my own perspective.

Counselling and psychotherapy as evidence-based interventions

Another burning issue amongst SLPs has been whether or not counselling or psychotherapy meet the criteria for empirically supported interventions. In the current climate of imperatives for evidence-based practice (EBP) against a background of managed care, medical model thinking, and tick-the-box clinical competencies during therapist training, the concerns are pertinent.

These questions have led to a number of lively and passionate discussions amongst academics and clinicians, during which they continue to reflect upon rather narrow interpretations of what was originally meant by EBP, and whether randomised control trials (RCT) alone adequately capture what is involved in the therapeutic processes of 'treatments' such as counselling and psychotherapy (DiLollo & Neimeyer, 2014; Levy & Ablon, 2010; S. D. Miller *et al.*, 2014; Sullivan, 2008). These authors acknowledge that RCTs are considered to be the gold standard for intervention and outcome studies, but they also emphasise how this methodology fails to account for what is happening 'in between'. It misses out on how this result was achieved, with whom, under what circumstances, and why the change took place. Furthermore, when the contribution of the therapeutic relationship is taken into account, they suggest that an effective outcome may be as much to do with the person of the therapist, as the models or strategies used. In order to understand these factors that are so much more difficult to quantify, the authors cited above have also urged practitioners to consider qualitative methodologies that would enable these interpersonal processes, along with the meanings attributed to them, to be explored more effectively.

Several decades of research have clearly established the efficacy of different models of counselling and psychotherapy as bona fide treatments (Duncan, Miller, Wampold, & Hubble, 2010; Levy & Ablon, 2010; Wampold, 2001). Somewhat paradoxically, the findings from several meta-analyses of numerous outcome studies have revealed that no particular model of counselling or psychotherapy is any more effective than another, and that hallmark strategies and techniques of particular models only account for between 5–15% of the variance (Beutler & Harwood, 2002). Other findings have shown that the *quality of the therapeutic relationship* and the *therapist's way of being* are the more significant factors in determining outcomes. As a consequence of these trends, more recent efforts to substantiate the effectiveness of counselling and psychotherapy have focused on *principles of therapy* and the *person of the therapist*, rather than particular theories, models, and techniques.

In the field of neuroscience, recent functional imaging studies are revealing neural correlates of mental disorders such as anxiety and depression, and there is now clear neurophysiological evidence for changes in the brain in response to psychotherapy. In a fascinating overview of this field of research, Roffman and Gerber (2010) discuss the evidence for changes in the brain that have been demonstrated with both interpersonal therapy and medications, or when comparing different therapeutic models with one another such as cognitive behavior therapy (CBT) and psychodynamic psychotherapy. They also refer to several studies exploring the more discrete interpersonal processes such as *empathy*, where specific neurophysiological changes have been shown to take place in the *insula* and *anterior cingulate cortex* (Lamm, Batson, & Decety, 2007; Shamay-Tsoory, H., & Chisin, 2005; Singer, 2006). This capacity to be empathic is closely aligned with the constructs related to 'the quality of therapeutic relationship' and the therapist's 'way of being' that play a pivotal role in effective counselling and psychotherapy (Crago, 2012; Etkin, Pittenger, Polan, & Kandel, 2005; Fuchs, 2004).

The evidence leading to a meta-model of therapy-assisted change

In response to a number of meta-analyses of any common factors likely to facilitate change in counselling and psychotherapy, Fife *et al.* (2014) recently highlighted the following elements: the *effective presentation of knowledge*, *application of techniques and strategies* pertinent to the particular problem; the *hope, trust, expectancy*, and *motivation* of the client; the *therapeutic alliance* between client and therapist; *therapist confidence*; and the therapist's *way of being*. On the basis of these findings, theauthors have recently proposed *a meta-model* to reflect the trends represented in the form of *The Therapeutic Pyramid* (Fig. 9.3).

The model incorporates features, previously identified throughout the literature, known to contribute to positive therapeutic outcomes, and gives emphasis to three key elements shown to be the most influential: *skills and techniques*; *the quality of the therapeutic alliance*; and the therapist's *way of being*. The authors propose a hierarchical inter-relationship between these three factors, 'where essential skills and techniques are seen to rest upon the therapeutic relationship, and these in turn, are both grounded in 'the way of being' of the therapist' (p 22). While the primary focus is on the clinical relevance of this meta-model, consideration is also given to training and research implications.

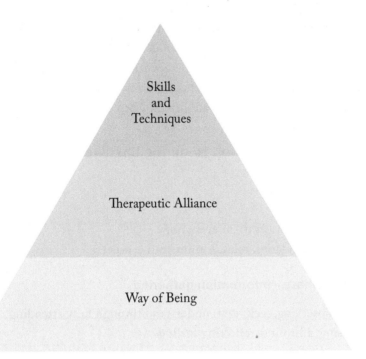

Fig. 9.3 The therapeutic pyramid (Fife et al., 2014)

Reproduced courtesy Wiley

Skills and techniques

The Therapeutic Pyramid places skills and techniques at the apex, indicating that these elements will be embedded in and supported by those aspects that lie below. The authors refer to a number of meta-analyses of outcome studies for marital and family therapy, where only 5–15% of the variance was accounted for by specific model-based skills and techniques (Beutler & Harwood, 2002; Wampold, 2001). Fife *et al.* (2014) suggest that while these figures may lead clinicians to be dubious about the value of technical skills and strategies, it would be a mistake to underestimate their importance. Rather, they argue that the academic and clinical training across different models of family therapy is built upon strong foundations of knowledge and skills appropriate to working with individuals and families in distress. They propose further that provided there is a credible rationale for intervention in relation to a client's concerns or symptoms, then the judicious implementation of specific strategies remains both necessary and important. They urge practitioners to acknowledge 'that theoretical and technical mastery is therapeutic when grounded in factors related to the therapeutic alliance and the therapist's way of being' (p. 23). These are important considerations for practitioners incorporating counselling into traditional voice therapy approaches; the way in which this may be done will be addressed in Chapters 10–12. Many counselling skills and strategies that may be undertaken across the different therapeutic models have been described in detail throughout the literature, including texts devoted to counselling for communication disorders. Examples are listed in Box 9.3.

Box 9.3 Technical skills involved during the different stages of counselling

1. Initial phase

- Joining, conveying warmth, interest, hope
- Establishing boundaries, roles, administrative aspects

2. Exploration phase – information gathering

- Listening, observing, seeking to understand through fully attending
- Empathising, affirming, reflecting feelings
- Clarifying ideas, attitudes, beliefs, concerns with closed and open-ended questions
- Externalising the problem, reframing
- Summarising and contracting for changes in thinking, feelings, behaviours

3. Action phase

- Informing, explaining, teaching, advising
- Planning, setting goals, developing options
- Motivating, directing, suggesting options to achieve desired changes
- Recognizing and dealing with grief, restraints to change, confronting, challenging
- Use of the self and self-disclosure

4. Closing phase

- Consolidating, generalizing, evaluating gains
- Reflecting upon what has transpired, including therapeutic relationship
- Referring on, seeking second opinion, supervision where appropriate
- Ending therapy

(Corey, 2012; Crago & Gardner, 2012; DiLollo & Neimeyer, 2014; Egan, 2009; Fourie, 2011b; Gibney, 2010; Holland, 2007; Rhodes & Wallis, 2011; Rogers, 1961; Sullivan, 2008)

The therapeutic relationship and the therapeutic alliance

In the second part of *The Therapeutic Pyramid*, Fife *et al.* give emphasis to the importance of the *therapeutic relationship*, which refers to 'the feelings and attitudes the therapy participants have toward one another and the manner in which these are expressed' (Gelso & Samtag, 2008) (p.268). Integral to this relationship are influences from the client and the particular issues being brought to therapy, and the ways of relating between the therapist and client which include the *working alliance* and the *personal qualities of the therapist* (Fife *et al.*, 2014).

The *working alliance* accounts for approximately 50% of therapist-driven influences and it is the most important factor likely to determine outcomes (Zuroff, Kelly, Leybman, Blatt, & Wampold, 2010). It reflects the moment-to-moment attitude of the therapist towards the client and the collaboration that takes place as they reach a consensus about goals for change and how these might be achieved. Essentially, the working alliance includes 'all of the actions and conscious intentions of the participants that pertain directly to getting the work of therapy accomplished' (Gelso, 2009) (p. 257). Factors shown to contribute to the strength and effectiveness of the therapeutic alliance are listed in Box 9.4.

Box 9.4 Factors that determine the effectiveness of the working alliance

- Interpersonal liking, trust and respect
- Compatibility and congruence in attitudes, beliefs and world view
- Strength of the bond and attachment that develops in committing to the work
- The therapist's style of relating
- The ability of the therapist to communicate about relational issues

(Extrapolated from Fife *et al.*, 2014)

Fife *et al.* refer to numerous studies demonstrating that the personal qualities of the therapist directly contribute to the strength of the therapeutic alliance. This highlights the deeply personal nature of therapy, and that the person of the therapist is a major influence in shaping his or her professional role as counsellor or psychotherapist.

Gelso (2009) offers further support for this notion in a most interesting discussion paper about the psychotherapeutic relationship. Here, he proposes that the therapeutic relationship comprises three components: the *transference/ counter-transference* configuration, the *working alliance*, and the *real relationship*. Gelso suggests that the *real relationship* operates from the moment the therapist and client meet, and is not necessarily dependent upon the working alliance or embedded in transference/counter-transference issues. It is characterised by 'realism' and 'genuineness' and may be defined as 'the personal relationship existing between two or more people as reflected in the degree to which each is genuine with the other and perceives and experiences the other in ways that befit the other' (p. 255). Empirical data from his study show that the strength of the real relationship is more likely to predict treatment progress than the working alliance, therapist empathy, or client-therapist attachment patterns. Findings from an earlier study also indicated that *self-disclosure* on the part of the therapist strengthened the real relationship by permitting clients to appreciate their therapists as more real and human (Knox, Hess, Petersen, & Hill, 1997).

Therapist self-disclosure is generally viewed with concern as this may 'violate client-therapist boundaries' and may be seen to be self-serving or even manipulative (Audet, 2011). However, in some cases it may also remove barriers and in my experience, judicious self-disclosure can enhance the real relationship and strengthen the working alliance with positive therapeutic outcomes. Several clinical examples of therapist self-disclosure to the benefit of the client are given in Chapters 10–12.

Personal qualities of the therapist and the therapist's way of being

The third part of *The Therapeutic Pyramid* refers to particular *personal qualities* of the clinician and the therapist's *way of being*. This is considered to be the bedrock for most aspects of effective therapy (Fife *et al.*, 2014).

In developing this third level of the model, Fife *et al.* refer to the early work of Martin Buber (1958), who differentiated between those who relate to others with an *I-It* frame of mind and those who relate with an *I-Thou* philosophical stance. As proposed by Buber, the *I-It* orientation makes us more likely to view another as an object, or as belonging to a category. Alternatively, the *I-Thou* stance opens the therapist to the reality of 'the other', and to appreciate that this person has thoughts, feelings, and aspirations unique to his or her circumstances. Other practitioners refer to features such as placing of the client's needs as the foremost consideration, the humanity of the therapist, and the authenticity of a real relationship, all of which are conveyed to the client through attitude, tone of voice, body language, and overall demeanour.

As defined most effectively by Anderson (2006), 'the therapist's 'way of being' conveys to the other that they are valued as a unique human being and not as a category or people; that they have something worthy of saying and hearing; that you meet them without prior judgment' (p. 44). Fife *et al.* (2014) propose that a therapist's 'way of being' is not model-dependent, and while it might appear to play a more prominent role in the humanistic and relational therapies, it is just as important for practitioners in those models of counselling and psychotherapy that give emphasis to skills, strategies, and more instrumental interventions. This view was recently endorsed by the phoniatrician Jürgen Wendler in a keynote address at PEVOC in which he reflected upon changes taking place in approaches to voice therapy over the last century. On the basis of his extensive experience he concluded 'it is not the method that makes the difference, but the person who uses it, if several methods are in use for the same purpose' (Wendler, 2015) (p.62).

In addition to the therapist's *way of being*, Fife *et al.* distinguish other features that also shape the '*self of the therapist*', such as gender, race, cultural, and religious or educational factors. Therefore, in order to maintain a humane and responsible *I-Thou* stance, the therapist needs to remain vigilant about his/her own attitudes, beliefs, and potential for bias, to be self-reflective about any power differential and his/her contribution to the therapeutic process, and to act responsibly by undertaking appropriate supervision (Whiting, Oka, & Fife, 2012). Some of the personal qualities and 'ways of being' of competent therapists, and other features that are recognised in master clinicians are shown in Box 9.5.

Box 9.5 Personal qualities & 'ways of being' of competent therapists* & master clinicians**

Affective

- Warm, compassionate, sensitive, empathic, understanding and kind*
- Genuine, emotionally stable, integrated, positive, confident, inspiring*
- Express feelings appropriately and effectively*
- Emotionally aware of self and others**
- Prepared to work on one's own emotional well-being" **
- Overall affect reflecting graciousness and 'restorative poise'**

Relational

- Good interpersonal communication especially about relational issues*
- Respectful, trustworthy, generates a strong working alliance**
- Not afraid to deal with difficult emotions, including their own**
- Accept responsibility for actions**
- Seek and accept feedback, and deal with conflict**

Cognitive

- Understanding, open-minded, non-judgmental, accepting fair, flexible*
- Erudite, and able to explain complex issues easily*
- Lifelong learners who draw on practical and reflective experience**
- Values cognitive complexity and ambiguity**
- Highly observant and also intuitive**
- Deep knowledge of their field and practiced in doing the work**

(Extrapolated from Egan, 2009; Fife, Whiting, Bradford, & Davis, 2014; Fourie, 2011b; S. D. Miller, Hubble, Chow, & Seidel, 2014; Rogers, 1961; Sullivan, 2008)

Fife and colleagues propose that the 'personal qualities', 'ways of being' and 'self of the therapist', work together to create a strong foundation for the working alliance and a therapeutic relationship that is warm, compassionate, and non-judgmental. They argue just as strongly that there is a real place for *knowledge* and *proficiency in skills* and techniques, depending upon the problems being faced. Successful therapy is thus dependent upon the way in which a therapist attends to these three levels, recognising that at times the emphasis of the work may be more on one level than another. It is the ongoing interaction between these three key elements that fosters effective therapeutic outcomes. *The Therapeutic*

Pyramid, along with many of the interesting issues raised by Crago *et al.* (2000; 2012) as discussed in Chapter 9, provides a useful platform for us to consider how different levels of counselling along the helping continuum might be legitimately undertaken by the SLP or voice practitioner in conjunction with traditional voice therapy.

The aims of counselling in relation to voice and other communication disorders

In the sections below I refer to a number of general principles underpinning the aims and objectives that are common to many models of counselling and that may be appropriate for an integrated approach to the treatment of communication disorders, including disorders of the voice. These have been drawn from the counselling and psychotherapeutic literature, the voice therapy literature where many practitioners have strongly advocated for the judicious integration of counselling with direct approaches to voice therapy, and several excellent texts that offer a comprehensive account of ways in which the SLP may integrate counselling with communication disorders in general. These texts are listed in Box 9.6.

Box 9.6 Texts devoted to counselling in relation to communication disorders

1. Applications of Counseling in Speech-Language Pathology and Audiology (Crowe, 1997)
2. Psychology of Voice Disorders (Rosen & Sataloff, 1997)
3. Counseling in Communication Disorders (Holland, 2007)
4. Understanding and treating psychogenic voice disorder: A CBT framework (Butcher, Elias, & Cavalli, 2007)
5. Counselling persons with communication disorders and their families (D. M. Luterman, 2008)
6. Therapeutic Processes for Communication Disorders (Fourie, 2011b)
7. Counselling Skills for Speech-Language Pathologists and Audiologists (Flasher & Fogle, 2012);
8. Counseling in Speech-Language Pathology and Audiology (DiLollo & Neimeyer, 2014)

Counselling enhances the experience of speech-language therapy

'Appropriate counseling greatly increases the opportunity for an optimal outcome for clients, whether this involves resolving a specific disorder or maximizing quality of life by means of coping and adjustment techniques' (Holland, 2007) (p.1).

In all the texts cited above, the authors emphasise the way in which advanced knowledge of and training in generic counselling skills adds to and enriches the experience of therapy for the patient or client, and expands upon the therapist's pre-existing disorder-specific knowledge and approaches to intervention. It is appropriate for clients of all ages and across all stages of the *family life cycle*. There is no sense that counselling is recommended as a substitute for traditional SLP treatment, or that it is intended to supplant skills, techniques, and strategies appropriate to specific disorder groups. Rather, the purpose of integrating counselling with SLP approaches is intended to enhance the patient's experience by: improving their knowledge about their condition; understanding the clinician's rationale for the interventions being recommended; helping them to be open to making changes; and supporting them in embracing alternative ways of coping. This perspective reflects that of Fife *et al.* (2012), as shown in their *Therapeutic Pyramid*, where skills and techniques pertaining to particular models of counselling are seen as 'essential but not necessarily sufficient', and are more likely to be successful if based upon relational aspects of the therapeutic process with attention to the therapeutic alliance and the therapist's 'way of being'.

Of course the primary objective of counselling is for the benefit of the client seeking assistance. However, it is evident from reports of therapists that their experience of the process is also deeply affecting. Fourie (2011a) has highlighted how 'meaningful dialogue' in the context of an equal and mutual therapeutic relationship process becomes transformative for both client and therapist. Christina Shewell (1998) has described this process as being like a travelling companion of the person dealing with his or her communication disorder, where the therapist benefits from this journey as much as the client. It has often been my experience that each journey is unique, often fun as well as purposeful and serious, and we are never quite sure where it may take us both.

Counselling draws upon existing skills, strengths, insights, and resilience

Another interesting phenomenon is that most patients presenting with communication disorders do not generally present with a serious psychopathology that meets the criteria for psychiatric diagnosis. As highlighted in Chapter 6 of this book, individuals with voice disorders may present with elevated levels of anxiety, emotional maladjustment and vulnerability to tensional or somatic symptoms, and low mood but again, these may not meet the threshold for clinical diagnosis (Baker, 2008; Baker, Ben-Tovim, Butcher, Esterman, & McLaughlin, 2013). They are more likely to be individuals who have been dealing with normal life stresses reasonably well, at least up until the onset of their condition. For these reasons, a number of voice therapists advocate positive solution-focused approaches to counselling such as cognitive behaviour therapy (CBT). This enables clients and their families to recognise their psychological and emotional strengths and to draw upon these resources to sustain their motivation in attempting new ways of thinking, feeling, or behaving (Butcher *et al.*, 2007; Deary & Miller, 2011; O'Hara, Miller, Carding, Wilson, & Deary, 2011). Counselling assists clients to harness these same strengths and insights to develop their *resilience*, and to learn more *effective ways of coping* with the voice problem. In the longer term this integrated process is intended to help patients improve their quality of life and achieve their lifelong aspirations (DiLollo & Neimeyer, 2014; Holland, 2007).

Counselling enables clients to grieve what may have been lost

For many individuals with voice and other communication disorders, emotional reactions of grief, fear, anger, confusion, or even resentment are often at the forefront, especially during the early phases of assessment. These negative emotions can block a person's concentration or diminish their ability to hear information or recommendations for change. Counselling helps to create the psychological space for these activities to be effective (Shewell, 1998).

David Luterman (2011) proposes that one of the key purposes of counsellling is to assist a person in *grieving what may have been lost* as a result of his or her communication difficulty. He also emphasises that clients may be 'emotionally upset' but not necessarily 'emotionally disturbed', and that the experience of painful feelings and grief is an inevitable and normal response 'when confronted with a life challenge for which there is no preparation' (p.3). He also suggests it is impossible for people to process information or to engage fully in activities involving change when they are emotionally distraught. Therefore, from the earliest phases during the initial consultation and assessment, there needs to be the time and space within the context of the therapeutic relationship for acknowledging this sense of loss. This is when healing begins.

Counselling provides a theoretical framework that broadens the scope of questions and depth of conversations in relation to the communication or voice disorder

A constant theme throughout the literature is the emphasis on counselling as 'a way of thinking' as much as it is a set of strategies and techniques. This is achieved through *therapeutic conversations* that encourage clients to consider their communication or voice disorder in relation to their wider context, to reflect upon the impact that their problem is having upon their lives and those around them, and the implications of their condition. Some only want to work practically and concretely but for others, counselling enables individuals to go beyond a focus on signs, symptoms and behaviours. Through therapeutic conversations that can be exploratory, supportive, and even challenging or confronting, this generates deeper insights. These processes allow new perspectives on the meaning of their communication or voice disorder with further options for coping or adapting.

As further emphasised in the texts cited above, counselling is not a separate strategy or intervention tacked onto the treatment plan as an after-thought. Rather, it is integral to the whole therapeutic process. While for some it may play a major role, especially during particular phases of clinical management such as coming to terms with progressive deterioration or residual disability, it does not necessarily need to take a long time, or to be complex. In fact, it often takes the form of 'a counselling moment' or a conversation within structured activities. Alternatively, it may occur following a spontaneous comment made by a patient and develop into a deeper exploratory conversation that reveals new insights for both client and clinician. What matters is that the therapist has the knowledge and experience to form judgments about which levels of counselling are most appropriate at the various stages of intervention (DiLollo & Neimeyer, 2014; Holland, 2007).

Different levels of counselling and therapeutic engagement

Across the mental health literature, practitioners have recognised different stages within the counselling process, with each requiring different levels of intensity and therapeutic engagement. To some extent, the ways in which these stages are construed relates to the position within the continuum along which the different models of counselling and psychotherapy may lie. For instance, in many professional counselling texts it has been suggested there are essentially four stages: *the initial phase; the exploratory phase; the action phase;* and *the closing phase* (Egan, 2009; Sullivan, 2008). These nominal stages do not have fixed boundaries and are not necessarily sequential. Rather, in the context of the therapeutic reality, they operate in a flexible manner, 'as more of a spiral process where different phases are repeated and revisited as new depths are reached' (Sullivan, 2008) (p. 130).

The four stages are well suited to the more pragmatic models of counselling that are more content driven and where the psychological work is likely to be problem or solution-focused (Crago, 2000; Crago & Gardner, 2012), and they are often taught in undergraduate programmes for SLP. Here, the emphasis is given to drawing upon the positive strengths and resources of the individual, and therapist interventions are aimed towards recommending strategies for behavioural action and change. These four stages and some of the different interventions associated with each are shown in Box 9.7.

Box 9.7 Different stages within the counselling process

1. Initial phase

- Greetings, role definitions, limitations to confidentiality
- Administrative aspects and contracting the relationship

2. Exploration phase

- Information gathering including details of person's wider context
- Hearing the client's story

3. Action phase

- Setting goals and seeking solutions
- Planning strategies and developing options

4. Closing phase

- Consolidating, generalising, summarising, evaluating gains
- Reflecting upon therapeutic relationship
- (Extrapolated from Egan, 2009 and Sullivan, 2008, p. 130)

DiLollo and Neimeyer (2014) also propose four levels of counselling intervention for SLP and audiologists (albeit with a different emphasis), with clinical examples to illustrate these different stages. They suggest: that counselling need not necessarily be complicated, and that it is more 'a way of thinking'; that valuable *transformative moments* can follow brief counselling conversations; that in some cases longer sessions devoted specifically to psychologically challenging issues will be required; and that *attention to meaning* at all levels of the therapeutic encounter really matters. Their four levels of counselling and some of the therapeutic processes involved at each level are listed in Box 9.8.

Box 9.8 Levels of counselling intervention for SLP and audiologists

1. Person-centered thinking

- Influences ways of listening, engaging in conversation
- Focus is on contextual features and meaning of communication disorder
- Guides giving of information, education, therapeutic decision-making

2. Enhancing conventional therapies

- Assists with 'making sense' of behavioural change
- Leads to understanding of the meaning behind difficulties in generalising

3. Changing identities

- Facilitates changes in beliefs, attitudes that may be constraining progress
- Encourages alternative ways of thinking about the problem
- Enables new behaviours and improvements to overall quality of life

4. Recognising limits

- Identifies psychological problems that are beyond the scope of the therapist
- Recognises religious, cultural or moral issues that create conflict of interest
- Makes referrals to appropriately qualified mental health professionals

(Extrapolated from DiLollo and Neimeyer, 2014, pp. 18–26)

When turning to the relational models of psychotherapy, Gibney (2010) proposes the following four levels of intensity and associated processes. Level One: *therapeutic engagement*; Level Two: *problem solving or solution focused therapy*; Level Three: *the therapeutic relationship* as the consciously perceived nexus of change; and Level Four: *transformative therapy* in the presence of an implicated witness. These are shown in Box 9.9.

Box 9.9 Levels of therapeutic engagement and processes involved

1. Of engagement

- Is therapy wanted, needed, or appropriate at this time?
- Is client a 'visitor', voluntary or involuntary?
- Clarification of attitudes or expectations about approaches to therapy
- Brief-strategic-problem or solution focus
- Longer-term existential meaning or relational focus

2. A form of problem solving or solution-focused therapy

- Specific problem requiring strategic assistance – problem to be fixed
- No real desire for insight or focus on therapeutic relationship
- Problem is externalised-alternative narratives supplied by therapist
- Challenges to beliefs, attitudes feelings to enable changes in behaviours

3. The therapeutic relationship as the consciously perceived nexus of change

- Therapist has dual tasks
- To offer practical and strategic help to deal with crisis
- To provide a 'holding environment' that enables change to take place within the safety of the therapeutic relationship
- 4. Transformative therapy in the presence of an implicated witness
- Willing client motivated with sense of urgency to uncover issues
- Transformation occurs within mutual process of therapeutic relationship
- Therapist is witness to client's transformation rather than instrumental
- Client and therapist developed through energy and intensity of exchange

(Extrapolated from Gibney, 2010, pp. 81–89)

In describing activities during the different levels of therapeutic engagement Gibney also challenges notions that assume a sequential process of moving logically from one level to another. He suggests that in clinical practice, there may be some clients wanting practical strategies, others who are motivated to explore and understand their past and how this is impacting upon their current relationships, or others who clearly wish to enter into longer-term psychotherapy. Furthermore, during individual work with any given client, the co-evolving nature of the therapeutic process will often require the therapist to shift between the different levels of therapeutic engagement, even within the session itself. To some extent the levels of therapeutic engagement may be determined by the client's personality and preferences, but for the deeper work, the skills and capacity of the therapist will be a crucial factor. 'The emotional holding required in the reconstitution of self is only able to be offered by therapists who have experienced this for themselves'(Gibney, 2010) (p. 89).

Clearly, some of the processes of therapeutic engagement in Gibney's Levels Three and Four are more closely related to the practice of psychotherapy and may not lie within the scope of practice for the SLP or voice therapist unless they have qualifications in psychotherapy. However, I have included these levels requiring deeper engagement here because there is much for us to learn about the importance of the therapeutic relationship in supporting clients making changes concerning specific problems.

For instance, Gibney (2010) proposes that when clients seek help it is often following a series of events or a crisis 'that facilitates a disorienting change in a person's sense of self' (p. 85). This may be due to external factors such a loss of employment, but it may also be due to interpersonal issues involving betrayal and loss of trust, or the shattering of firmly held beliefs about close family members and others highly revered. He suggests that during crises that threaten a person's 'sense of self', while problem solving and solution-focused approaches would certainly be necessary, the therapeutic relationship becomes just as important, if not more so, than strategies and instrumental interventions alone. His reasons for this are that when a person's 'sense of self' is threatened, he or she is particularly vulnerable, and basic trust in others as well as the self has often been challenged. Furthermore, since 'one's original and ongoing reality is created in relationship and dialogue' (p. 86), if there is to be a new sense of reality, this will need to be created through a meaningful relationship based upon trust and dialogue once again.

This resonates strongly with what may happen in relation to disorders of the voice. As outlined in Chapter 5, stressful life events such as the ones described above have been shown to precede the onset of both FVD and OVD. Furthermore, as highlighted in Chapter 7, many of the more profound psychosocial impacts of a voice disorder can destabilise a person's equilibrium; they may also threaten their identity and lead to *a compromised sense of self* (Jacobs & van Biene, 2015). This is particularly relevant to professional voice users, such as singers or actors, when they experience loss or profound changes to their voices (Baker, 1999, 2002; Rosen & Sataloff, 1997; Shewell, 2009). It has also been shown that when individuals undergo a total laryngectomy and loss of voice, they are catapulted into a crisis that can best be described as '*an altered sense of self*' (Bickford, Coveney, Baker, & Hersh, 2013).

In Level Four, Gibney describes those relatively rare situations where a client enters into therapy, transforms before our eyes with his or her self-directed search for insight and meaning, and where we as therapists may not really know what we have done to make this possible. He suggests that this transformation can only happen 'if the therapist has a sense of mutual process and of the literal or metaphorical interplay with the client' (p. 88). I understand this to mean that the therapist's 'way of being' can help to create the psychological space for this mutuality, and through this process, *transformation and healing* can take place. Significantly too, in being witness to the transformation, this also promotes the growth and development of the therapist.

Conclusion

In concluding this chapter, it is important to emphasise once more that the purpose of undertaking different levels of counselling in conjunction with direct approaches to voice therapy is to enable deeper insights, and to enhance the experience for the client. This begins at the outset during the initial consultation, psychosocial interview, and assessment phases, through all the subsequent stages of intervention that also includes ending therapy. It is proposed that the different levels of counselling within the context of a warm, empathic,, and supportive therapeutic relationship help to create the psychological space necessary for the changes in thoughts, feelings, and new behaviours to take place. In those rare circumstances where a client's psychological distress signals the need for deeper levels of engagement, the clinician's knowledge and awareness of different models and levels of counselling enables the referral for other forms of medical or psychological intervention. In such cases psychotherapy, where the therapeutic relationship operates as the 'nexus of change', may be recommended (Gibney, 2010). It is also proposed that when effective counselling is combined with voice therapy it enables competent treatment and technical proficiency to be elevated to an experience of 'psychotherapeutic value', and one in which healing and even transformation can take place.

References

Anderson, H. (2006). The heart and spirit of collaborative therapy: The philosophical stance – a "way of being" in relationship and conversation. In H. Anderson & D. Gerhart (Eds.), *Collaborative therapy: Relationships that make a difference* (pp. 43–59). New York: Routledge.

Aronson, A. E. (1990). Importance of the psychosocial interview in the diagnosis and treatment of "functional" voice disorders. *Journal of Voice, 4*(4), 287–289.

Aronson, A. E., & Bless, D. M. (2009). *Clinical voice disorders* (4th ed.). New York: Thieme.

Audet, C. T. (2011). Client perspectives of therapist self-disclosure: Violating boundaries or removing barriers. *Counselling Psychology Quarterly, 24*(2), 85–100.

Aybek, S., Nicholson, T. R., Zelaya, F., O'Daly, O. G., Craig, T. K., David, A. S., & Kanaan, R. A. (2013). Neural correlates of recall of life events in conversion disorder. *JAMA Psychiatry.* doi:10.1001/jamapsychiatry.2013.2842

Baker, J. (1998). Psychogenic dysphonia: Peeling back the layers. *Journal of Voice, 12*(4), 527–535.

Baker, J. (1999). Changes to women's voices following hormonal therapy. A report on alterations to the speaking and singing voices of four women. *Journal of Voice, 13*(4), 496–507.

Baker, J. (2002). Persistent dysphonia in two performers affecting the singing and projected speaking voice: A report on a collaborative approach to management. *Logopedics, Phoniatrics, Vocology, 27*, 179–187.

Baker, J. (2003). Psychogenic voice disorders and traumatic stress experience: A discussion paper with two case reports. *Journal of Voice, 17*(3), 308–318.

Baker, J. (2008). The role of psychogenic and psychosocial factors in the development of functional voice disorders. *International Journal of Speech-Language Pathology, 10*(4), 210–230.

Baker, J. (2010). Women's voices: Lost or mislaid, stolen or strayed? *International Journal of Speech-Language Pathology, 12*(2), 94–106.

Baker, J., Ben-Tovim, D. I., Butcher, A., Esterman, A., & McLaughlin, K. (2013). Psychosocial risk factors which may differentiate between women with functional voice disorder, organic voice disorder, and control group. *International Journal of Speech-Language Pathology, 15*(6), 547–563.

Beck, A. T. (1979). *Cognitive therapy and the emotional disorders.* Madison USA: Penguin.

Beck, A. T., & Weishaar, E. (2014). Cognitive therapy. In D. Wedding & R. J. Corsini (Eds.), *Current psychotherapies.* Belmont: Thomson Brooks Cole.

Beutler, L. E., & Harwood, T. M. (2002). What is and can be attributed to the therapeutic relationship? *Journal of Contemporary Psychotherapy, 32*(1), 25–33.

Bickford, J., Coveney, J., Baker, J., & Hersh, D. (2013). Living with the altered self. *International Journal of Speech-Language Pathology, 15*(3), 324–333.

Boscolo, L., Cecchin, G., Hoffman, L., & Penn, P. (1987). *Milan systemic family therapy.* New York: Basic Books.

Butcher, P., & Elias, A. (1983). Cognitive-behavioural therapy with dysphonic patients: An exploratory investigation. *The Royal College of Speech & Language Therapists Bulletin*(377), 1–3.

Butcher, P., Elias, A., & Cavalli, L. (2007). *Understanding and treating psychogenic voice disorder: A CBT framework.* Chichester: Wiley.

Carding, P., Deary, V., & Miller, T. (2013). Cognitive behavioural therapy in the treatment of functional dysphonia in the United Kingdom. In E. M.-L. Yiu (Ed.), *International perspectives on voice disorders* (pp. 133–148). Bristol: Multilingual Matters/Channel View Publications.

Cavalli, L., Butcher, A., & Elias, A. (2009). *Incorporating Cognitive Behaviour Therapy principles and skills into the clinical practice of SLT's working with Psychogenic Voice Disorders: A partnership approach* Paper presented at the RCSLT Scientific Conference, London.

Cohn, F. (2001). Existential medicine: Martin Buber and physician-patient relationships. *Journal of Continuing Education in the Health Professions, 21*(3), 170–181.

Corey, G. (2012). *Theory and practice of counselling and psychotherapy* (9th ed.). Belmont: Brooks Cole/Cengage Learning Inc.

Crago, H. (2000). Counselling and psychotherapy: Is there a difference? Does it matter? *Australian and New Zealand Journal of family Therapy, 21*(2), 73–80.

Crago, H. (2012). A tale of two hemispheres: Psychotherapy, psychology and the divided brain. *Psychotherapy in Australia, 18*(4), 58–65.

Crago, H., & Gardner, P. (2012). *A safe place for change. Skills and capacities for counselling and therapy.* Melbourne: IP Communications.

Crowe, T. A. (Ed.). (1997). *Applications of counselling in speech–language pathology and audiology.* Baltimore: Williams & Wilkins

Daniilidou, P., Carding, P., Wilson, J., Drinnan, M., & Deary, V. (2007). Cognitive behavioural therapy for functional dysphonia: A pilot study. *Annals of Otology, Rhinology & Laryngology, 116*(10), 717–722.

de Shazer, S. (1982). *Patterns of brief family therapy.* New York: The Guilford Press.

de Shazer, S. (1985). *Keys to solution in brief therapy.* London: W.W Norton.

de Shazer, S. (1988). *Investigating solutions in brief therapy.* New York: W.W. Norton.

Deary, V., & Miller, T. (2011). Reconsidering the role of psychosocial factors in functional dysphonia. *Current Opinion in Otolaryngology and Head and Neck Surgery, 19*(3), 150–154.

Demmink-Geertman, L., & Dejonckere, P. H. (2010). Differential effects of voice therapies on neurovegetative symptoms and complaints. *Journal of Voice, 24*(5), 585–591.

DiLollo, A., & Neimeyer, R. A. (2014). *Counseling in Speech-language Pathology and Audiology.* San Diego: Plural Publishing.

Duncan, B. L., Miller, S. D., Wampold, B. E., & Hubble, M. A. (Eds.). (2010). *The heart and soul of change: Delivering what works in therapy* (2nd ed.). Washington: APA Press.

Eastwood, C., Madill, C., & McCabe, P. (2015). The behavioural treatment of muscle tension voice disorders: A systematic review. *International Journal of Speech-Language Pathology, 17*(3), 287–303.

Egan, G. (1997). *The skilled helper* (6th ed.). Pacific Grove: Brooks Cole.

Egan, G. (2009). *The skilled helper* (9th ed.). Belmont: Brooks Cole.

Egan, G. (2014). *The skilled helper: A problem-management and opportunity-development approach to helping* (10th ed.). Belmont: Brooks Cole/Cengage Learning Inc.

Elias, A., Raven, R., Butcher, P., & Littlejohns, D. (1989). Speech therapy for psychogenic voice disorder: A survey of current practice and training. *British Journal of Disorders of Communication, 24,* 61–76.

Etkin, A., Pittenger, C., Polan, H. J., & Kandel, E. R. (2005). Toward a neurobiology of psychotherapy: Basic science and clinical applications. *The Journal of Neuropsychiatry and Clinical Neurosciences, 17*(2), 145–158.

Fife, S. T., Whiting, J. B., Bradford, K., & Davis, S. (2014). The therapeutic pyramid: A common factors synthesis of techniques, alliance, and way of being. *Journal of Marital and Family Therapy, 40*(1), 20–33.

Flasher, L. V., & Fogle, P. T. (2012). *Counseling skills for speech-language pathologists and audiologists* (2nd ed.). Clifton Park: Delmar/Cengage Learning.

Fourie, R. J. (2011a). From alienation to therapeutic dialogue. In R. J. Fourie (Ed.), *Therapeutic processes for communication disorders.* New York: Psychology Press.

Fourie, R. J. (Ed.). (2011b). *Therapeutic processes for communication disorders.* New York: Psychology Press.

Freedman, J., & Combs, G. (1996). *Narrative therapy: The social construction of preferred realities.* New York: W.W. Norton.

Freud, A. (1954). The widening scope for indications for psychoanalysis: Discussion. *Journal of the American Psychoanalytic Association, 2,* 607–620.

Fuchs, T. (2004). Neurobiology and psychotherapy: An emerging dialogue. *Current Opinion in Psychiatry, 17,* 479–485.

Geldard, D., & Geldard, K. (2009). *Basic personal counselling* (6th ed.). Sydney: Pearson Prentice Hall.

Geller, E., & Foley, G. M. (2009). Expanding the "ports of entry" for speech-language pathologists: A relational and reflective model for clinical practice. *American Journal of Speech Language Pathology, 18*(1), 4–21.

Gelso, C. J. (2009). The real relationship in a postmodern world: Theoretical and empirical explorations. *Psychotherapy Research, 19*(3), 253–264.

Gelso, C. J., & Samtag, L. W. (2008). A tripartite model of the therapeutic relationship. In S. D. Brown & R. W. Lent (Eds.), *Handbook of counseling psychology* (pp. 267–283). New York: Wiley.

Gibney, P. (2010). *The pragmatics of therapeutic practice.* Melbourne: Psychoz Publications

Hackney, H. L., & Cormier, S. (2013). *The professional counselor* (7th ed.). Upper Saddle River: Pearson Education.

Hammarberg, B. (1987). Pitch and quality characteristics of mutational voice disorders before and after therapy. *Folia Phoniatrica, 39,* 204–216.

Hayley, J. (Ed.). (1971). *Changing families.* London: Grune & Stratton.

Holland, A. L. (2007). *Counselling in communication disorders*. San Diego: Plural Publishing.

Iwarsson, J. (2015). Reflections on clinical expertise and silent know-how in voice therapy. *Logopedics Phoniatrics Vocology, 40*, 60–71.

Jacobs, M., & van Biene, L. (2015). Psychogenic voice disorder: A view through the lens of self. *European Journal for Person Centered Healthcare, 3*(2).

Kaderavek, J. N., Laux, J. M., & Mills, N. H. (2004). A counseling training module for students of speech-language pathology training programs. *Contemporary Issues in Communication Science and Disorders, 31*, 153–161.

Kaplan, D. M., Tarvydas, V. M., & Gladding, S. T. (2014). 20/20: A vision for the future of counseling: The new consensus definition of counseling. *Journal of Counseling and Development, 92*, 366–372.

Knox, s., Hess, S. A., Petersen, D. A., & Hill, C. E. (1997). A qualitative analysis of client perceptions of the effects of helpful therapist self-disclosure in long-term therapy. *Journal of Counseling Psychology, 44*, 274–283.

Kollbrunner, J., Menet, A., & Seifert, E. (2010). Psychogenic aphonia: No fixation even after a lengthy period of aphonia. *Swiss Medical Weekly, 140*, 12–17.

Lamm, C., Batson, C. D., & Decety, J. (2007). The neural substrate of human empathy: Effects of perspective-taking and cognitive appraisal. *Journal of Cognitive Neuroscience, 19*(1), 42–58.

Levy, R. A., & Ablon, J. S. (Eds.). (2010). *Handbook of evidence-based psychodynamic psychotherapy: Bridging the gap between science and practice*. New York: Humana Press.

Luterman, D. (2011). Ruminations of an old man: A 50-year perspective on clinical practice. In R. J. Fourie (Ed.), *Therapeutic processes for communication disorders* (pp. 3–8). New York: Psychology Press.

Luterman, D. M. (2008). *Counselling persons with communication disorders and their families* (5th ed.). Austin: Pro-Ed, Inc.

MacKenzie, K., Millar, A., Wilson, J. A., Sellars, C., & Deary, I. J. (2001). Is voice therapy an effective treatment for dysphonia? *British Medical Journal, 2001*(323), 658–661.

Marzillier, J. (2004). The myth of evidence-based psychotherapy. *The Psychologist, 17*(7), 392–395.

McGilchrist, I. (2009). *The master and his emissary: The divided brain and the making of the Western world*. New Haven: Yale University Press.

Miller, S. D., Hubble, M. A., Chow, D. L., & Seidel, J. A. (2014). The outcome of psychotherapy: Yesterday, today and tomorrow. *Psychotherapy in Australia, 20*(3), 64–75.

Miller, W. R., & Rollnick, S. (Eds.). (2013). *Motivational interviewing* (3rd ed.). New York: The Guilford Press.

Minuchin, S. (1974). *Families and family therapy*. London: Tavistock Publications.

Nichol, H., Morrison, M. D., & Rammage, L. (1993). Interdisciplinary approach to functional voice disorders: The psychiatrist's role. *Otolaryngology-Head and Neck Surgery, 108*, 643–647.

O'Hara, J., Miller, T., Carding, P., Wilson, J., & Deary, V. (2011). Relationship between fatigue, perfectionism, and functional dysphonia. *Otolaryngology-Head and Neck Surgery, 144*(6), 921–926.

Papp, P. (1983). *The process of change*. New York: The Guilford Press.

Parkinson, K., & Rae, J. P. (1996). The understanding and use of counselling by speech and language therapists at different levels of experience. *British Journal of Disorders of Communication, 31*, 140–152.

Phillips, D., & Mendel, L. (2008). Counseling training in communicaiton disorders: A survey of clinical fellows. *Contemporary Issues in Communication Science and Disorders, 35*, 44–53.

Rammage, L. (2011). Emotional expression and voice dysfunction. *Perspectives on Voice and Voice Disorders, 21*(3), 8–16. doi: 10.1044/vvd 21.1.8

Rammage, L., Morrison, M., & Nichol, H. (2001). *Management of the voice and its disorders*. San Diego: Singular Publishing Group.

Rhodes, P., & Wallis, A. (Eds.). (2011). *A practical guide to family therapy*. Melbourne: IP Communications.

Riley, J. (2002). Counseling: An approach for speech-language pathologists. *Contemporary Issues in Communication Science and Disorders, 29*, 6–16.

Roffman, J. L., & Gerber, A. J. (2010). Neural models of psychodynamic concepts and treatments: Implications for psychodynamic psychotherapy. In R. A. Levy & J. S. Ablon (Eds.), *Evidence-based psychodynamic psychotherapy* (pp. 305–338). New York: Humana Press.

Rogers, C. R. (1951). *Client-centered therapy*. London: Constable.

Rogers, C. R. (1961). *On becoming a person*. New York: Houghton Miffin.

Rogers, C. R. (1980). *A way of being*. New York: Houghton Mifflin.

Rosen, D. C., & Sataloff, R. T. (1997). *Psychology of voice disorders*. San Diego: Singular Publishing Group.

Ruotsalainen, J. H., Sellman, J., Lehto, L., & Verbeek, J. H. (2008). Systematic review of the treatment of functional dysphonia and prevention of voice disorders. *Otolaryngology Head and Neck Surgery, 138*(5), 557–565.

Schoenberg, P., & Yakeley, J. (Eds.). (2014). *Learning about emotions in illness: Integrating psychotherapeutic teaching in medical education*. Hove: Routledge.

Shamay-Tsoory, S. G., H., L., & Chisin, R. (2005). The neural correlates of understanding the other's distress: A positron emission tomography investigation of accurate empathy. *NeuroImage, 27*(2), 468–472.

Shewell, C. (1998). The counsellor as travelling companion. *Speech and Language Therapy in Practice*(Summer), 8–10.

Shewell, C. (2009). *Voice work: Art and science in changing voices*. Chichester: Wiley-Blackwell.

Singer, T. (2006). The neuronal basis and ontogeny of empathy and mind reading: Review of literature and implications for future research. *Neuroscience and Biobehaviour Review 30*(6), 855–863.

Speyer, R. (2006). Effects of voice therapy: A systematic review. *Journal of Voice, 22*(5), 565–580.

Sudhir, P. M., Chandra, P. S., Shivashankar, N., & Yamini, B. K. (2009). Comprehensive management of psychogenic dysphonia: A case illustration. *Journal of Communication Disorders, 42*, 305–312.

Sullivan, B. (2008). *Counsellors and counselling: A new conversation.* Sydney: Pearson Education Australia.

Wampold, B. E. (2001). *The great psychotherapy debate: Models, methods, and findings.* Mahwah,: Erlbaum.

Wendler, J. (2015). Voice therapy: From past to the present from a phoniatrician's perspective. *Logopedics Phoniatrics Vocology, 40*(2), 56–63.

White, M. (1995). *Re-authoring lives: Interviews and essays.* Adelaide: Dulwich Centre.

White, M. (2011). *Narrative practice: Continuing conversations.* New York: WW Norton.

White, M., & Epston, D. (1990). *Narrative means to therapeutic ends.* New York: WW Norton.

Whiting, J. B., Oka, M., & Fife, S. T. (2012). Appraisal distrortions and intimate partner violence: Gender, power, and interaction. *Journal of Marital and Family Therapy, 38*, 133–149.

Winek, J. L. (2010). *Systemic family therapy: From theory to practice.* Thousand Oaks: Sage Publications Inc.

Yalom, I. D. (1970). *The theory and practice of group psychotherapy.* (2nd ed.). New York: Grune and Stratton.

Yalom, I. D. (1989). *Love's executioner and other tales of psychotherapy.* London: Penguin.

Yalom, I. D. (2002). *The gift of therapy: An open letter to a new generation of therapists and their patients.* London: Piatkus.

Zuroff, D., Kelly, A., Leybman, M., Blatt, S., & Wampold, B. E. (2010). Between-therapist and within-therapist differences in the quality of the therapeutic relationship. *Journal of Clinical Psychology, 66*, 681–697.

10

Theoretical constructs underpinning family therapy practice and applications to voice work

Introduction

My clinical, teaching, and supervisory work are strongly embedded in systems theory and the principles of family therapy, and while much of my work is with individuals, this in no way detracts from thinking in systemic terms. Further training and familiarity with other models of counselling and psychotherapy continue to inform my practice. These include analytical psychotherapy, Jungian psychotherapy, Rogerian person-centered therapy, attachment theory and relational approaches, existential therapy, transactional analysis (TA), gestalt therapy, Ericksonian hypnotherapy, neurolinguistic programming (NLP), bodywork approaches, wellness perspectives, narrative therapy, motivational interviewing, and cognitive behavior therapy (CBT). Some of these models are the preferred approaches to counselling for other speech-language pathologists (SLP) working with communication disorders in general (Crowe, 1997; DiLollo & Neimeyer, 2014; Flasher & Fogle, 2012; Fourie, 2011; Holland, 2007; D. M. Luterman, 2008); some are applied in relation to specific occupational groups such as professional voice users (Miller, 2003, 2008; Rosen & Sataloff, 1997); others are recommended for specific voice disorder groups such as psychogenic voice disorders (PVD) (Butcher, Elias, & Cavalli, 2007; Jacobs, 2011; Jacobs & van Biene, 2015).

In Chapter 2, several basic concepts in relation to systems theory and family therapy were introduced. These included notions from *cybernetics* and *information theories* that seek to explain how change takes place in living systems. For the purposes of this chapter, I review some of these constructs that now form a framework for thinking about the organisational structure and functioning of families across *the family lifecycle*, and how this may be reflected in perspectives on physical and mental health. This conceptual framework explains how properties inherent in all living systems are reflected in the *dynamics of the therapeutic relationship*, and that interpersonal communication is a *multilevel process*, all of which have implications for the *processes of change* during therapy.

My approach to the integration of counselling with voice work is guided by a number of principles that have been described by many distinguished family therapists and psychotherapists. As distilled by Catherine Sanders in an inspiring keynote address entitled *'What lies beneath: The hidden foundations of therapy'* (2012), she uses the evocative metaphor of tapestries to illustrate how theory underpins clinical practice at Bower Place. She reminds us that with all tapestries, it is the foundation canvas and *the warp* that supports the wonderfully different coloured threads of *the weft*, which then becomes the decorative pattern that we see. This is the case in therapy too. Sanders then draws upon the famous series of seven tapestries produced in the Southern Netherlands between 1495 and 1505 known as *The Hunt for the Unicorn* as a way of illustrating the constructs that inform their approach to therapy (s.ee Fig 10.1).

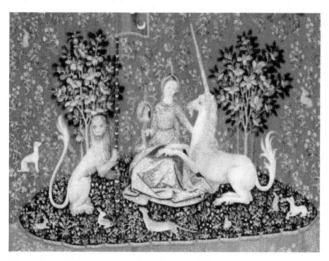

Fig. 10.1 The Hunt for the Unicorn Tapestries 1495–1505
(Source: imgarcade.com 960 x 714; publicly available)

'The dramatic and colourful picture that we create in sessions, the story we conjour, is underpinned by hidden and much less dramatic threads. Thus that which we see is supported by a hidden foundation which provides the basis on which the picture is constructed' (Catherine Sanders, personal communication 2012).

The clinical work at Bower Place is firmly supported by a *model of practice* and a clearly articulated *explanation for change* that incorporates both structural and systemic approaches to family therapy, with a strict adherence to their clearly stated *ethics and values*. These values include acknowledgement of the feminist and social constructionist critique of system theory that gives emphasis to therapists taking 'an active position against violence, abuse, and power dynamics' (Rhodes & Wallis, 2011) (p.22).

Of equal significance is their acknowledgment of the importance of the *therapeutic relationship*, and that one cannot underestimate the implicit influence of each therapist's *family of origin* or their *personal and professional history and experience*. Sanders and other practitioners give careful consideration to the *use of the self*, and even the place of *self-disclosure*, as this may contribute to a therapeutic relationship that is both *professional* and *real* (Audet, 2011; Flaskas, 2011; Gelso, 2009). The necessity for disciplined *reflective practice* is strongly advocated by these therapists, especially when individuals or families have reached an impasse, and 'attending to your use of self in therapeutic relating is part and parcel of all family therapy' (Flaskas, 2011) (p. 15). Flaskas proposes that 'the discipline of reflective practice is not an optional addition to the process of therapeutic relating, but rather sits at the centre of all good practice in the therapeutic relationship and use of the self' (p.15). In my opinion we should never underestimate the ways in which all of above factors interact to determine the course and outcome of voice therapy.

In addition to these crucial ingredients, Paul Gibney (2010) refers to a number of *loading parameters* that he considers to be fundamental to the dynamic structure of effective therapy. Two of these are highlighted for the purpose of this chapter because I have found them to be particularly pertinent to our work as voice therapists across the full range of voice disorders, and especially in relation to those with functional voice disorders (FVD). The first is the capacity of the therapist to offer *containment* and a suitable *holding environment* throughout the therapeutic process. The second relates to the clinical skills of *double description*, *reframing*, and *redefining*.

Gibney strongly asserts that while experienced therapists offer treatment that is shaped by their years of practice and wisdom, it is also the case 'that unique therapies are created consciously or unconsciously by how the practitioner allows the parameters of the dynamic structure of psychotherapy to 'line up' and interact to meet the unique requirements of *this* client and *this* context' (p.7). Integral to the dynamic structure of therapy then is the principle that *the needs of the client are primary over the demands of the theory*, and that while practitioners need to know the theories, they also need to forget them as soon as the patient walks through the door and to be able to construct a unique therapy for each client (Jung, 1934; Yalom, 2002).

This is salutary advice for student clinicians armed with the obligatory structured treatment plans that they have scrutinised the night before clinical placement. There is much here as well that can be extrapolated into our work as experienced voice practitioners, where we might be tempted to believe there is only one theoretical model or one regime of clinical practice that is the correct and right way to approach voice therapy.

Systems theory, principles of family therapy, and explanations for change

'Contemporary systemic family therapy encompasses a broad range of theoretical influences including attachment, neurobiology, and psychodynamic theories, but began in the twentieth century with two primary influences, systems theory and cybernetics' (Rhodes & Wallis, 2011) (p. 16).

'General systems theory is based on the concept that the whole entity, as a system, is greater than the sum of its parts' (Rhodes & Wallis, 2011) (p. 78).

'Cybernetics is the study of communication, particularly as it applies to self-regulated systems or mechanical systems in which feedback from one part of the system generates an action in another part of the system automatically' (Rhodes & Wallis, 2011) (p. 17).

Family therapy draws upon *general systems theory* and *cybernetics* as its primary theoretical framework. Since the literature on systems theory and cybernetics can be as thrilling to the eager mind as Chomsky before bed, I begin by highlighting some of these constructs by referring to a somewhat 'tongue in cheek' conversation that I had with an experienced family therapist, Margaret Burrell. This took place prior to a speech pathology conference presentation reporting upon my abject failure when treating a boy with vocal nodules with traditional approaches to voice therapy, and where the integration of family therapy helped the boy and his family to make the necessary changes. I asked for her help in explaining these constructs briefly, but in a way that would bring the ideas to life and in a manner that would be memorable. This is how our conversation went.

"Margaret, could you help me with a simple straightforward explanation of systems theory and cybernetics in about two paragraphs and don't forget this is for a very sophisticated and scientific audience?" In making such a request at this early stage of my family therapy training I was embarrassingly naïve to the complexities of this vast topic.

At the mention of 'sophisticated' and 'scientific' a mild glint appeared in my colleague's eye.

"Sure" and she smiling graciously. "Are you ready? Do you remember the last time you saw a film about the early American pioneers traveling across the continent? " (see Fig. 10.2).

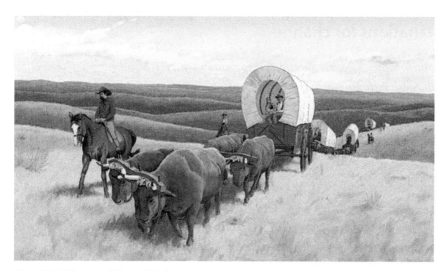

Fig. 10.2 Pioneer Wagon Trains
(Source: jpeg jhessesmadhouse.blogspot.com; publicly available)

"Oh no", I said, "I can't possibly do this – not for speech pathologists – they will think I've lost the plot or that I am treating them like children".

She replied, "Do you want to help them understand systems theory or not?"

"Go on", I said immediately regretting my ridiculous request.

"Well, do you recall seeing scenes of the wagons pulled by team of horses and cattle across the prairies with a couple of drivers at the helm and a bundle of wives, children and chattels in the back?"

"Uh huh", I groaned.

"Well, could you tell me what may have been the major restraints governing the speed at which the wagons travelled? Just the obvious things will do?"

"Restraints? Restraints to the speed of the wagon such as the weather, the tortuous terrain of the canyons, the negotiations they needed to make with traditional land owners who may well have felt very threatened by their presence?"

"Yes that's right, the external environment through which they would be travelling is one, and of course other people in the vicinity is definitely another".

"I guess other restraints would have been the skill and co-operation of the drivers, the fitness of the horses, perhaps their experience in working as a team, the number of passengers on board, and the actual structure of the wagon".

"And what would happen if a wheel were to begin rattling about?" she asked.

"Well on the one hand it could begin to *distract the drivers*, or they might *ignore it* and *drive the horses harder to compensate*. It could, I suppose, even *split the drivers* if one kept mentioning it while the other refused to notice it at all. If neither of them recognised it as a problem, *maybe one of the children* would notice and even *do the worrying for the drivers* – perhaps *try to catch their attention* by clowning around or trying to warn them".

" And what if the wheel fell off?"

"Well *that would be a major problem that no one could ignore*!! Not only for that particular wagon, but the whole wagon train would have to stop".

"And so now you see that *if one small part of the wagon changes it affects the functioning of the whole*"."Well of course" I said, "it's so obvious". But then I couldn't help thinking if it's so obvious, why had it taken me, and I presume so many others in my profession, so long to work with whole families, or at the very least to think about disorders of the voice and other aspects of communication more systemically. And how was it possible that so many courses on clinical methods and the importance of the therapeutic relationship had never alluded to systems theory as these ideas may help to explain interactions, communication and change in living systems?

"Go on" I said.

"That's it", said Margaret, "that is the crux of systems theory".

"But surely I need to explain **the links between systems and cybernetics theory** and that the family is like any living system that has the characteristics of organisation and energy? Don't I need to say that the family is *a system of interacting individuals* with a *mechanism for self-regulation and change* in the form of *positive and negative feedback loops*? These feedback loops act to *maintain the homeostatic balance,* and yet *permit change under limited conditions*. I'll have to explain how *information gets into the system from the outside,* and that the system makes a choice about *whether the new information makes any difference*.

For instance, if we give a child and his parents specific counselling about vocal abuse, such new information can be used by the system to promote learning and better coping mechanisms or it might pass through unnoticed".

"And importantly too, they need to understand that the family will *react to, or resist any change or challenge which threatens the stability of their system.* These challenges may come from inside, such as a child reaching adolescence, or from the outside, such as the sudden unemployment of a parent, even the intervention of a speech pathologist. And even while asking for help, a family may appear to resist the very change they say they want".

"Surely it needs to be pointed out that *if families didn't have restraints to change* and were too flexible *acting upon advice from all and sundry* then the system might disintegrate into chaos. Or, if they *never reacted to any new information,* they would be unlikely to learn, grow or adapt, and we might describe such a family as rather *rigid* or *stuck.* Surely I have to explain all of this?"

"Well yes," said my colleague yawning sleepily, "I do have a science degree too Jan, but I'll bet you ten to one, that what they remember is the wagon, and that if one part is affected it influences the whole".

A number of these precepts are summarised in point form in Box 10.1.

Box 10.1 Properties inherent in all living systems

Wholeness and organisation with divisions into subsystems

- Boundaries
- Hierarchy and roles
- Relationship – interacting parts influence one another and system as a whole

Drives towards both growth and control resulting in dynamic steady state

- Homeostasis maintained by positive and negative feedback loops
- Living systems also evolve and are capable of transformation

Cybernetics as applied to communication and change in living systems

- Feedback in one part of system generates action elsewhere in the system
- Communication and causality are circular rather than linear
- Influencing and being influenced is a recursive process
- Mutual influence via feedback loops explains change or lack of in systems

Change in living systems and the role of new information

- Systems seek growth and development
- Systems invite change but also thrive on equilibrium and status quo
- Systems need new information or energy in order to change
- Events of high probability carry little information
- Events that are unexpected carry much more information
- The new information needs to be sufficient to create 'news of difference'
- Some systems react and respond to the new input, re-organise and transform
- Some systems adapt to discomfort rather than change
- Systems are restrained from changing due to internal or external influences

(Extrapolated from the original writings of Bateson, 1972; Shannon & Weaver, 1963; von Bertalanffy, 1968; Weiner, 1961)

Early conceptual contributions to understanding families and family therapy

'The central insight which intellectually united the pioneers of family therapy movement was that human problems are essentially interpersonal, not intrapersonal, and so their resolution requires an approach to intervention which directly addresses relationships between people' (Carr, 2012) (p. 54).

As proposed by anthropologist Gregory Bateson (Bateson, 1972, 1979; Bateson & Ruesch, 1951) along with the many psychotherapy collaborators who went on to form the Mental Research Institute in the USA, these constructs from general systems theory and cybernetics offered new perspectives on the structure, organisation, and changes that take place within families and their development over time. Further, in noticing the complex and paradoxical patterns of communication in families presenting with clinical problems, Bateson and his collaborators also proposed that *interpersonal communication* is a *multi-level process* involving both verbal and non-verbal messages. In many families presenting with problems, they observed that while the words spoken represented one level of meaning, the non-verbal or *meta-communications* reflected more implicit aspects of the communication, such as hierarchical differences in roles, authority, or power differentials.

This recognition of the multi-level processes involved in interpersonal communication was strongly influenced by the work of the renowned hypnotherapist Milton Erickson, whose therapeutic work was documented extensively by the family therapist Jay Hayley (1985). Erickson often dealt with a patient's resistance to change by giving a *double-bind message* which simultaneously addressed the patient's conscious mind while also addressing his unconscious mind. For instance, while the message to the conscious mind invited change, the message to the unconscious mind anticipated resistance to such change. Alan Carr (2012) suggests an example of such a double-bind message: 'Your conscious mind might be ready to make progress but your unconscious mind might be wary of the dangers of this; the wisdom of both the conscious and unconscious minds needs to be respected' (p. 64).

Similar notions with respect to communication being a multi-level process have been incorporated into the psychotherapeutic fields of TA and NLP, where it has been proposed that there are essentially two levels to all interpersonal transactions (Lankton, Lankton, & Brown, 1981). The first is the *social level message* contained in the consciously chosen spoken words; the second is the more implicit or *psychological level message* that reflects the truly intended meaning.

Applications to voice work

When we think about these constructs from our perspectives as voice practitioners, we recognise that verbal communication via speech contains the social level aspects of the message such as intentions, thoughts, and ideas, but that it is the voice of a person and their patterns of intonation that may portray the more basic emotions of anger, sadness, fear, and joy, and with further refinements, the more subtly nuanced emotions of shame, humiliation, derision, uneasiness, affection, and humour (Mathieson, 2001). In this sense, our voice constitutes a form of meta-communication that carries the psychological levels of meaning and what is truly meant, often belying the ostensible message conveyed through our carefully chosen words. Alan Carr (2012) provides a comprehensive overview of these foundation propositions drawn from systems theory, cybernetics, and the multi-level processes involved in communication in his excellent text. The key tenets as summarised by this author are shown in Table 10.1.

Table 10.1 Propositions from systems theory and cybernetics on which family therapy was based

Domain	Propositions
Boundaries	The family is a *system with boundaries* and is organized into *subsystems* The boundary around the family sets it apart from the wider social system, of which it is one subsystem The boundary around the family must be *semi-permeable* to ensure adaptation and survival.
Patterns	The behavior of each family member, and each family subsystem, is determined by the pattern of interactions that connects all family members. Patterns of family interaction are rule-governed and *recursive*. These rules may be inferred from observing repeated episodes of family interaction. Circular causality should be used when describing or explaining family interaction.
Stability & change	Within family systems, there are processes which both prevent and promote change. These are morphostasis (or homeostasis) and morphogenesis.
Stability	Within a family system, one member – the identified patient – may develop problematic behaviour when the family lacks the resources for morphogenesis. The symptom of the identified patient serves the positive function of maintaining family homeostasis. Negative feedback or deviation-reducing feedback maintains homeostasis and subserves morphostasis.
Change	Positive feedback or deviation-amplifying feedback subserves morphogenesis and may lead to a runaway or snowball effect. Individuals and factions within systems may show symmetrical behavior patterns and complementary behavior patterns, which if left unchecked may fragment the system. Positive and negative feedback is new information, and new information involves news of difference. A distinction may be made between first-and second-order change: between behaving differently according to the system's rules, and changing the rules.
Complexity	Within systems theory, a distinction may be made between first- and second-order cybernetics: between observed and observing systems. Within social systems, recursive patterns present in one part of the system replicate isomorphically in other parts of the system. Only probabilistic statements may be made about the impact of interventions on social systems.

Reproduced with permission Alan Carr (2012, pp. 73–74) Courtesy-Wiley Blackwell

Systems theory and cybernetics in relation to physical and mental health

In earlier bio-medical models the primary emphasis was given to linear notions of causality that located a range of physiological, emotional, and behavioural problems firmly in the psychopathology of the individual. The constructs extrapolated from general systems theory and cybernetics have now transformed the ways in which many medical practitioners and therapists think about physical and mental health. For instance, it is now recognised that communications and feedback loops that take place between parts of living systems are reciprocal, that if change occurs in any one sub-system it will impact on the functioning of other sub-systems, and that causality is circular rather than linear.

As a consequence, when individuals present to physicians or therapists with problems, contemporary approaches to intervention no longer focus upon the problem alone or the individual in isolation. They are more likely to take into account the inter-relationships between one neurophysiological sub-system and another, between the person with the problem and significant others in the patient's immediate or extended family, and significantly too, between the person and his/her social network that may extend to friends, the workplace, and the wider community (Carr, 2012). In addition to attention to contextual factors impacting upon the patient, Paul Gibney highlights the importance of recognising the context under which therapy services may be offered, the context of the therapist in any multi-disciplinary or hierarchical structure, and the context of different approaches to therapy in the current social and political culture (Gibney, 2010).

A number of excellent texts that have integrated these constructs from systems theory, cybernetics, and the multi-level nature of communication into dynamic theoretical frameworks for the different models of family therapy, are listed below in Box 10.2.

Box 10.2 Excellent texts integrating core concepts into theoretical framework

- A Safe Place to Change (Crago & Gardner, 2012)
- Family Therapy: Concepts, Process and Practice (Carr, 2012)
- The Pragmatics of Therapeutic Practice (Gibney, 2010)
- A Practical Guide to Family Therapy (Rhodes & Wallis, 2011)

The family lifecycle Many family therapists find it helpful to think about how problematic emotional and behavioural issues may be construed throughout the various stages of the family lifecycle. These stages as originally described typically reflected the structures and trajectories of more traditional nuclear families in Western cultures, but it is now recognised that with marked changes to the way in which couples and families are formed and fractured, these stages are no longer necessarily the norm (McGoldrick et al., 2011).

This has led to a strong critique of the earlier family lifecycle constructs, where it has been emphasised that: individual family experiences 'are inextricably tied to the socioeconomic and cultural sociopolitical context of the family' (Falicov, 2011) (p. 339); lifecycle stages 'are not necessarily predictable, universal or cumulative'(p. 339); and issues such as gender, racial oppression, cultural diversity, and the powerful impact of migration on families need to be taken into account. At this time when such traumatic mass migrations are taking place across the world, this issue is particularly pertinent. However, while keeping these important caveats in mind, an appreciation of the different stages that generally do occur in families can provide therapists with a preliminary context for any therapeutic encounter, whether it is with an individual or their family, and regardless of the presenting problem. The *key stages in the family lifecycle* along with the *emotional transition processes* and *tasks* that are considered essential for developmental progression have been described by a number of authors (Carr, 2012; McGoldrick *et al.*, 2011). The key stages are highlighted in Box 10.3.

Box 10.3 Stages in the Expanded Family Lifecycle

- Leaving home
- Forming a couple
- Families with young children
- Families with adolescents
- Launching children and moving into midlife
- Families with parents in late middle age
- Families with parents nearing end of life

(Extrapolated from McGoldrick, Carter & Garcia-Preto, 2011 and Carr, 2012)

The family lifecycle and applications to voice work

In my work as an SLP and clinical educator of both student and experienced clinicians, I have found it very helpful to consider ways in which both OVD and FVD may be experienced by individuals in the context of the different family lifecycle transitions (Vetere & Dallos, 2008). For instance, in the case of a patient presenting with a sudden onset of PVD following of an acutely stressful event and psychological threat, it can be readily appreciated that numerous systems and sub-systems within the body will be affected. As discussed in Chapter 8, this may begin with heightened arousal at the level of the limbic and endocrine systems with rapidly re-routed messages to the cerebral cortex to stimulate a readiness for action. This will have a flow-on effect leading to changes in levels of activity in the extrinsic and intrinsic laryngeal musculature that in turn may be reflected in different degrees of behavioural inhibition, presenting as either hyperfunctional or hypofunctional attempts to phonate (Roy & Bless, 2000a, 2000b).

While interventions will inevitably focus on modifying muscle tension patterns as these affect respiratory, vocal fold and supraglottic behaviours, approaches informed by systemic thinking will also take a range of other factors into account. These will include aspects of the person's physical and mental health, and dispositional features such as his or her habitual coping style in the face of anxiety and threat. The person's age and gender, current place within the context of the their family lifecycle, and whether others in the immediate or extended family are able to offer appropriate support, will also need to be considered. This may extend to gathering information about the person's religious, cultural, or community network, and the work environment to which he or she will be returning when the voice disorder has resolved.

Two case examples of patients diagnosed with a psychogenic voice disorder (PVD) in the form of a *puberphonia* are described. These very different cases illustrate how attention to the stages of the family lifecycle will influence *hypotheses about causality*, and how these may then determine the different levels of counselling that would be most appropriate to integrate with direct voice work for long-term resolution of the dysphonia (see Case examples 10.1).

Case example 10.1 Puberphonia: Two males in different family lifecycle stages

Example 1: Family with adolescents

A boy aged 16 years (S) presents with a 6 month history of PVD diagnosed as *puberphonia* or *mutational falsetto* characterised by high-pitched falsetto phonation with embarrassing pitch breaks and difficulty projecting his voice. S is an only child, and both his parents attend for the initial consultation because they are concerned about the degree to which their son is being teased at school and the fact that he is having trouble sleeping at night. They have noticed that his unstable voice and the teasing from school mates have contributed to his recent loss of confidence, and they are worried about how this will affect his exams and choice of occupation.

Example 2: Family with parents moving into late middle age

A man aged 50 years (S) presents with a sudden onset of *conversion reaction puberphonia* shortly after being informed that he will be made redundant with the pending collapse of the motorcar manufacturing industry. He is advised to consider seeking another job in the near future. S is married with three children, two of whom are still in high school. The third child, his eldest son, is half way through a trade school apprenticeship, with the intention of following his father into the same industry. All three young people are living at home. His wife works part-time on shifts, and together they support his mother, who has poorly controlled brittle diabetes, and her father who has relatively early onset of Alzheimer's disease with moderate cognitive decline.

Comment

It can be seen from Case examples 10.1 that although both of these male patients have been diagnosed with a PVD in the form of a puberphonia, it will be important for therapists to recognise the very different psychological issues that will be arising as a consequence of their respective family lifecycle stages. For instance, in the case of the 16 year-old boy, the counselling work is likely to focus on issues related to an adolescent transitioning into physical maturity and manhood with all that this involves. This would naturally generate conversations in relation to psychosexual development and maturity, establishing and holding one's identity with peers in view of the unusual changes taking place with his voice, and balancing the needs for more independence with greater degrees of separation from parents while still needing practical and financial support. With more significant degrees of distress in relation to the particular features of the dysphonia, it might require the therapist to be alert to reports of school avoidance, subtle signs of elevated anxiety or low mood and in extreme cases, suicidal ideation and evidence of clinical depression. Under these circumstances, referral to a mental health practitioner would be necessary.

In the case of the middle-aged man with sudden onset of a conversion reaction puberphonia, the counselling work may need to focus on issues related to a husband and father facing a redundancy that may threaten his sense-of-self and his very existence, with his significant financial and social responsibilities for his immediate and extended family. There are elements here too that may challenge his identity as an effective role model for his son, who is undertaking training to follow in his father's footsteps, and with respect to his wife whose sense of security may be threatened.

Equally confronting would be the ongoing stress of continuing to actually go to work each day where this particular work environment is a strongly male-dominated occupation and where his high-pitched falsetto phonation with unexpected pitch breaks would make him an easy butt of ridicule. He would also be facing additional psychological pressures if attending interviews for a new position in another male-dominated 'blue collar' working environment, where his unusual voice symptoms would be exposed. As discussed in earlier chapters, these issues related to *anticipatory stress* coupled with the *evaluative threat* and critical judgement of those in power can contribute to the experience of *chronic stress* and may even make this man vulnerable to the development of a *clinical depression*. If this occurred, it would take the counselling work outside the domain of the SLP, and referral to a mental health professional would be appropriate.

Systems theory and cybernetics in relation to the therapeutic relationship

The *therapeutic relationship* also exhibits all the *properties of living systems*. For example, at the organisational level, the therapeutic relationship has an observable structure with sub-systems established by both explicit and implicit semi-permeable boundaries that reflect degrees of hierarchy, roles and rules that establish appropriate levels of engagement. Further, the changes that take place within the context of the therapeutic relationship reflect many of the qualities of other living systems with *positive and negative feedback loops* in response to inputs from outside and within. These dynamic processes impact not only upon the patient and the therapist as individuals, but also on the therapeutic relationship as a whole, with implications for outcomes.

For example, these constructs influence the priorities that the therapist and client may give to what needs to change. This may also involve decisions, even if only considered subliminally, around whether it is sufficient for the emotional or behavioural difficulties to be resolved at a symptomatic level (*first order change*), or whether resolution would be more complete with change to the rules governing the patterns of problematic behaviours. This would involve a deeper level of insight and appreciation of meaning (*second-order change*) (Rhodes & Wallis, 2011).

First and second-order cybernetics as this influences the processes of change

Significantly, these constructs enable us to consider the impact of the therapeutic relationship on the change process. For instance, earlier models of psychotherapy and family therapy construed the therapist as being 'an independent or objective observer', looking in from the outside upon another with his or her patterns of problems. The therapist was seen as being able to alter the family system 'while remaining separate from and unaffected by the system' (first order cybernetics) (Carr, 2012) (p. 78). However, Rhodes and Wallis (2011) raise two important questions about these earlier assumptions that are also important for voice practitioners to consider. First, 'Do therapist's views exert an influence?' (p.19). Secondly, 'How do we actually separate our own family experiences, culture, and social position from what we observe?' (p. 19). Catherine Sanders suggests:

> '*We also bring our own personal experience, as sons and daughters, mothers and fathers, husbands and wives, friends and lovers, our gender, class, sexuality and circumstance. We, like our clients, are also shaped by this experience we call living and even the most junior of practitioners will have a wealth of both formal and informal wisdom to bring to the process*' (Personal Communication, Sanders, 2012).

Therefore, more contemporary approaches to family therapy would argue that once a therapist has entered into any form of relationship with clients to help them solve a problem, a new system has formed and the therapist has become part of that new dynamic system (*second order cybernetics*). The implications of this are that as a result of *mutual influence* upon one another, a therapist may help a person or a family to change and to resolve the stated problem. Alternatively, the influence of the therapist may inadvertently facilitate responses that serve to maintain the status quo and prevent resolution. This is a confronting notion to think about and one that every voice practitioner needs to keep in mind, especially in those cases where there is no change and where one might be tempted to persevere for far too long, or to keep doing more of the same. Ways in which the therapeutic relationship reflects the properties of living systems and acts as a powerful determinant in the change process are shown in Box 10.4.

Box 10.4 The therapeutic relationship reflects the properties of living systems

The therapeutic relationship has organisation

- Structure with boundaries to delineate sub-systems, hierarchy, rules and roles

The therapeutic relationship reflects the qualities of a dynamic steady state

- Drives towards homeostasis, equilibrium, status quo
- Drives towards change, growth and development and transformation

First-order cybernetics and the role of the therapeutic relationship in change:

- Assumptions that therapist can change a family system 'while remaining separate from and unaffected by the system'

Second-order cybernetics and the role of the therapeutic relationship in change

- When therapist joins with client and/or family she becomes part of the system
- Therapist and client influences are recursive and mutual
- The therapeutic relationship may act as a facilitator of change (*morphogenesis*)
- The therapeutic relationship may act as restraint to change (*morphostasis*)
- By entering the system the therapist creates some imbalance or discomfort
- Feedback from one part of the system facilitates response in another part
- By offering new information this enables the system to change
- This information must be perceived as *difference that makes a difference* sometimes referred to as *news of difference*

First-order change

• Change in the presenting symptoms in the form of altered behaviours

Second-order change

• Change involving deeper insight and understanding and changes to rules governing pattern of relationships in systems

(Extrapolated from Bateson, 1979; Carr, 2012; Crago & Gardner, 2012; Gibney, 2010; and Rhodes & Wallis, 2011)

Key elements underpinning the dynamic structure of effective therapy

As previously mentioned in Chapter 9, there are many skills, techniques and therapeutic qualities that have been shown to be helpful across all models of counselling and psychotherapy. However, there are a number of elements operating 'that may not be accessible to the practitioner's or the client's conscious awareness' (Gibney, 2010) (p. 6). This author refers to these elements as 'loading parameters' that interact to form the dynamics of individual therapy. They are: containment; double description; context; inclusion; levels of therapeutic engagement; time orientation; timing; language; inter-subjectivity; and the juxtaposition of meaning and strategy. Some of these loading parameters have been mentioned in a number of the counselling texts for SLP (DiLollo & Neimeyer, 2014; Fourie, 2011; Holland, 2007). For the purposes of this discussion I have chosen to highlight the first two of these: 1) the therapist's capacity to develop an appropriate holding environment or sense of containment that is appropriate to the nature of the concerns being expressed; 2) the therapist's ability to engage with the client in the process of double description and reframing. Both of these processes generate different perspectives to a problem and the options for new solutions. Brief reference is made to the ways in which these elements are relevant to voice therapy. (Clinical examples that illustrate how these factors may be incorporated during the different phases of intervention are described in Chapters 11 and 12.)

Containment and the capacity to create a holding environment

'The skills of holding are basic to virtually all forms of counselling and psychotherapy. They lay the foundations for a helpful relationship with a client. Holding skills allow the client to talk freely, and encourage them to say more about what they have already said' (Crago & Gardner, 2012) (p. 21).

The metaphor of the therapeutic holding environment derives from observations of the paediatrician and psychoanalyst, Donald Winnicott (Winnicott, 1982), who noted how mothers or other primary care givers hold their infants during their early childhood development. Winnicott observed the different ways in which mothers demonstrated 'sensitivity and emotional attunement' to their infants, protecting them against stresses from the outside world and keeping them as physically and emotionally as safe as possible. In this sense, the mother, or care giver, was seen as a *container* and the infant as experiencing the feeling of *being held* in a safe and protective space (Geller & Foley, 2009).

Winnicott also highlighted similarities and parallels between the *client-analyst relationship* and the *mother-infant relationship*, proposing that the practitioner has to display all the patience, tolerance, and reliability observed in a mother's devotion to her child. He described the holding environment as 'that atmosphere of safety and trust that the parent provides for the child and analogously, the therapist provides for the patient' (Winnicott, 1982).

In all forms of therapy, creating a sense of containment is reflected in 'an exquisite empathy and thoughtfulness with which the therapist responds to the client throughout the session' (Gibney, 2010) (p. 46). This requires the practitioners to manage their own feelings as well as those of their clients and families 'through containing and holding the gamut of emotional reactions, impulses, and feelings that often get triggered during clinical work' (Geller, 2011) (p. 208).

Practitioners can develop the capacity for creating a holding environment through both verbal and non-verbal means. The verbal approaches may include thoughtful *paraphrasing, summarising,* and *empathic reflections,* all of which are intended to show an understanding and recognition of the client. They are also intended for the client to understand and recognise themselves with an added insight that helps them to move forward (Gibney, 2010). These verbal ways of creating a holding environment are comprehensively described in the general counselling texts and those related to counselling for communication disorders, previously cited in Chapter 9.

Containment and the development of a holding environment is also achieved through non-verbal means, which is exemplified in the 'non-anxious presence' of the therapist who is able to join at the emotional level of the client and listen carefully before responding (Baker & Lane, 2009; Crago & Gardner, 2012). Here, the emphasis is on 'being with' rather than 'doing', and for those of us in professions that depend upon our asking a lot of questions, and where there are high expectations for us to be proactive in our work, this may not initially seem to have a good fit. However, holding skills that involve *saying little* and *doing less* can be very effective across all models of therapy, requiring *a particular quality of listening* and the *purposeful use of silence*. It is these more subtle and elusive skills and therapeutic ways of being that are highlighted below.

A particular quality of listening and the purposeful use of silence

'The goal of counselling after all is not to fill space with sound but to fill space with sound interaction' (Holland, 2007) (p.83).

One way in which we may offer *non-verbal holding* is through listening intently to what the client is saying, and to avoid intruding too much with frequent questions or comments. This may involve the purposeful use of silence and although this sounds simple, it requires considerable poise on the part of the practitioner to stay out of the way and to allow this to happen (Crago & Gardner, 2012). A therapist's choice to use silence might depend to some extent on the personality of the client, where prolonged silence may lead to doubts about the competence of the therapist, or where it might prompt the client to imagine that the therapist is forming a negative judgement about them. Equally, it may also depend on the personality, level of maturity, and confidence of the therapist because undoubtedly, being able to allow the space for silence develops with practice and experience. It requires a balance between a silence that is comfortable and therapeutic, and is not one that resembles some interminable parody of earlier psychoanalytic models.

As proposed by the authors above, learning to wait before responding, and remaining silent, enables the client 'to hear themselves', to tell their story and to think about what they have just said. The implicit permission to tell one's story is more cathartic than we may realise, and even before the therapist responds with words or other verbal ways of holding, such as with empathic reflections, the client begins to feel they are being understood. This purposeful use of silence gives the client the opportunity to determine the content of the session. It provides the space for the client to say more about what has already been said and to think about deeper feelings.

Applications to voice work

When these constructs are applied to the integration of counselling across the full range of communication disorders (and here I am including disorders of the voice), this special quality of listening and the capacity to tolerate silence is often pinpointed as the most important skill underpinning this work (DiLollo & Neimeyer, 2014; Holland, 2007; D. Luterman, 2011). Whether the struggle with words or the voice is physical or psychological, there needs to be time and space for the speaker to find a way through.

In working with students, I have found that they often need a lot of encouragement to allow silence in sessions. On one of my good days this would entail hands tied behind their backs and masking tape across their mouths! They find it virtually impossible to refrain from leaping in with more information, questions, and activities to meet their pre-planned therapy objectives. For experienced therapists too, it takes real courage and presence of mind to tolerate silence. However, this role as listener and silent witness is crucial as a counselling skill, and while it may only appear to manifest as a thoughtful pausing, such a subtle intervention allows patients to gather their thoughts and move on to the next thing they would like to share (Shewell, 1998).

The rehabilitation audiologist David Luterman (2011) cautions therapists to avoid the natural impulse to show how one is 'on top of the problem' by prematurely rushing in with education, advice, and ready options for new ways of thinking, feeling, and behaving. Further, in reflecting upon his own remarkable career, he notes that the more accomplished he has become the less he does and as a consequence, the more the client can learn. He states paradoxically *'I had to learn to cultivate the art of not doing and at the same time being present for the client'* (p. 5). Audrey Holland (2007) echoes these same sentiments when she proposes that much of what is beneficial in counselling actually occurs during the silences: *'It is one thing to know what to say. It is quite another to know when to say nothing at all'* (p. 83). These observations are all the more significant in the light of recent perspectives on the *principles of perceptuo-motor learning* whereby voice practitioners helping patients to modify vocal behaviours are now encouraged to hold back from offering feedback too soon or too often, and 'getting in the way' of a patient's learning experience (Titze & Verdolini Abbott, 2012).

Allowing for silence may also indicate to the patient that the therapist is thinking carefully about what has just been said. For instance, I will sometimes tell the patient that this is what I am doing, and when a patient hears this transparent explanation it has a powerful impact. It is also my impression that when we attend so deeply to a person, and when the sound of silence can be tolerated, it is as if the therapist is 'listening' with her eyes as well as her ears. When we do this it enables us to sense multiple meanings, perhaps without knowing how we are doing this. This is possibly the basis of intuition (discussed further in Chapter 11), and echoes the clinical observation of the psychotherapist Eric Berne who suggested that if you squint at the patient you will see his child (Berne, 1977). The renowned Australian author, Tim Winton, captures these phenomena in the marvellous piece of poetic writing in his recent book *Island Home* (2015), when explaining how he tried, as a young boy, to understand the natural world. Although the context of his discussion is entirely different to that being addressed here, it speaks to these issues of listening and looking deeply, and perhaps also to the facility for intuition. He says:

'Like any kid I was told not to stare. But I stared all the time – and at the oddest things. I found if you gazed hard enough at a handful of sand the individual grains became enormous; you could see cavernous spaces between them…When you looked at things long enough your gaze seemed to alter what you were looking at. It felt like a quirk of optics, a sleepy trick' (Winton, 2015) (p.86).

He then goes on to say:

'But young or old, stare as we might, much of what we learn about the objects of our attention in the natural world seems to come from out of the corner of the eye. When you're not trying to dig a place up with your eyes, a feeling for what's present will creep up on you, seep into vision and consciousness. Sometimes seeing is about duration and experience' (p.86).

Double description

The notion of *double description* and as this may translate to the clinical skill of *reframing* underpins all psychotherapeutic processes regardless of the theoretical models and orientation. It enables a person to have a different perspective on a problem with options for new solutions. Paul Gibney (2010) points out that earliest construction of this process was proposed by Carl Jung when he described psychotherapy as enabling 'a healing fiction' that was co-created by client and therapist in place of 'a pathologising fiction'. To some extent this is now reflected in the *narrative therapy movement* of family therapy (White & Epston, 1990), and more recently it has been most effectively proposed as a suitable model of counselling in the text *Counselling in Speech-Language Pathology and Audiology: Reconstructing Personal Narratives* (DiLollo & Neimeyer, 2014).

Gibney also notes that the construct of double description was later used as a possible explanation for the emotional changes that occurred during therapy. This draws on the work of analysts Alexander and French (1946) who controversially challenged the notion that it was *insight* alone that cured the patient. They proposed instead that change occurred as a result of the *corrective emotional experience* when a client felt and recognised the difference between what they expected to receive when they came to therapy and what they actually received. They maintained that when a therapist attended deeply to the client and his or her problem, this offered a stronger sense of being recognised than they may have experienced before. It was the *emotional impact* that this had on the person that was instrumental in facilitating change. These notions have since been captured by Gregory Bateson's two major constructs that now underpin the family therapy movement. These are: *new information creates a difference*, and 'it is the difference that makes the difference' (Bateson, 1979) (p. 99).

Applications to voice work

I have found these different perspectives on how change might be occurring in therapy as a revelation. For all voice practitioners, whether in the clinical field of SLP or the different domains of vocal pedagogy for the speaking and singing voice, these ideas emphasise that our interventions constitute a form of double description. However we choose to intervene, we need to enable a healing fiction that focusses on a person's strengths and resources rather than on a narrative that draws attention to the person's pathology and deficiencies. The use of double description needs to offer a curative emotional experience that clearly differs from previous experiences, and should be done in such a way that it provides new information and in a manner that makes a difference. This might entail very practical and behavioural changes; it might involve reflective conversations about attitudes or beliefs and ironically, it might, on some occasions, mean withdrawing effort and doing very little or nothing at all. Even abstaining from striving to make something better can constitute new information and make a difference. Another way that has been found to be particularly effective in facilitating a process of double description and changes in therapy is through reframing or redefining problems.

Reframing and redefining

'To reframe means to change the conceptual or emotional setting or viewpoint in relationship to which a situation is experienced and to place it in another frame which fits the 'facts' or the same concrete situation equally well or even better, or thereby changes its entire meaning' (Watzlawick, Weakland, & Fisch, 1974) (p. 95).

Reframing refers to 'the positive re-description of a complex behaviour pattern, described originally by clients in negative terms' (Carr, 2012) (p. 105).

The construct of double description as it may influence change in therapy is integral to the clinical skills involved in *reframing and redefining*. As explained by the authors above, in order to apply the technique a therapist needs to be able to distinguish between the reality of the 'observable facts' or sequence of events that could be agreed upon by anyone witnessing the situation, and then the reality of 'interpretation and new meanings' that each observer might place on that set of events.

In recent teaching seminars on the theoretical and clinical principles behind reframing (Personal communication Malcolm Robinson, 2012), trainee therapists were encouraged to recognise that when people first come to therapy they are often deeply pre-occupied with the problems they are facing. Robinson suggests that the client's psychological space is often overwhelmingly crowded or constricted by their concerns and preconceptions about what is wrong, or their failed attempts to make things better. There is little space for more hopeful explanations to appear, leading to a feeling of being stuck and perpetuating worries that their problems may be insurmountable. The purpose of reframing is to help to create the psychological space for different thoughts, feelings, and behaviours that will take into account the client's model of the world while also linking it to developmental, genetic, dispositional, and relational aspects of their life. Reframing is also intended to enhance the clients' awareness of their inherent skills, strengths, and resources that have been useful in solving problems in the past.

These experienced clinicians reassure others that even with the best will in the world practitioners do not always make an effective reframe. However, they also observe that in general, clients are very forgiving and appreciate knowing that another person is trying to come to a deeper understanding of who they are and what is going on. In a similar vein Paul Gibney (2010) proposes that it is not essential that clients agree with the reframe, rather that they will think about it, even question it, and through this process alone may alter their perspective on the problem and their responses to it. However, as also emphasised by Gibney, for a reframe or redefinition of a problem to be effective, any new meaning contained within the reframe needs to be 'more compelling, more therapeutic and contain more options' (p.66) than that originally expressed by the client.

Reframing is suitable for use with children as well as with adults; it can be 'playful, engaging, and non-blaming of the child', where the reframe not only gives a different meaning to problematic behaviours but also contains within it 'an implicit alternative response' that the family might be able to practise with this new way of thinking (Rhodes & Wallis, 2011). For instance, these authors give an example of a positive reframe where a therapist might say: "He's not bad, he's not mad, he's just young". This carries with it 'the message of hope that the child can grow up and the expectation that parents may need to set firmer limits in order for him to do so' (p. 136). Similarly, Alan Carr (2012) stresses that whether a therapist is working with an individual or members of a family, the problem needs to be reframed in interactional terms, with an emphasis on possible solutions rather than intractable difficulties, and with a clear acknowledgement that problematic behaviors are motivated by positive rather than negative intentions.

Applications to voice work

Reframing or refining a problem has direct application to voice work, whether early on in the process where a patient may be very concerned about their recent medical diagnosis, or subsequently in therapeutic conversations focusing upon changes to aspects of their thoughts, feelings, and behaviour. A brief clinical example of a positive reframe and redefining for a 21 year-old classically trained singer diagnosed with a MTVD and early vocal nodule formation is described. It is designed to illustrate how knowledge of the observable facts helps a therapist to offer a reframe that presents 'a different interpretation' with a 'new meaning' to the rather anxiety-provoking perspective that weighs heavily on this young person. It highlights the fundamental tenet that a therapist's appreciation of context is crucial (see Case example 10.2).

Case example 10.2 Reframing with a young singer with MTVD and early vocal nodules

A 21 year-old woman (S) studying classical singing at a conservatorium presents at initial consultation declaring guiltily that the medical assessment and laryngoscopy showed inflammation of the vocal folds and early indications of vocal nodules. S is a soprano and expectations of her course include individual singing lessons, performance at lieder class, jazz choir, chamber choir and preparation of a recital programme for a pending examination. She reports noticing sensations of vocal fatigue and strain in her upper range after several weeks of attending three compulsory rehearsals a week in preparation for a performance of Beethoven's Ninth Symphony in addition to her other commitments.

Patient S: *"I have been told that these nodules have been caused by blatant vocal abuse, and that I am constricting my laryngeal muscles. I was also told that I probably have poor vocal technique that needs urgent attention if I am to continue singing".*

Possible reframe by therapist: "This certainly is a very heavy vocal load for a young singer to be carrying and it is actually a credit to you, your vocal teacher and your vocal technique that you are managing as well as you have so far. It may well have led to some undue patterns of effort and strain that we can now address.

Comment

The choral work in the Ninth Symphony (see Case example 10.2) is challenging for the sopranos and places considerable vocal demands on a singer's technique and stamina. In some sections of the chorus work it requires the sopranos to sing towards the top of their range for over 40–50 consecutive bars. Even the most experienced singers with well-established vocal technique find it really difficult (Jean Callaghan, Singing Voice Consultant, personal communication, March 30th, 2016). Furthermore, for such a young singer, her overall vocal load is very high, requiring her to move between different styles of singing throughout the week that may range from choral work to solo work, from classical repertoire to jazz voice, all of which place different demands on the voice and on any singer's vocal technique. Diagnostic terminology such as 'blatant vocal abuse' carries with it the imputation that the person has not been sufficiently careful about their voice, which for young singers at a conservatorium is rarely true. Moreover, the suggestion that her vocal technique is in question, although accurate to a point, does not take into account what is being demanded of her at this very formative stage. Realising that better management of her vocal load (which frankly is unreasonable), and learning new ways to avoid compensatory patterns of muscle tension as this affects both her speaking and singing voice, is more likely to offer a *healing narrative* or *corrective emotional experience* than one that blames or engenders guilt and self doubt. This reframe is also intended to generate hope, which for many patients is a state of mind that is energising and motivating.

In my opinion, this final element of the positive reframe that gives recognition to problematic behaviours being motivated by good intentions is possibly the most potent aspect of reframing that will be therapeutic and likely to promote healing. It lies at the heart of helping people to save face and to avoid humiliation, which in many cultures is one of the most negative emotions of all. We never forget what it feels like to be humiliated, what was done, what was said, and who said it. As originally stated by the Chilean biologist Humberto Maturana (1988) 'words are not trivial, for they have both healing and damaging capacities and that to be human means to live in language'. Paul Gibney adds further that 'reframing grasps those truths and sets out to heal humanely through a language of more compassionate and varied realities in which people can live' (Gibney, 2010) (p. 66). Reframing or redefining a problem is a very powerful intervention and as expressed so strongly by Malcolm Robinson, *when reframing works, the client can never see this situation the same way again*' (Personal communication, 2012).

A summary of the key clinical processes of containment and double description as described by Paul Gibney (2010), and as supported by many other experienced practitioners cited in this chapter, is presented in Box 10.5.

Box 10.5 Key elements underpinning the dynamic structure of effective therapy

1. Containment and the capacity to create a holding environment

- Verbal means
  - Paraphrasing, empathic reflecting and summarising
- Non-verbal means
  - Non-anxious presence of therapist
  - Joining at emotional level of patient
  - Being with rather than doing
  - A particular quality of listening and purposeful use of silence

2. Double description-that may be offered in the forms of:

- A healing narrative
  - Focus is on strengths, resources, and new possible solutions
- A corrective emotional experience
  - Therapeutic intervention differs from expectations
  - Offers new *information* in a way that makes a difference
    - In the form of strategies to promote behavioural change
    - In the form of reflective conversation and insight
    - In the form of doing less or even nothing
- Positive reframing that offers new meanings to observable facts
  - States facts and new meanings in interactional terms
  - Creates psychological space for new solution
  - Recognises motivations for problematic behaviours are well-intended and generally positive

Conclusion

In conclusion, the focus of this chapter has been on a number of theoretical constructs and clinical processes that underpin systemic thinking and family therapy practice. Many of these principles are integral to all models of counselling and psychotherapy, and translate most effectively into the clinical management of voice disorders. While the emphasis from the family therapy literature is generally on working with couples or families, it is important to stress that much of the work undertaken by voice specialists from different disciplines is generally carried out with individuals. However, this in no way detracts from the primary emphasis of this particular chapter and the text in general, which is that *systemic thinking* and a constant *attention to context* are relevant to all aspects of our work, whether we are working with one person or the entire family. This includes our perspective on the physical and mental health of the individual, the development and the lifecycle of the family, the therapeutic relationship, and the processes involved in change.

All of these theoretical constructs provide a strong foundation for approaching the initial consultation and voice assessment, and then the subsequent phases of therapeutic intervention.

References

Alexander, F., & French, T. M. (1946). *Psychoanalytic therapy*. New York: Ronald Press.

Audet, C. T. (2011). Client perspectives of therapist self-disclosure: Violating boundaries or removing barriers. *Counselling Psychology Quarterly, 24*(2), 85–100.

Baker, J., & Lane, R. D. (2009). Emotion processing deficits in functional voice disorders. In K. Izdebski (Ed.), *Emotions in the human voice* (Vol. 3, pp. 105–136). San Diego: Plural Publishing.

Bateson, G. (1972). *Steps to an ecology of mind: Collected essays in anthropology, psychiatry, evolution, and epistemology*. New York: Ballantine Books.

Bateson, G. (1979). *Mind and nature: A necessary unity*. New York: Dutton.

Bateson, G., & Ruesch, J. (1951). *Communication: The social matrix of psychiatry*. New York: Norton.

Berne, E. (1977). *Intuition and ego states*: San Francisco: T.A. Press.

Butcher, P., Elias, A., & Cavalli, L. (2007). *Understanding and treating psychogenic voice disorder: A CBT framework*. Chichester: Wiley.

Carr, A. (2012). *Family Therapy: Concepts, process and practice*. Chichester: Wiley-Blackwell.

Crago, H., & Gardner, P. (2012). *A safe place for change. Skills and capacities for counselling and therapy*. Melbourne: IP Communications.

Crowe, T. A. (Ed.). (1997). *Applications of counselling in speech-language pathology and audiology*. Baltimore: Williams & Wilkins

DiLollo, A., & Neimeyer, R. A. (2014). *Counseling in Speech-language Pathology and Audiology*. San Diego: Plural Publishing.

Falicov, C. J. (2011). Migration and the family life cycle. In M. McGoldrick, N. Garcia-Preto & B. Carter (Eds.), *The expanded family life cycle: Individual, family and social perspectives* (4th ed., pp. 336–347). Massachusetts: Allyn & Bacon.

Flasher, L. V., & Fogle, P. T. (2012). *Counseling skills for speech-language pathologists and audiologists* (2nd ed.). NY: Delmar, Cengage Learning.

Flaskas, C. (2011). The therapeutic relationship and use of the self. In P. Rhodes & A. Wallis (Eds.), *A practical guide to family therapy* (pp. 1–15). Melbourne: IP Communications.

Fourie, R. J. (Ed.). (2011). *Therapeutic processes for communication disorders*. New York: Psychology Press.

Geller, E. (2011). Using oneself as a vehicle for change in relational and reflective practice. In R. J. Fourie (Ed.), *Therapeutic processes for communcication diosrders* (pp. 195–212). New York: Psychology Press.

Geller, E., & Foley, G. M. (2009). Expanding the "ports of entry" for speech-language pathologists: A relational and reflective model for clinical practice. *American Journal of Speech Language Pathology, 18*(1), 4–21.

Gelso, C. J. (2009). The real relationship in a postmodern world: Theoretical and empirical explorations. *Psychotherapy Research, 19*(3), 253–264.

Gibney, P. (2010). *The pragmatics of therapeutic practice*. Melbourne: Psychoz Publications

Hayley, J. (1985). *Conversations with Milton H. Erickson, MD. Volume 1. Changing individuals*. New York: Norton.

Holland, A. L. (2007). *Counselling in communication disorders*. San Diego: Plural Publishing.

Jacobs, M. (2011). *Psychogenic voice disorder and a compromised sense of self.* (Master of Science in Medicine (Psychotherapy) dissertation), University of Sydney.

Jacobs, M., & van Biene, L. (2015). Psychogenic voice disorder: A view through the lens of self. *European Journal for Person Centered Healthcare, 3*(2).

Jung, C. G. (1934). *Collected works of C.G. Jung: Civilization in transition* London: Routledge & Kegan Paul.

Lankton, S. R., Lankton, C. H., & Brown, M. (1981). Psychological level communication in Transactional Analysis. *Transactional Analysis Journal, 11*(4), 287–299.

Luterman, D. (2011). Ruminations of an old man: A 50-year perspective on clinical practice. In R. J. Fourie (Ed.), *Therapeutic processes for communication disorders* (pp. 3–8). New York: Psychology Press.

Luterman, D. M. (2008). *Counselling persons with communication disorders and their families* (5th ed.). Austin: Pro-Ed, Inc.

Mathieson, L. (2001). *Greene and Mathieson's: The voice and its disorders.* (6th ed.). London: Whurr Publishing.

Maturana, H. (1988). Reality: The search for objectivity or the quest for a compelling argument. *The Irish Journal of Psychology, 9*(1), 25–82.

McGoldrick, M., Carter, B., & Garcia-Preto, N. (2011). *The expanded family lifecycle. Individual, family and social perspectives* (4th ed.). Boston: Allyn & Bacon.

Miller, J. (2003). The crashed voice – a potential for change: A psychotherapeutic view. *Logopedics Phoniatrics Vocology, 28*, 41–45.

Miller, J. (2008). *The creative feminine and her discontents. Psychotherapy, art, and destruction.* London: Karnac Books.

Rhodes, P., & Wallis, A. (Eds.). (2011). *A practical guide to family therapy.* Melbourne: IP Communications.

Rosen, D. C., & Sataloff, R. T. (1997). *Psychology of voice disorders.* San Diego: Singular Publishing Group.

Roy, N., & Bless, D. M. (2000a). Toward a theory of the dispositional bases of functional dysphonia and vocal nodules: Exploring the role of personality and emotional adjustment. In R. D. Kent & M. J. Ball (Eds.), *The handbook of voice quality measurement.* (pp. 461–481). San Diego: Singular Publishing Group.

Roy, N., & Bless, D. M. (2000b). Personality traits and psychological factors in voice pathology: A foundation for future research. *Journal of Speech, Language, and Hearing Research, 43*, 737–748.

Sanders, C. (2012). *What lies beneath – The hidden foundations of family therapy.* Paper presented at the AAFT Family Therapy Conference, Perth.

Shannon, C. E., & Weaver, W. W. (1963). *The mathematical theory of communication.* Urbana: Univeristy of Illinois.

Shewell, C. (1998). The counsellor as travelling companion. *Speech and Language Therapy in Practice* (Summer), 8–10.

Titze, I. R., & Verdolini Abbott, K. (2012). *Vocology. The science and practice of voice habilitation.* Salt Lake City: National Center for Voice and Speech.

Vetere, A., & Dallos, R. (2008). Systemic therapy and attachment narratives. *Journal of Family Therapy, 30*(4), 374–386.

von Bertalanffy, L. (1968). *General systems theory: Foundation, development, application.* New York: Braziller.

Watzlawick, P., Weakland, J., & Fisch, R. (1974). *Change. Principles of problem formation and problem resolution.* New York: Norton.

Weiner, N. (1961). *Cybernetics.* Cambridge, MA: MIT Press.

White, M., & Epston, D. (1990). *Narrative means to therapeutic ends.* New York: WW Norton & Co.

Winnicott, D. (1982). *The Maturational processes and the facilitating environment.* London: Hogarth Press.

Winton, T. (2015). *Island home: A landscape memoir* Melbourne: Hamish Hamilton, Penguin.

Yalom, I. D. (2002). *The gift of therapy: An open letter to a new generation of therapists and their patients.* London: Piatkus.

11

Initial consultation and psychosocial interview

Introduction

The first session for any patient with a voice disorder is the most important one. It is crucial. And while it is generally anticipated that patients with voice disorders will need to attend for several sessions in order to achieve resolution of a problem, anecdotal evidence suggests that many voice patients only attend for one session. A similar finding has been reported for patients coming for psychotherapy (Talmon, 1990). This makes it all the more important that the first session is a significant and positive therapeutic experience. It is more likely to be so if the patient actively participates in finding a solution to his/her problems (Amini & Woolley, 2011). Even if patients decide not to return, it is important that each person feels they have been heard and understood, that they can now think about things differently, and that there is some hope for improvement. Whatever their decision, we should never underestimate the impact of the initial session – both good and bad.

Assessment and interventions are often reciprocally linked during the initial phase; during the later stages they are focused more directly on change, so any delineation between the different processes seems rather arbitrary. For instance, it would be the normal practice for many voice practitioners during the *initial consultation* to undertake a number of strategies to help the patient achieve some improvement in phonation. For those with psychogenic voice disorders (PVD), this would involve activities to confirm *symptom reversibility* and where possible, to restore normal phonation before the patient leaves the session.

However, for the purposes of this chapter, the emphasis is centered on the first two stages of intervention, as described in Chapter 9, which include Stage 1: Consideration of the referral letter, greeting and joining, and Stage 2: The exploration and gathering of information that includes the case history, and psychosocial interview. In Chapter 12, I address ways of integrating counselling with voice work for patients with more complex psychological issues in relation to their vocal difficulties. This discussion focuses on Stage 3: The action phase which includes setting goals, exploring ways to improve or restore phonation, seeking solutions, and gaining further insights into the vocal problem, and Stage 4: The closing phase which involves consolidating, generalising and ending therapy.

In this current chapter, the *general principles of counselling* including those related to systems thinking and family therapy that shape the *initial consultation* are discussed. I also introduce several additional constructs derived from the post-Milan schools of family therapy. These relate to *hypothesising*, *circularity* and *neutrality* (Selvini Palazzoli, Boscolo, Cecchin, & Prata, 1980) and to the notion of *interventive interviewing* (Tomm, 1987a, 1987b, 1988). These clinical constructs influence: the way in which the therapist approaches the original referral; greets and joins with the patient; gathers early biographical information; invites the patient to tell his/her story; and undertakes a psychosocial interview. It is proposed that these theoretical and clinical principles will be reflected in the therapist's 'way of thinking', as 'counselling moments on the fly' (Holland, 2007), or in the form of *embedded counselling* appropriate to the practitioner's work context and levels of experience (McLeod & McLeod, 2015).

Reference is made to the *key purposes* generally anticipated during Stage 1 and Stage 2, the *different intensities of therapeutic engagement* that might be appropriate throughout this process, and a number of *skills*, *qualities* and *ways of being* often demonstrated by effective therapists during these activities. Some will include more formalised strategies and rational qualities typically associated with left cerebral hemisphere functioning. Others will be reflected in the clinician's capacity for *practical wisdom*, *humour* and *intuition* generally originating from the right hemisphere, and often surprising the therapist as much as the patient (Crago & Gardner, 2012; McGilchrist, 2009; Schore, 2012). (The distinctions between these two different ways of thinking about information and communicating were discussed in Chapter 9.) It is proposed that when therapists can permit these left and right brain processes to flourish in an integrated and dynamic way, they become the therapists whom others may recognise as *master clinicians*. A tantalising question hangs in the air: "Do you have these skills and qualities, do I have them, and if not, can they be learnt?"

Stage 1: The initial phase of the first session

The primary purpose of the initial stage of the first session is to consider *the referral*, and to join and engage with clients in such a way that they feel able to express their concerns so that they may anticipate an in-depth exploration and assessment of their voice disorder. As proposed by Rhodes and Wallis (2011) 'The first session is critical to ensuring that a family returns, providing hope that things can change, and developing their commitment to work with the therapist towards their goals' (p. 20).

Considering the nature, source and implications of the referral

'...a therapeutic reality is constructed from the first words a client and therapist utter to each other. By extension then, even the messy initial contacts with the agency or the referring party are the beginnings of a psychotherapeutic contract' (Gibney, 2010) (p. 9).

Counselling in relation to the clinical management of voice disorders begins with the referral. From the moment the first spoken or written contact is made, the therapist begins to think about the person and the problem that they might bring to therapy. Depending on the source and nature of the referral, questions may arise about whether or not the person is a willing client, having acknowledged that there is a problem with a need for change. Alternatively, the person may be an involuntary 'visitor' who comes only in order to satisfy the expectations of someone else, and where the perceptions of the referring source may differ from those of the client.

Under these circumstances the person may be rather reluctant to come at all, bringing with him/her a preconceived sense of indignation or an intention to complain that others are responsible for the current situation. This may go hand in hand with a strong sense of entitlement about what their employers or others may owe them, and with total insistence that the responsibilities for all aspects of their problem lie elsewhere (Cade & O'Hanlon, 1993; Hutchins & Cole, 1992; Watzlawick, Weakland, & Fisch, 1974). Some *medico-legal referrals* requesting second opinion for work-related voice disorders may generate these 'complainant' attitudes along with large folders of documents related to worker's compensation. When these are placed firmly on the table between patient and therapist before even a word is spoken my heart sinks. (Case examples with complex psychosocial issues associated with worker's compensation are discussed in Chapter 12.)

With all referrals, tentative hypotheses about aetiology may hover in the back of the mind and in some cases, the therapist might begin to consider possible approaches to intervention. Even at this early stage, one might begin to ask oneself if it is appropriate to take on the case, if this may be a situation where *collaboration* with another therapist, or *mentoring* from a colleague may be advisable, or if more *formal supervision* is likely to be required (Flasher & Fogle, 2012).

These processes, even if only subliminal, will be based upon the nature and source of the referral and the firm foundations of the therapist's discipline-specific knowledge. They will also be influenced by preliminary statements made by the patient or others about their hopes and expectations, the fundamental principles underpinning the therapist's preferred models of counselling, and, not to be forgotten, the clinical experience of each practitioner (Baker, 2012). Aspects of this process, such as the mental preparation in response to the referral and the ways in which this may shape our joining with the patient, are highlighted below.

The referral

> *'Dear Jan,*
> *Another teacher with vocal nodules, please treat as you see fit,*
> *Yours faithfully'*

This tiny referral letter has loomed large in my amused professional memory more vividly than any other. In saying so little it says so much. Without the reader knowing anything about the referring specialist we can assume he has total trust in the therapist. That's nice. We can surmise that the otolaryngologist considers vocal nodules to be rather trivial as a form of vocal pathology, and the use of the phrase 'another teacher' suggests a commonality about these individuals, with a rather weary anticipation of possible medico-legal issues related to worker's compensation. If for a moment we avoid leaping into sanctimony and outrage at the brevity and tone of the letter, some practitioners might admit to sharing these sentiments. Others may challenge the assumptions being made.

For instance, the referral implies that the SLP's intervention for teachers across the country will be as straightforward as opening up a step-by-step-how-to-treat-nodules manual, and to use an Australian colloquial phrase, getting rid of vocal nodules will be 'as easy as falling off a log'. However, falling off a log, even in Australia, is not as easy as it sounds. The way in which we fall will depend upon how big the log is, how far it is to fall and where it is in relation to the terrain above and below. It will be influenced by our experience of the local flora and fauna, and the likelihood of our being attacked by a ferocious koala or kangaroo on the way down, or snapped up by a carnivorous crocodile when we get there. Most importantly of all, it will depend upon whether we know how to fall, even though our gold standard evidence-based recipe book has mapped out exactly what we need to do.

Furthermore, many of us recognise that it is one thing to read about how others do it, but it is another thing to do it ourselves, especially if we have never had the opportunity to observe someone else falling effectively, or if we have never had any practice (Lindhe & Hartelius, 2009). In addition, while there will be optimism and excitement about undertaking this seemingly simple task, there may inevitably be some anxiety about being a bit clumsy, even some concern about causing some harm to anyone else who may be taking the fall with us. Such concern is good.. These are all important things to remember when reflecting on this referral letter because experienced practitioners recognise that not all teachers are the same, the clinical presentations and severity of dysphonia arising in response to vocal nodules in individual cases are by no means identical, and 'getting rid of vocal nodules' is not always simple, especially when issues related to occupational health and worker's compensation lurk in the background.

In addition, treatment manuals with neatly signposted micro-steps are not necessarily easy to follow. This is particularly so when confronting different patterns of onset, the vocal load being demanded of each person, and a range of external and internal psychosocial factors that may have contributed to the onset or aggravation of the problem, or arisen in response to the condition. As highlighted in the different theoretical models for FVD discussed in Chapter 8, these external factors might include: recent experiences of acutely stressful life events; longer-term difficulties leading to chronic or accumulated stress; situations characterised by conflict over speaking out (COSO) and powerlessness in the system (PITS); or troubling circumstances where anticipatory stress in the face of evaluative judgment and threat to the person's integrity and identity begins to manifest in changes to physical and mental health.

Some of the internal factors may be associated with the person's current family and family life cycle situation, their prior or current physical and mental health, dispositional features such as personality and stress reactivity, and their emotional expressiveness and ways of coping. These in turn will be influenced by their attachment style as reflected in patterns of forming and maintaining intimate relationships with partners and others close to them, and in seeking social support. These psychosocial factors may then influence a person's level of motivation, inner resources, and development of resilience in meeting the challenges ahead, as illustrated in *The Interactive Psychosocial Model of Resilience* previously discussed in Chapter 2. Best laid plans as mapped out in treatment manuals will also need to take into account the clinical reality of different practice settings, the skills, qualities and 'ways of being' of the therapist, the strength of the therapeutic alliance forged between the patient and therapist, and the wider contextual factors that will determine the possible levels of therapeutic engagement.

The map is not the territory

While holding onto our somewhat minimalist referral, and keeping in mind all the factors above, it is relevant to recall the famous quotation often attributed to Gregory Bateson (1987). When considering the processes involved in teaching and learning he said, "The map is not the territory. The name is not the thing named" (p. 21) (see Fig. 11.1).

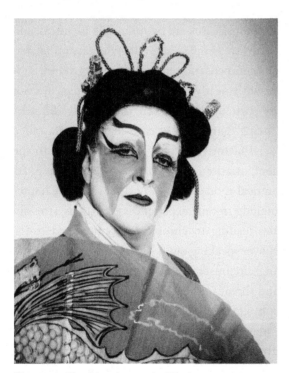

Fig. 11.1 The Map is not the Territory

"Adelaide Mezzo Soprano Jan Baker in the role of Katisha in the Mikado G&S Society. (Source, Adelaide Advertiser, The Arts Pages, October 1991)
"No, no, no, it's Roy Rene, Drag Queen in Chinese opera drag". (Source Peter Goers, Arts critic with a sting in his tail, Sunday Mail, The Arts Pages, October 1991).

This famous sentence was originally proffered by the philosopher Alfred Korzybski (1933), who suggested that words are not the objects that they represent. He used the metaphor of the map to illustrate this notion and in a more complete statement he said: 'A map is not the territory it represents, but if correct, it has a similar structure to the territory, which accounts for its usefulness' (p. 58). He emphasised that provided the map has structural integrity it can be both relevant and valuable. He also argued that if the map becomes disconnected in structure from the underlying territory that it is meant to represent, it could be 'misguiding, wasteful of effort … and in the case of emergencies, it might be seriously harmful' (p. 750). Both aspects of this original proposal have significant relevance to our work.

For instance, when applying these notions to communication and counselling the metaphor has been used to explain how a map is only a condensed representation of reality, and that there can be many different maps for the same location. These will differ in scale, emphasis, and detail depending on the primary purpose of the map; it will be influenced by the perceptual, cognitive and affective filters of the person creating it and those trying to follow it. Each map will offer different perspectives on the terrain to be traversed, with some well suited to the knowledge, experience, and skills of one traveller but not so readily understood by another. Some maps may be appropriate for one stage in the journey, while others will be more relevant at a later stage.

A time and place for practical wisdom

I further suggest that under some circumstances it might be better to put aside someone else's prescriptive map altogether and rely on what Aristotle referred to as one's own phronetic judgment. In his original text entitled Nicomachean Ethics, written in 350 BCE and now translated in The Complete Works of Aristotle (Barnes, 1985), Aristotle proposed two highly desirable intellectual virtues which he referred to as episteme (knowing: our analytical and scientific knowledge) and techne (our technical skills and expertise required to achieve a particular goal). However, he later introduced the concept of phronesis. This refers to a form of practical wisdom or common sense and the capacity to make prudent decisions in any given moment in relation to human problems with attention to values, context, and alternative perspectives. In applying this construct to the practice of counselling it has been suggested that we should not underestimate the power and importance of our practical wisdom, which not only incorporates our knowledge, skills, and techniques but also, fosters the awareness and integration of thinking and feeling (Sullivan, 2008). These notions, which encourage therapists to allow their practical wisdom to stand with equal footing alongside the highly revered intellectual virtues of knowledge and technical know-how, are integral to our work as clinician scientists and voice therapists. This sentiment is captured in the sage advice of Lewis Carroll (Box 11.1).

Box 11.1 Sage advice on the use of our practical wisdom

"That's another thing we've learned from **your** nation", said Mein Herr, "map-making. But we've carried it much further than you. What do you consider the largest map that would be really useful?"

"About six inches to the mile."

"Only six inches?" exclaimed Mein Herr. "We very soon got to the six **yards** to the mile. Then we tried a **hundred** yards to the mile. And then came the grandest idea of all! We actually made a map of the country, on the scale of **a mile to the mile!**"

"Have you used it much?" I enquired.

"It has never been spread out, yet," said Mein Herr: "The farmers objected: they said it would cover the whole country, and shut out the sunlight! So we now use the country itself, as its own map, and I assure you it does nearly as well."

(From *Sylvie and Bruno Concluded* (Carroll, 1893)).

Greeting, engaging and joining

The *joining process* entails making some form of connection with each person who attends for this first session, and finding a way to show that he or she has been heard. It is a special time in the therapeutic relationship and draws upon every therapist's keen observations skills and finely honed attention to verbal and non-verbal cues, with opportunities to show respectful curiosity and caring. This early joining phase may also incorporate a brief overview of the way in which the therapist intends to proceed with the assessment and interview, and what the patient might anticipate by the end of the first session. Such a conversation would be offered from a position of warmth and respect for the well-being of the patient and may include reference to administrative aspects. Clarification of roles and *professional boundaries* will be outlined, and assurances about *confidentiality*, with explanations about situations where limitations to confidentiality may apply, will be explained. These formal processes of *greeting and joining* are described in excellent detail in many of the counselling texts already cited.

Welcoming and joining is serious business and requires that therapists greet and respond to each person with appropriate respect for cultural norms regarding age, gender, hierarchy, and roles, with due attention to the person's concerns. However, it is also a very enjoyable process and provides opportunities for therapists to follow their intuition, to reveal their sense of humour and occasionally, to disclose unexpected aspects of their knowledge and life experience. These informal approaches can be just as effective in putting patients at their ease and enabling joining to take place; it may happen in ways that seem to defy logical explanation, with a depth of connection that goes beyond words alone.

One explanation for this might be that joining with the patient is mistakenly construed as a professional responsibility that is both structured and initiated solely by the therapist. However, it is often as much to do with what the patient offers to the therapist. Two such examples of joining between therapist and patients are presented below. The first involved a young woman with an organic voice disorder (OVD) of neurological origin leading to a severe dysarthrophonia, and the second was a frail elderly woman with a conversion reaction psychogenic voice disorder (PVD) (see case examples 11.1 and 11.2).

Case Example 11.1 Mental preparation following referral that shaped therapeutic joining

A 19-year-old woman (S) was referred for a second opinion with a traumatic brain injury following a car accident, leaving her with severe impairments across all areas of functioning including communication. Medical and neurological reports highlighted the extent and severity of the diffuse cortical and cerebellar damage incurred, suggesting that it was most unlikely that S would ever walk, communicate or function independently again.

Assessment revealed that S was able to comprehend basic conversational speech, but she was completely anarthric and aphonic, and deeply frustrated at being unable to communicate other than with a spelling board. She wanted this to be shredded as soon as possible.

Oral examination revealed flaccidity and minimal movement of lips and tongue with a paralysed soft palate. Her respiratory flow on expiration was so severely limited that she was unable to blow a feather, even with her nose blocked. She was able to swallow slowly but with frequent episodes of aspiration and coughing. She was unable to articulate words even with a silent whisper and no voluntary or involuntary phonation had been heard by anyone. She was inclined to emotional lability but she listened avidly to her mother's explanation of her difficulties and she watched me closely during our mutual efforts to clarify what she was able and unable to do, and what she was experiencing.

My mental preparation following receipt of the referral involved accessing medical records and setting up conversations with the referring SLP and physiotherapists. The accident and tragic outcomes for this young woman S had been widely reported in the media so other preparations involved finding out a little more about the family situation. This revealed that S was one of three children, her parents were widely recognised in the community, and the young woman herself was very popular and socially sophisticated with lively interests in public relations, journalism and a flair for fashion.

I noted earlier media references and photographs of S attending fashion parades, and chose my one and only designer outfit on the morning of that first interview with this background knowledge in mind.

Despite the extent and severity of the brain injury, the hopes and expectations of this family were very high. Their courage, determination and motivation were palpable, and no reasoned caution from previous medical specialists about limited prospects would be entertained. I experienced all of these pressures as being very challenging, and even during this preliminary stage of the first session as I sought information and informally assessed various aspects of S's communication, I began to have serious doubts that I would be able to help. This echoed the experiences of others who had been involved with her care before me. While S attempted every activity I asked her to try as best she could, it was impossible to elicit any whisper, articulation or phonation at all during these tasks. As the session progressed I was undecided about whether or not to offer a trial period of diagnostic therapy sessions in case this led to false hopes. During one of these equivocating moments, I made one of those 'out-of-right-brain' comments as a way of continuing to join with this young woman who was young enough to be my daughter, with an attempt to touch on her knowledge of fashion and to share my sense of humour in the hope it might tap into hers too. I said, "I hope you notice that I chose an outfit today that was designed by two of your favourite fashion designers". With the nearest approximation to a facial expression that she had made in that hour, her knowing eyes lit up, she grabbed her spelling board and with ataxic fervour she jabbed out *"Old model"*!

What could one say? *"Old model clothes, old model therapist"*, whichever one of these she meant, I roared with laughter, her head and body arched back into a reflex inspiratory laugh, and we were hooked. On the meeting ground of a hideous banana-coloured trouser suit that I thought was simply splendiferous at the time, we had joined in a long, difficult and mutually gratifying journey that led to her being able to speak again some years later.

Case Example 11.2 Joining that involved both left and right brain interventions with appropriate use of the self for the well-being of the patient

A 75-year-old woman (S) presented for second opinion at the request of her treating therapist who had been working with this patient for several weeks but with no improvements. S had a 10 month history of PVD in the form of a conversion reaction aphonia. She attended with her treating therapist and her son who regularly took time out from work to bring his mother to medical appointments in view of her difficulties with English as a second language.

Brief medical history revealed S had been completely aphonic all of this time, and no voluntary phonation had been heard during daily activities, or even leaking inadvertently while laughing, crying, or coughing during the previous therapy sessions. S was physically very frail, with multiple serious medical conditions, all of which required numerous medical specialist appointments. She reported being more devastated than anything about her inability to communicate using her voice. She appeared extremely desperate and anxious, perhaps because a more experienced therapist had been consulted, but her facial expression and body language also suggested an acute sense of anticipation and readiness to participate. This heightened sense of hope and expectation following months of serious illnesses and aphonia gave the woman the appearance of being both physically and psychologically fragile, and I noted she was close to tears throughout the early part of this encounter. As time was a constraint, we moved swiftly into reviewing some basic details about the history of her vocal disorder and some facilitating techniques known to effective in demonstrating symptom reversibility. All of these efforts were unsuccessful and I sensed her feelings of desperation as we attempted activities that others may have tried before, and that might well have been experienced as 'more of the same.'

At this point I made an intuitive decision to change direction. I commented with genuine interest upon her Christian name and how fascinating to be meeting someone of this name, given that Verdi's Italian opera *Nabucco* was being performed in our city at the time.

At the mention of an Italian composer from her native country who was well known to her, and the fact that I had made the link between her name and a leading character in an opera, her eyes widened with a different kind of attention and she momentarily lost the strained and anxious look of pleading. Then without knowing quite why I chose the next intervention, I began to hum the opening lines of *The Chorus of the Hebrew Slaves* from *Nabucco.* With no prompting at all, she then began to hum along with me, singing softly with a perfectly normal voice albeit rather waveringly, until we had completed the entire chorus. Her eyes filled with tears, her son's eyes filled with tears, and he then explained that their family had always loved classical music and that his mother had long been involved in choral singing. This was the first time they had heard her voice in 10 months. I then began to sing one of the early Vaccai Italian songs that we had all had to learn as part of our early 'Bel Canto' singing training at the conservatorium, hoping that with this brief diagnostic therapeutic intervention S might begin to sing along with the Italian words if they were familiar to her. Although she did not know the song, on hearing her native language, S appeared deeply affected, moved forward in her chair, took my hand, and smiled broadly. We had inadvertently entered into a different space.

I then asked if there was any particular Italian song that she loved, and she immediately began to hum her favourite song with a tentative but perfectly normal voice. The beautiful song was not familiar to me, so I asked her to teach it to me right there and then. **Here she took charge**, shifted from merely humming to singing gently with the words, and as she led me into learning the first two or three stanzas of her Italian folk song, together we knew that she felt safe enough to stay and to embark on therapy. There was no illusion on my part that her PVD had resolved. Rather, that in demonstrating the reversibility of her symptoms and that normal phonation during singing was possible, joining had taken place with sufficient 'holding' to enable trust and hope to develop. The sense of safety and 'containment' that had been generated via this intuitive intervention of self-disclosure by my singing had opened up opportunities for a deeper level of therapeutic engagement.

Comment upon different ways of joining, judicious self-disclosure and intuition

These two case examples highlight several interesting issues. The first is that joining is a two way process involving contributions from both parties and in some cases, there may even be an element of daring and risk for both patient and therapist. Secondly, it is not only patients who may be required to release information about themselves. For instance, when therapists share aspects of their life experience, albeit with the well-being of the patient in mind, it can open the door to humour and may actively strengthen the therapeutic alliance, even at this very early stage (Geller, 2011). Thirdly, while some insightful comments, use of *humour* or *self-disclosure* may be consciously calculated interventions with a strategic intent, at other times they may emerge spontaneously as *intuitive gestures* emerging from sub-conscious observations derived from *right brain processing*. Under these circumstances the therapist seems to draw upon intuitive knowledge gleaned from the experience of being with the patient 'that represents knowledge without knowing how she knows' (Berne 1977).

The role of intuition

> *'There is a time for scientific method and a time for intuition, the one brings with it more certainty, the other offers more possibilities'* (Berne, 1977).

Intuition, derived from the Latin *intuir*, refers to 'knowledge from within'. It has been the subject of debate since 200 BC when Aristotle alluded to 'intuitive induction', a process whereby man's perceptions were sensed, stored, and organised systematically for later retrieval. Throughout the philosophical literature, intuition has been likened to 'insight', inspiration', 'empathy', 'sixth sense', 'hunch', 'hypothesis', 'guesswork', 'mind reading', and 'whatever it is women use in place of reasoning and logic'!

Eric Berne, who was reputed to be highly intuitive, wrote six papers concerning the nature of intuition, highlighting its relevance to diagnosis and psychotherapy. These ideas led to his concept of the three ego states, the Parent, the Adult, and the Child, and were eventually consolidated into his theory of Transactional Analysis (Berne, 1977).

He maintained that *intuition* resided in the Child ego state which was characteristically spontaneous, free and impulsive, exploring, curious and creative, and capable of wisdom. He proposed that intuitive knowledge is to a great extent derived from the 'latent communications' that include impressions from non-verbal behaviours and attitudes expressed sub-consciously by the patient. He suggested that in order to recognise such stimuli, the therapist must be receptive to an overall impression and open to the imagery which arises sub-consciously both from patient and therapist in response to each other. He concluded that intuiting comprises two processes: an automatic sorting of perception into an integrated final impression, which he called subconscious perception, and the communication of this knowledge to himself or others, which he called conscious verbalisation of knowledge.

In a most interesting chapter entitled '*Intuition versus rationality and how to become really good at what you do*', Massimo Pigliucci (2012) highlights the cognitive processes that distinguish between the non-conscious cognitive and affective processes of intuition generated primarily from the right cerebral hemisphere, and the more deliberately considered thoughts and conscious processes articulated in words that derive primarily from the left cerebral hemisphere. According to Pigliucci, neurophysiological studies reveal that in addition to the *right hemisphere dominance for intuitive processes*, other areas of the brain most involved with intuition include the amygdala, the basal ganglia, the nucleus accumbens, the lateral temporal cortex, and the ventromedial prefrontal cortex, highlighting the well-recognised association between the amygdala and emotions.

In drawing further distinctions between intuitive versus more rational cognitive processes, Pigliucci explains 'intuition works in an associative manner: it feels effortless (even though it does use a significant amount of brain power), and it's fast. Rational thinking, on the contrary, is analytical, requires effort, and is slow' (p. 94). Like Eric Berne, he cautions that although intuition operates very swiftly and often provides helpful hypotheses, it is not necessarily infallible and a more studied rational consideration is also needed to support these provisional hypotheses.

The question that often arises for students and even experienced therapists is whether or not being intuitive is an innate gift, and if so, do the rest of us give up now, or is it something that can be learned. I suggest that *intuitive competence*, just like linguistic competence, is latent in us all and can be developed if we are open to doing so (Boeckx & Longa, 2011; Lenneberg, 1967). Pigliucci has highlighted a number of interesting features about intuition that might be reassuring to those practitioners who are intent upon developing their intuitive competence.

For instance, research shows that no person is intuitive about everything, and that intuition is definitely 'domain specific', with individuals being particularly intuitive in one area but not necessarily in another (e.g. in medicine, or chess, or ballgames). He stresses that the key cognitive process that underpins 'intuition' is *the brain's ability to recognise certain recurring patterns* and that intuition, like other skilled behaviours, improves with practice. Moreover, only after deliberate, mindful practice over an extensive period of time (10 years is generally required to become and 'expert' in any intellectual or physical pursuit) does the recognition of relevant patterns become automatic and internalised.

Pigliucci suggests that once this has occurred, a practitioner shifts from the more naive level of knowledge of 'the amateur', where understanding is often limited to one causal explanation or 'a failure to appreciate the intricacies of the system' (p.105), to a deeper field of the *structured knowledge* of 'the expert'. It is this structured knowledge based upon the ability to recognise recurring patterns, to anticipate problems, and to describe 'multiple causal pathways', that sets the *expert practitioner* apart from the novice (Hmelo-Silver & Pfeffer, 2004). Having acquired this deeper structured knowledge and the capacity to anticipate problems more rapidly, the 'expert' is in a stronger position to rapidly generate solutions to the current problem, whatever their domain of practice.

Setting the scene for gathering of information and psychosocial interview

In the discussions above, a number of processes involved in the initial phase of the first session, such as attention to the referral and different ways of joining between therapist and patient, have been described. It has been suggested that these activities may be highly structured and rather formal; alternatively, other ways of joining might include intuitive interventions, spontaneous humour, and judicious self-disclosure. It is proposed that effective joining sets the scene for the deeper levels of engagement required for the more formal gathering of information and voice assessment that will involve exploring the concerns of the patient and, in some cases, lead to undertaking a more comprehensive psychosocial interview. A summary of the counselling processes that may be involved in the initial stage of joining are shown in Box 11.2.

Box 11.2 Stage 1: The initial phase of the first session

Main aims

- To consider the nature, source and implications of the referral
- To greet, engage, and join with the client which may include his/her family
- To set the scene for further inquiry, assessment, and psychosocial interview

Levels of counselling

- Respectful, person-centered thinking with attention to context and meaning
- Curious, supportive, empathic listening, seeking to understand
- Clarification of administrative processes

Different intensities of therapeutic engagement

- Joins at the emotional level of the client
- Initiates a 'holding environment' or one of 'containment'
- Pre-empts the gathering of information phase, deeper psychosocial interview

Therapist skills, strategies, qualities and 'ways of being'

- Thorough mental preparation in relation to the referral
- Begins to formulate hypotheses based upon knowledge, skills, experience
- Vigilant observation of verbal and non-verbal cues of client & family
- Allows intuition and 'right brain processing' to facilitate some interventions
- Demonstrates confidence and sense of authority
- Creates a sense of safety that enables the person to begin to discuss concerns
- Reflects qualities that are gracious, erudite, soothing, and empowering
- Reveals sense of humour and a preparedness for self-disclosure if appropriate

Stage 2. Exploration, information gathering and psychosocial interview

The primary purpose of this next phase of the initial session is for the therapist 'to meet the challenge of the case' (Winnicott, 1982). This entails reaching an understanding about the nature of the voice disorder that is meaningful to both patient and therapist, acknowledging the strengths and resources of the client, and offering some form of help.

This will begin with an exploration of the patient's perspective on their voice disorder, including the perspectives of others. In addition to the traditional case history and voice assessment, which generally entails strategies to facilitate improved phonation, the therapist may decide to conduct a *psychosocial interview* that will focus attention on contextual issues related to interpersonal relationships, the immediate and extended family, work obligations, or factors related to the patient's wider social network. This often leads to reflections about the *emotional impact* and practical implications the voice disorder is having on the person's life, and on those close to him or her.

Integral to this process will be the formulation of a number of *hypotheses about causal factors* that might be contributing to the onset, maintenance, or aggravation of the voice disorder. Both the external situations preceding onset and the internal dispositional factors that determine different ways of coping will need to be taken into account. This will enable the therapist to offer an *assessment* and *diagnostic explanation* that makes sense, and at the same time provide hope for improvement and a way forward. At this point the therapist and client can *decide whether therapy is warranted* and if so, what form this might take. They can then discuss *a contract for change* that reflects their mutual expectations and refers to their respective responsibilities in the process ahead. These processes may take place during brief counselling moments embedded within the traditional assessment and case history procedures, or as focused conversations and strategies within the context of the psychosocial interview and diagnostic explanation phase that follows.

To inquire about the nature of the problem as experienced by patient and others

In all general counselling texts, including those devoted to communication disorders, emphasis is given to the need for therapists to try to understand the nature of the problem from the *perspective of the client*, then as judged by others and finally, from their own professional viewpoint. This requires a mind-set that takes into account the motivation and intent of the person attending for the first time. For instance, self-referred patients may have a definite idea about what needs to change with their voice; they may imagine enthusiastically what is likely to happen with voice practitioners of different persuasions when they get there, and then discover that not all voice work is as exciting as it was trumped-up to be (see Fig. 11.2).

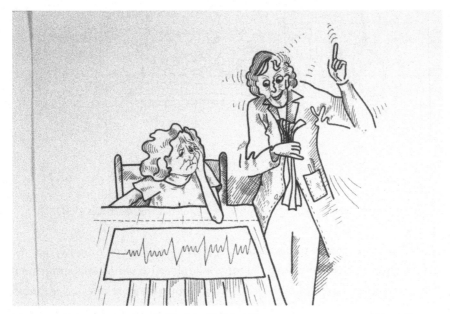

Fig 11.2 "Oh ecstasy, the thrill of facilitating formants one, two and three!"
Cartoon created by a patient for JB in preparation for a conference paper (Baker, 1981).

Those assessed by an otolaryngologist generally attend willingly, even if they are somewhat bemused about why they have been referred to the SLP. This will be particularly puzzling for those diagnosed with FVD, where on a very busy day the full extent of the explanation might include a sentence such as "Your vocal folds are absolutely fine" (see Fig. 11.3).

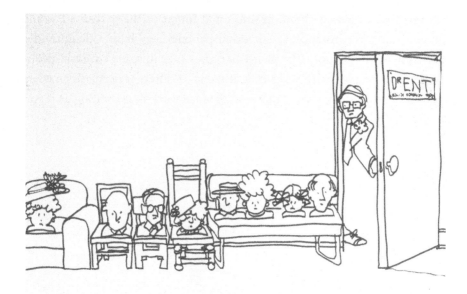

Fig. 11.3 "Next"!

Cartoon created by a patient for JB in preparation for a conference paper (Baker, 1981).

Some patients only attend to please others, such as children coming in response to the demands of their concerned parents, or adults with strong encouragement from partners, friends, or colleagues. A further group may present under duress. This might occur when the referral has been instigated by a third party for a second opinion, for medico-legal assessment with pending financial implications, or with respect to worker's compensation and occupational health issues.

Whether the patient appears to be willing and voluntary, sceptical and ambivalent, or in some cases, clearly hostile and involuntary, it is crucial at this very early stage to recognise any discrepancy between the patient's perspective on their voice problem and that of others who may be either directly or indirectly involved. Inevitably, this will have a direct impact on motivation and application to whatever may be required in therapy. Such differences in perspectives might relate to the perceived severity of the dysphonia as reflected in the auditory-perceptual quality of the voice, or the effect that the dysphonia is having on day-to-day communication or work responsibilities. As emphasised by many experienced practitioners, genuine respect for the patient involves acknowledging that he/she is the expert on themselves (DiLollo & Neimeyer, 2014; Holland, 2007; Rogers, 1951).

These different perspectives may also highlight the hidden agendas of others who create subtle and not so subtle pressures on the therapeutic process. These pressures may be reflected in the inordinately high expectations of what needs to be done and how quickly it needs to be achieved. For instance, a parent might demand a particular approach to therapy for a family member suffering dysphonia in association with a progressive neurological disorder for which there is no evidence to support its effectiveness. Alternatively, the singing teacher of a seriously dysphonic young tenor, with an A-grade passion and a D-grade talent, might make extreme demands on the therapist to help a student reduce his Reinke's oedema in time for auditions where *The X Factor* awaits (Fig. 11.4).

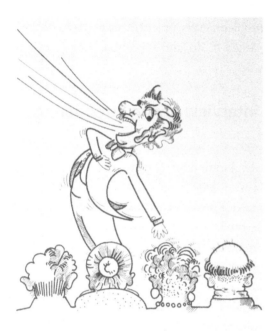

Fig. 11.4 "Who me? A-grade passion and D-grade talent?"

Cartoon created by a patient for JB in preparation for a conference paper (Baker, 1981).

On a more serious note, these different perspectives and pressures may also come from other health professionals with well-founded concerns about the status or progress of a patient, or from employing bodies and larger institutions in relation to medico-legal matters or their financial obligations to a patient. When these pressures are substantial, it is important to be able to answer some tough questions. One of these might be "Who is my client/patient?" Another might be "To whom am I accountable and ultimately responsible?"

These may seem rather strange questions to have to consider and even discuss with the patient because one's first impulse is always to say "The person with me right now, the person with the voice problem is my patient". But in the reality of clinical practice, where the concerns of parents or close others may be very acute, with the hovering constraints of managed care being imposed on many individuals or employees, and with third party involvement in many referrals that often involves financial support for the treatment being offered, it is not quite so simple. This can have significant implications for ethical issues to do with confidentiality, the kind of material that we include in our written reports, who may be permitted to have access to our clinical records, and for what purpose that may be. In the final analysis, when considering different perspectives on the nature and severity of the voice problem, every practitioner needs to be very clear about what he or she is being asked to do, and for whom. Every patient deserves to know where our loyalties lie.

To conduct a psychosocial interview giving attention to the wider social context

The gathering of information and exploration of a patient's voice problem generally begins with a traditional case history and voice assessment by the otolaryngologist and SLP. These procedures are extensively documented in a number of excellent seminal texts devoted to the full range of voice disorders and therefore, they will not be reiterated here (Aronson & Bless, 2009; Colton, Casper, & Leonard, 2006; Mathieson, 2001; Rammage, Morrison, & Nichol, 2001; Stemple, Roy, & Klaben, 2014; Titze & Verdolini Abbott, 2012). During these standard approaches, different levels of educational, *person-centered* or *supportive counselling* are generally undertaken by the SLP.

However, more sensitive psychosocial factors that emerge during the standard case history may need to be explored more thoroughly. These factors may have contributed to onset, or they may now be perpetuating the problem, even creating risk for recurrence of symptoms after intervention. Under these circumstances, an *expanded case history* in the form of a psychosocial interview that involves deeper levels of counselling and therapeutic engagement may be considered. In the discussion below I refer to the rationale for integrating a more comprehensive psychosocial interview into voice work as proposed by a number of practitioners, followed by those aspects of the patient's life that may be explored and how this sensitive information can be elicited.

Rationale for a psychosocial interview

One of the strongest proponents of the SLP undertaking the psychosocial interview is Arnold Aronson. He has been, and currently remains, one of the most highly respected clinicians, educators, and scholars in the world of SLP and otolaryngology, and over the last four decades he has continued to urge our profession to be both willing and able to conduct a 'psychodiagnostic' or 'psychosocial' interview during the initial consultation or assessment phase for patients with voice disorders (Aronson, 1973, 1990; Aronson & Bless, 2009). He argues that in view of the strong evidence for causal associations between stressful life events, interpersonal conflicts, dispositional factors, and the clear links between anxiety and depression, often seen as an outcome of vocal problems, this is an aspect of our work that cannot and must not be ignored.

In anticipation of anxious questions about the psychosocial interview being within the scope of practice for the SLP (questions I have addressed in Chapter 9), Aronson and Bless reassure clinicians that they are not recommending that the SLP conducts psychotherapy 'but rather that they obtain background information to identify aetiology and to relieve acute psychological distress by providing psychologic support' (p.194). They explain that the primary aim of the psychosocial interview is 'to aid them in determining the presence of emotional factors and the extent to which they are instrumental in causing or perpetuating voice disorder' (p. 194). Such a process involves being able to recognise those patients who may need referral to a mental health professional for deeper psychological work, and in order to do so *we need to consider our training incomplete until we have learned the basic skills of psychologic interviewing and counselling* (Aronson & Bless, 2009) (p. 194). These sentiments are strongly supported by a number of SLP working with communication disorders (DiLollo & Neimeyer, 2014; Fourie, 2011b; Geller & Foley, 2009; Holland, 2007). They are also reflected in the work of others specialising in the area of voice disorders (Baker *et al.*, 2013; Baker & Lane, 2009; Butcher, Elias, & Cavalli, 2007; Cavalli, 2009; Kollbrunner & Seifert, 2015; T. Miller, Deary, & Patterson, 2014; Rosen & Sataloff, 1997).

These practitioners openly acknowledge that depending on the nature and severity of the voice disorder, not all patients will necessarily need a broader *psychosocial history* to be taken. Moreover, even if psychosocial issues do seem to be relevant, not all patients want to explore them, either on their own or with another, and this view needs to be respected. Some may feel somewhat threatened at the suggestion that this deeper form of inquiry is going to be part of the SLP assessment, conjuring up clichéd visions of the psychiatrist's couch and being lowered down the proverbial well (see Fig. 11.5).

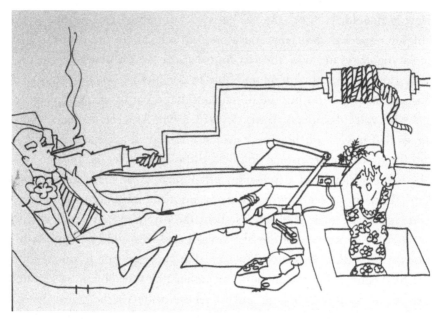

Fig. 11.5 "The psychosocial interview and down the well we go!"
Cartoon created by a patient for JB in preparation for a conference paper (Baker, 1981).

Here, the importance of the therapeutic relationship is crucial and in my clinical experience, if we are genuinely sensitive to these concerns and at the same time able to explain to a person in a transparent manner why additional questions about psychosocial issues might be relevant, this can alleviate the anxiety. When it is explained that part of the process involves identifying any patterns that may be connected, it then becomes clear that such an approach will lead to a more holistic appraisal of the voice problem, and may help the patient to construe their vocal symptoms in a more meaningful way.

While practitioners may approach the gathering of this additional information from the perspectives of different theoretical models, as suggested by Kolbrunner and Seifert (2015) *'this enhancement of psychosocial orientation and formation is possible under the basic principles of most different schools of psychotherapy. If learned in a responsible way, therapeutic techniques of cognitive behaviour therapy (CBT), psychodynamic therapy, systemic family therapy, or humanistic therapy can be used'* (p. 3).

The psychosocial interview begins with biographical information

To some extent the nature and extent of the *biographical information* gathered for any voice patient will depend on the work setting of the voice practitioner and the key purpose of the assessment or intervention being sought. This is not to imply that obtaining detailed biographical information about one person with a dysphonia is any more important than it is for another. Rather, it is a matter of relevance, timing, and context. For instance, in a voice analysis clinic specialising in care of the professional voice, the biographical information might initially be limited to that which is relevant to an urgent assessment and decision about whether it is safe for a singer to perform that night. In a community health setting, where many referrals to the SLP are for children with FVD, more details related to the immediate and extended family constellation would be important. Alternatively, in a clinic where the patients may be predominantly teachers with muscle tension dysphonia (MTVD), or adults and adolescents with psychogenic voice disorders (PVD), the biographical information would need to be more extensive.

In some of these settings, such as in a teaching hospital, a standardised approach to gathering information before the person arrives for their first session may be the norm. This may involve seeking personal details with a tick-the-box form that also asks for details about the nature of the voice disorder that is of concern. This may be done as a way of ensuring that there is consistent data for all patients using a particular service for auditing purposes, or in the interests of saving time. In other situations, this approach may be used for large population research projects where it is the most efficient way to gather large amounts of epidemiological data.

However, for the purposes of clinical practice and for research projects too if possible, I consider it preferable to gather this biographical information *face-to-face*. A research protocol may require that all questions are answered regardless of how sensitive or relevant they may seem, and under these circumstances, being face-to-face offers an excellent opportunity to observe how a person responds even at this very basic level of inquiry. Alternatively, in the clinical setting, this approach enables the therapist to decide which information is reasonable to gather on the first occasion, or if some information might be more appropriately pursued at a later date. For instance, deeply sensitive issues related to a previous or recent experience of violence or sexual abuse may only be raised by a SLP on very rare occasions. This would be if clues are given in the psychosocial interview suggesting that such incidents had occurred, or if the clinical presentation of the voice disorder is such that this may be suspected as being relevant. This more personal approach also offers the therapist an early opportunity to engage in *educational counselling* where he/she might choose to explain why this information is being sought, and how it is intended to help them both understand the nature of the voice problem and the implications that it has for the person. It is during this seemingly simple process of gathering even the most basic biographical information that joining and the therapeutic relationship begins. Some of the key domains of biographical information that are very informative in both research and clinical settings are shown below. It is suggested that it would be up to the discretion of each therapist to decide whether some or all of this information was appropriate according to the clinical setting and patient population (see Box 11.3).

Box 11.3 Biographical information for individuals with voice disorders

Name: **Age:**   **DOB:**   **Gender**

Country of birth: Year the person arrived in this county; language spoken at home

Education: Highest level of education reached

Occupation: Current occupation and how long in present occupation

Employment status: How long in present job, hours working

If unemployed or if retired: Previous occupation

Medico-legal matters: Workers compensation

Relationship status: Committed relationship, Divorced, Separated, Single, Widowed

Partner: Education, occupation, employment status of partner if relevant

Children: Number of children, Ages, Gender, (Miscarriages)

Family of origin and extended family (alive and deceased): Parents, Grandparents, Siblings

Confidantes/supports: How many, how often seen, if likely to contact if in trouble

Sexual abuse, violence and/or strangulation*: Lifetime or recent experience*

(*It is not recommended that this information would be sought routinely by the SLP)

(Extrapolated from Demographic and Biographic Data Form (Baker, Ben-Tovim, Butcher, Esterman, & McLaughlin, 2013))

Social support and confidantes

Any aspects of this biographical information can also be extended in order to gain a clearer picture of the patient's important social context. For instance, one area that may be relevant for some patients relates to *social supports* and *close confidantes*. A format for collecting this additional biographical information is shown in Box 11.4.

Box 11.4 Social support and intimacy context form

Household Members

Relationship   Name   Age

Occupation/school/university

_____

Social contacts

Other relatives/in-laws

               Approximate frequency of contact

Relationship   Visual   Non-visual   Location

_____

Friends, acquaintances, work associates, neighbours you see regularly

Relationship   Visual   Non-visual   Location

_____

Intimacy Context

If you had a problem of some sort who would be the first person you would want to discuss it with? Who else? _____
_____

If you had been asked this question a year ago, would there have been anyone else you might have mentioned then? _____
_____

Total number of social supports_____

(As developed by Brown & Harris, 1978 and as used by Baker *et al.*, 2013).

Some voice practitioners might find this area of inquiry a little unusual. However, the quality of social supports and the opportunity for confiding in a trusted friend has been shown to contribute to an individual's overall sense of well-being and includes feelings of intimacy, belonging, social acceptance, and approval, as well as feeling able to depend on others for help (Bowling, 1995). The number and quality of social supports are often reflected in a person's *overall attachment style* (secure versus insecure), and are also associated with resilience and healthy coping. Significantly, too, *loss of key social supports* or close confidantes has been found to be a contributing factor to development of mental health disorders, such as anxiety or depression in women, when occurring in the 12 months prior to onset (Bifulco, Moran, Ball, & Bernazzani, 2002; Brown & Harris, 1989b). As also shown in our own study, women with FVD had *fewer social supports* and were more likely to report an *insecure attachment style* with a predominance of an *anxious attachment profile* than those in the OVD and control groups (Baker *et al.*, 2013). Many reported that whereas previously they would have described themselves as being likely to trust others and seek support, following events or difficulties that involved loss of close support figures through betrayal (as opposed to death or simply moving away geographically) they were now much less likely to do so.

The psychosocial interview as an extended traditional case history for voice disorders

Butcher *et al.* (2007) have developed a comprehensive framework for a standard case history in relation to assessment of psychogenic voice disorders (PVD) which includes detailed descriptions of topics to be explored in an extended psychosocial interview. Their overall approach to counselling is founded upon principles of cognitive behavioural therapy (CBT). However, this clinical team also puts a strong emphasis on relational issues and systemic factors that include the patient's wider social context. Their detailed framework for inquiry reflects the current empirical evidence for a number of *predisposing, precipitating, and perpetuating aetiologic factors* commonly associated with the onset of FVD and in particular the PVD sub-group. (See Chapters 4–6 for an account of this empirical evidence.) These theoretical foundations have 'a good fit' with my own approach to integrating systemic thinking, principles of family therapy, and relational practices with voice work. The expanded voice case history that emphasises screening for psychosocial issues is shown in Table 11.1.

Table 11.1 Voice case history extended for full psychosocial assessment

Standard (with Psychosocial Prompts)	**Presenting voice disorder** • Onset and history of voice problem including any history of previous voice disturbance • Description of present problem, variation of problem, triggers • Description of voice use. Hobbies, sports and interests
	Related health issues • Medical information • Suggestions of anxiety symptoms • General health, including depression or lowered mood
	Voice assessment • Including observation of breathing, posture, and tension sites as well as assessment of voice • Assessment/palpation of laryngeal muscles to detect musculoskeletal tension
Extended	**Family background** • Relationship with mother and father, type of person, current contact • Family tree, number of siblings, type of relationship(s), current contact • General home environment • Other significant figures e.g. grandparents, aunts, foster parents, carers • Family life events e.g. separation/divorce of parents, death of siblings/parents, relocation
	Personal history • Early development, family, cultural background and social relationships • Personality as a child e.g. shy/outgoing, confident/nervous • Transition to adulthood; identify changes, leaving home • Personality prior to symptom onset e.g. assertiveness/ability to express views and emotions, tendency to suppress anger and frustration • Events around time of onset of voice disorder • Significant life stresses e.g. bereavement, changes in job or at home, changes in responsibilities • Marriage(s) and children • Important relationships, including relationships where there may be a difficulty in voicing feelings, unresolved conflicts or imbalance of power; evidence of 'conflict over speaking out' • Current social circumstances • Employment history • Use of leisure time, ability to relax or pace oneself • Juggling responsibilities or carrying a burden of responsibility including ability to set limits or invite support • Self-esteem and feelings of self-worth

As represented in Table 4.3 (Butcher et al., 2007), (p. 72)

Reproduced with kind permission Butcher, P., Elias, A. & Cavalli, L. (2007), Courtesy Wiley

Relevance of the psychosocial interview to both functional and organic voice disorders

It can be seen that the emphasis of the psychosocial assessment above is primarily on causal factors that may be associated with PVD. I have also found that exploration of many of these broad areas can be helpful in appreciating the context in which other voice disorders may develop, including MTVD and in some cases, those belonging to the OVD classification (Baker, Ben-Tovim, Butcher, Esterman, & McLaughlin, 2007). This is based on our findings that women with MTVD experienced as many severely stressful incidents in the 12 months prior to onset as those diagnosed with PVD and surprisingly, just as many situations imbued with *conflict over speaking out (COSO)*. This was unexpected and has highlighted the relevance of offering a more comprehensive psychosocial interview for this group of patients in some cases.

In addition, while it is recognised that psychosocial issues are not generally related to the development of organic or neurological voice disorders to the same extent, there is both clinical and empirical evidence suggesting that stressful life events and difficulties may act as 'trigger events' prior to onset (Aronson & Bless, 2009; Baker *et al.*, 2013). Further, it has been clearly established that psychosocial factors, such as symptoms of anxiety and depression, often develop in response to these organic conditions as well as those classified as FVD. (See Chapter 7 for a comprehensive discussion of these issues.) For these reasons, I suggest it is important to be at least open to the idea of exploring psychosocial issues with all voice patients while recognising that the degree to which one pursues the issues will be determined by the nature and severity of the disorder, the clues that emerge in the context of the traditional case history, and the clinical judgment of the therapist about how significant these issues might be in the overall scheme of things.

Theoretical principles that may guide how we might gather this information

In addition to the fundamental constructs underpinning systemic and other approaches to counselling and psychotherapy (Chapters 9 and 10), there are several other principles that may guide the way in which voice practitioners elicit the biographical information and integrate this exploration of psychosocial issues. As derived primarily from the post-Milan school of systemic family therapy, three of these core concepts are *hypothesising*, *neutrality*, and *circularity* (Selvini Palazzoli *et al.*, 1980). Another is related to the proposition that asking different kinds of questions constitutes a form of *interventive interviewing* (Tomm, 1987a, 1987b, 1988). These clinical principles can be applied during the first session, but subsequently too during the later stages of intervention. The constructs are described briefly below.

Hypothesising, neutrality and circularity

Hypothesising in this context refers to the way in which a therapist thinks about the possible meaning of the symptom for a person or family, and how it might be functioning for that person, within the family, or in the wider social system. Systemic therapists would argue that hypotheses need to be formulated in relational terms, and although they do not have to be true or false, they do need to be relevant and 'more or less useful' to the person. Importantly too, they do need to stimulate further inquiry and testing out that will result in being confirmed or refuted.

Neutrality refers to an attitude of impartiality that reflects a stance of being open to each person's point of view and to different hypotheses generated by the information that each person brings to the conversation. This means that the therapist avoids siding with one person or another, with the intention of enabling each person to express their beliefs and attitudes. As originally proposed by Selvini-Palazzoli *et al.* (1980), neutrality refers to a 'specific pragmatic effect' that the therapist's behaviour has on the person or family. They also point out that during any session, a therapist may seem to be more allied to one person than another, especially if seeking information about one family member's perception of the problem. However, when the attention is then given to gathering information from another member, it can be seen that the alliance has shifted. These authors stress that by the end of the session, the therapist should be judged as being 'allied with everyone and no one at the same time' (p. 11). A corollary to this is the firm ethical stance, that *neutrality* does not mean that a therapist has no opinion, and does not imply remaining morally neutral to issues such as intra-familial sexual abuse or domestic violence (Carr, 2012; Rhodes & Wallis, 2011).

Circularity refers to 'the capacity of the therapist to conduct his investigation on the basis of feedback from the individual and other family members in response to the information he solicits about relationships and therefore, about difference and change' (Selvini Palazzoli *et al.*, 1980) (p. 8). When this term is used in relation to causality, problem behaviours can generally be observed as 'interactional patterns' where one factor influences another; this in turn has an effect on the next and then comes full circle to impact on the earlier components. In reflecting upon the ways in which circular assumptions might be demonstrated in the context of a therapeutic conversation, it is helpful to be reminded of Karl Tomm's seminal paper where he proposed that 'the kinds of questions a therapist chooses to ask depends on what kinds of answers the therapist would like to have heard. One has to bear in mind that to a significant degree, the question "pre-figures" the response in that it structures the domain of an "appropriate answer"' (Tomm, 1988) (p. 14).

Different styles of questions and interventive interviewing

As also emphasised by Karl Tomm (1988), while many informal conversations with friends, colleagues, or others can be therapeutic in their effect, it is the professional responsibility of the therapist to guide the conversation in such a way that it is both therapeutic and healing for any patient who is seeking help with personal problems or interpersonal difficulties. In being a witness to the therapeutic session of many therapists, he has observed that the communication style of effective therapists needs to 'contribute intentionally toward a constructive change in the problematic experiences and behaviour of clients' (1988) (p. 1). At the very least, this involves the therapist offering statements and generating questions with the need for a delicate balance between the two. While there are times when numerous questions will be appropriate and even anticipated, the therapist should avoid setting up a pattern that feels more like a one-way inquisition. This is less likely to happen if he or she also contributes statements or makes comments in relation to the patient's answers.

Applications to voice work

When thinking about this in relation to the processes of integrating counselling with traditional approaches to voice work, the interchange between statements with questions is fundamental. This would come naturally to many experienced clinicians. However, in my experience, it is evident that student clinicians are more reticent to combine comments or statements with questions. I suggest that when this is done effectively, it strengthens the authenticity of the conversation because it reveals something of the therapist's knowledge and authority over aspects of the topic, gives a sense of their perspective on issues, and importantly too, reveals something of his or her personality. This then facilitates a stronger sense of the patient being heard and enables a deeper level of therapeutic engagement. It also contributes to the development of 'a real relationship' (Gelso, 2009) (see Case example 11.3).

Case Example 11.3 Combining questions and contributing comments

A 72-year-old woman (S) presented with a sudden onset of high-pitched falsetto phonation diagnosed initially as MTVD – my own diagnosis – PVD. After a number of the usual case history questions this further exchange took place:

T: "Has anyone suggested how this might have developed at this time?"

S: *"Some people have said it was doing too much singing lately – you know, lots of community singing – we did do a lot of performances".*

T: "Did that make sense for you?"

S: *"Well no, not really. I have been in that choir for years, and it's never gone like this before. Bob and I think maybe it was something else. You know, stress. There were some worrying things that had been going on just before my voice went.*

T: "Well I agree. I think judging by the sound of your voice, this unusual falsetto quality that you call your 'Micky Mouse voice' doesn't really fit with a strained voice after too much singing. You are right – I think it might well be more to do with some others things that were happening at the time. Can we talk about that now?"

In his further observations of therapeutic conversations, Tomm noted that effective therapists tend to ask different kinds of questions. The four different groups of questions as outlined below accordingly:

1. *Lineal questions* designed to orient the therapist to the patient's particular problem
2. *Circular questions* that allow exploration of mental and interpersonal phenomena
3. *Strategic questions* that are designed to be corrective and to influence
4. *Reflexive questions* that are designed to facilitate different ways of thinking about the issues by reflecting upon current perceptions and behaviours and considering new options in a hypothetical manner. (See Box 11.5 for examples.)

He maintains that the choice of questions will be driven by a therapist's 'lineal' or 'circular' assumptions around causality and will also be guided by the therapist's specific intent. The primary intent of some questions will be to orient the therapists and to help them to understand the perspective of the patient. The key intent of others will be to influence the patient in the direction of change. His conceptual map depicting how these different types of questions are linked to linear and circular assumptions about causality is shown in Fig. 11. 6.

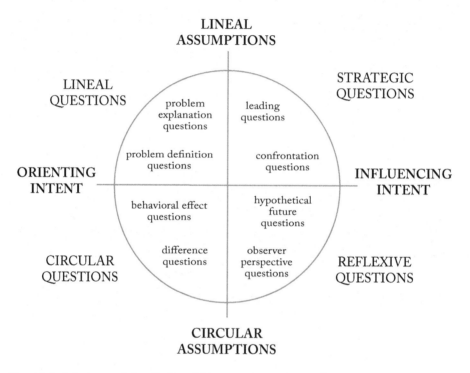

Fig. 11.6 A framework for distinguishing 4 major groups of questions

Tomm (1988) (p. 6). Reproduced with kind permission and Courtesy Wiley On-line

In addition to his distinctions between a therapist's *intent* that motivates the choice of particular groups of questions, Tomm highlights the way in which specific questions can have *distinctive effects* on both the patient and the therapist. For instance, some questions, such as lineal or strategic questions, will place *constraints on the conversation*; others, such as the circular or reflexive questions, will *expand the discourse* in a way that can be liberating and enable new insights. He stresses that there is a time and place for all of these different kinds of questions, and that the way they are interpreted will also be strongly influenced by tone of voice and other non-verbal aspects of a therapist's demeanour. His conceptual figure (Fig. 11.7) shows the predominant intent and probable effects of asking different kinds of questions.

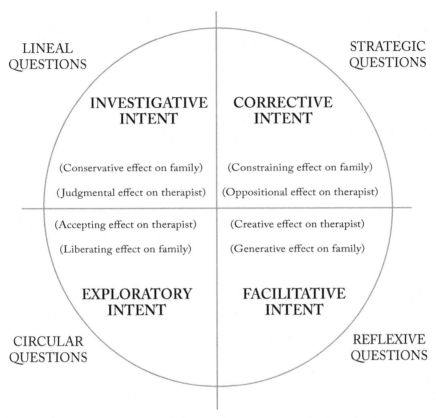

Fig. 11.7 Predominant intent and probable effects of differing questions (Tomm, 1988) (p. 13). Reproduced with kind permission and courtesy Wiley on Line

Applications to voice work

These systemic constructs in relation to hypothesising, neutrality, and circularity, and the notion of *interventive interviewing*, can be most effectively extrapolated into the clinical management of voice disorders. They are relevant to the way in which we may approach the initial consultation, and they are applicable throughout the subsequent stages of therapeutic intervention. Other therapists have referred to this approach as '*curious questioning*' with the clinician taking the role of an *interested conversational partner*(DiLollo, 2014) (p. 141).

I would also suggest that by the very nature of the work of the voice practitioners, lineal questions are often entirely appropriate in the early phases of the first session. This basic information is essential and the patient expects such a level of inquiry. Furthermore, strategic questions seem to come easily to SLPs who are mindful of outcome measures and the intent to influence patient attitudes, beliefs, and behaviours. What may be less familiar are the circular or reflexive questions that are designed to clarify and extend the patient's and the therapist's perspectives. As explained by Allan Carr (2012), circular questions help to modify hypotheses so that they take all the members or parts of the system into account. Circular questions can therefore seek to clarify:

1. The various sequences of interaction – what happened first, then next etc.
2. Comparisons in perspectives between different members of a system
3. Degrees of agreement or disagreement between the person and related parties
4. Explanations and interpretations of explanations from different sources
5. Futures predictions

Reflexive questions on the other hand give more emphasis to the way in which the person may perceive the situation now, how it might change in the future with new insights or different perspectives, and whether they are able to draw upon their own problem solving resources. These reflexive questions often prompt patients to suggest how they might think, feel, or act differently if this or that aspect of their situation changed. In this sense, while the therapist is maintaining a position of neutrality about the direction that the person might take, these questions show a respect for the ingenuity and inner resources of the individuals to generate solutions for themselves, even if only hypothetically at first. Some examples of the different types of questions that may be used to clarify and extend the patient and therapist perspectives in relation to voice disorders are shown in Box 11.5.

Box 11.5 Different kinds of questions and predominant intent that may be used to clarify psychosocial issues in relation to voice disorders

Lineal – Orienting and investigative intent

- What was the first sign of trouble with your voice?
- When did it first change?
- Where were you at the time?
- What did it feel like – sound like?

Circular – Orienting and exploratory intent

- Sequences of interaction
  - What happened next?
  - When she showed her worry, how did this affect you?
- Comparisons
  - Do you think she worried more than you?
  - Who might worry the least in your family?
- Agreement
  - Who else has noticed these changes in your voice?
  - Who would agree that it is different – and who might disagree?
- Explanations
  - What explanation do you have – does he/she have?
  - How does your explanation fit with these other explanations?
- Future
  - If this can be resolved how will this affect your plans for the next year?

Strategic – Influencing and corrective intent

- Has it occurred to you that you can do this differently?
- What has stopped you from doing something about it?
- What made you decide to wait 9 weeks before coming?

Reflexive – Influencing and facilitative intent

- If your voice came back now, what would you like to say?
- If your boss knew how worried you were about your voice how would that help?
- If they were willing to make changes in their behavior what would help you most?
- Would he feel able to seek help any earlier next time?

(Examples of questions as extrapolated from Tomm, 1988 and Carr, 2012).

The genogram and recording of relevant psychosocial factors

Generally speaking, while children or young adolescents may attend for their first consultation with one or both parents, most adult voice patients present on their own, or possibly with a partner. However, the application of these clinical principles, even if the patient comes alone, can facilitate the views of others significant in the person's life, such as their immediate and extended family members, colleagues at work, or even the institution to which he or she belongs. Through the processes of interventive interviewing or curious questioning, these other individuals can be 'brought into the room'.

An effective way to record and then hold much of this complex information is to create a *genogram* that is meaningful for both patient and therapist. The use of the genogram is a well-established practice across the different models of counselling and psychotherapy and it can be both informative and therapeutic to construct this map together. One way to do this is by using a large piece of paper shared by the patient and therapist on a table where both can record the information as the interview proceeds. Another approach is to use the much-maligned white board.

Either of these visual methods can create a very different ambiance in the room from one where the client may be responding obediently to standardised questions, and where the other is discretely writing on a well-concealed foolscap pad. This also models what is often said when therapists assure people that it will be an interactive process. Further, after creating a genogram together with the patient, the details seem to be more readily recalled and if not, they are readily accessible at a glance. Importantly too, if the genogram is shown to somebody else, patterns and trends can be readily visualised and often without the need for laborious explanation.

The information gathered for the genogram may include biographical information related to the person, their current and extended family constellation, and details of age, gender, marital status, and occupation. It may also include significant dates, family life cycle transitions, breaks in relationships such as separations or divorce, anniversary phenomena related to deaths, significant changes to health, and trans-generational patterns that are being repeated. In observing any trends and recursive patterns it readily opens up *counselling conversations* about how the person may have coped in the past, what strengths they have drawn upon on previous occasion, and whether or not the strategy seems to be working this time.

Mapping out stressful life events and longer-term difficulties

In addition to the genogram, it is also helpful to record and track the number and nature of stressful incidents that the patient reports to have occurred in the months preceding onset. For some patients, it can be the first time that they have taken stock of all they have been through. For many, this process creates the psychological space for the therapist and patient to reflect upon the possible consequences that these events or difficulties may have had on the person.

As highlighted in Chapter 5, there are different ways to elicit this kind of information, some with *tick-the-box checklists* and others via *semi-structured interviews* across key domains of inquiry. This is the preference of many clinicians because it facilitates an evaluation of the contextual features around the stressful incident, such as who else was involved, the nature of the relationship, and what the consequences of this incident were. For instance, there may be a question on a standardised form such as "Has there been a death in your family in the last 12 months?" If the answer is 'Yes', it in no way takes into account the *psychosocial context* of the incident. It fails to indicate which member of the family had died, how close the patient was to this person, how often the patient had seen this relative and under what circumstances (i.e., duty or pleasure), whether the relative had been suffering from a long illness and if so, was the death anticipated and what were the implications of this relative's death for the patient.

Alternatively, when this kind of information is elicited during a face-to-face interview, such as the *Psychosocial Assessment for Voice Disorders* as shown in Table 11.1 or the *Life Events and Difficulties Schedule (LEDS)* (Brown & Harris, 1978), contextual features play a major part in determining the degree of threat and severity of such an event. For example, as determined by the LEDS, the contextual criteria for rating a death as a 'severe event' require that this incident involves one of the patient's closest ties, such as a partner, a child, a parent, or a sibling, with additional details about how often they were seen, the quality of the relationship and the implications for the loss of the person at this time.

It is also important to mention that in some cases, no incidents of psychological significance are reported. This may be the case despite such incidents being suspected, and when the clinical presentation of the dysphonia, such as a sudden onset of PVD, suggests that this is likely (Baker, 2003; Baker & Lane, 2009). In these same cases, the dysphonia might even resolve without any stressful incidents ever coming to light. Similar phenomena have also been recognised in relation to *functional neurologic disorders* such as psychogenic or conversion reaction movement disorders, and it is important to note that the most recent changes to the DSM-V(American Psychiatric Association, 2013), the diagnostic criteria for these conditions, no longer require the evidence of, or even the reporting of, a psychologically stressful event prior to onset (Stone *et al.*, 2011).

Ways of accounting for those instances where no stressful incidents have been reported include the suggestion that the right questions have not been asked, that the timing of the questions may not be appropriate, or that the manner in which the questions have been asked is not conducive to divulging sensitive personal material. Another explanation might be that in instances of extreme psychological threat, such incidents are temporarily suppressed or may have been repressed (Baker, 2003). A third and less palatable explanation might be that current neuroscientific knowledge cannot always explain what is happening during the development and resolution of some 'functional symptoms', and we may have to tolerate 'not knowing'.

In the same way that the genogram offers an immediate visual impression of the immediate family and wider social context, it is illuminating to create a visual record of the events and difficulties across various domains of interest over time. This visual record may include a careful chronology of incidents, who else was involved, the length of time the longer term difficulties continued to impact upon the person, and additional ratings for conflict over speaking out (COSO) or a sense of powerlessness in the system (PITS) (Baker *et al.*, 2013). (See Chapter 5 for discussion of these features.)

When mapped out in this way, it is possible to see how certain events triggered longer term difficulties, how some stressful situations may have been running parallel with one another, and how these patterns may have contributed to both cumulative and chronic stress for that person. The implications of cumulative and chronic stress and its effects on the immune system leading to vulnerability for physical and mental health conditions have been discussed in Chapter 3. Once these incidents are viewed alongside the biographical information and key family connections as mapped out on the genogram, it creates the opportunity to develop *systemic hypotheses* about the symptom development. It affords the patient and therapist the opportunity to shift the focus from *'Another teacher with vocal nodules'*, to a person in the context of the family and the wider social context.

The genogram for a 47-year-old high school teacher diagnosed with MTVD and early vocal nodule formation is shown in Figure 11.8, with a *summary of the severe life events and major difficulties* that occurred in the 12 months prior to onset of her vocal disorder (Table 11.2).

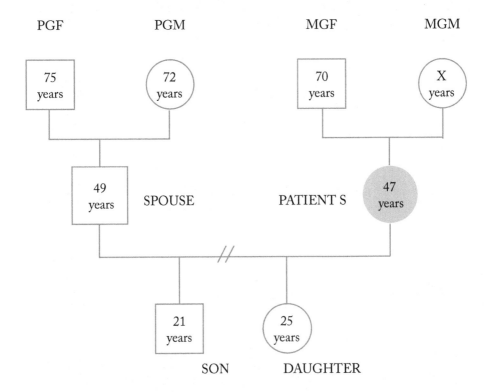

PGF = Parental Grandfather; PGM = Parental Grandmother
MGF = Maternal Grandfather; MGM = Maternal Grandmother

Fig. 11.8 Patient S genogram

Table 11.2 Summary of life events and difficulties experienced by a patient in the 12 months prior to diagnosis of a MTVD

	Jan	Feb	Mar	Apr	May	Jun	July	Aug	Sep	Oct	Nov	Dec
0 Education												
1 Work												
2 Reproduction												
3 Housing						House on market		House sold	Moved to a unit			
4 Finance			D-Financial difficulty									
5 Crime legal			Lawyer >	D-acrimonious divorce proceedings						Divorce Final		
6 Health				S-Clinical depression >	D-low mood affecting work & other relationships					Son Accident on bike		Diagnosis MTVD
7 Marital	S Learns of infidelity >	S Separates >	D-COSO in confronting truth, humiliation, PITS with constant denial despite evidence to the contrary									
8 Other relationships			S + Close friend – Betrayal >		D-COSO S discovers closest confidante implicated with husband in betraying S for many months							
9 Misc/Pets												

S=47yrs of age; Married 28 years; Children: Son 21yrs living at home; Daughter 25yrs living nearby.

S is a high-school teacher in the public sector with 25 years experience and prior to this period never experienced problems with her voice.

ENT Diagnosis=MTVD + early nodule formation

E=Severe Events rated for impact up to 14 days in relation to both reported threat and contextual threat. Severe events relate to the person and jointly with close ties

D=Major Difficulties rated for impact for at least 4 weeks or more and related to the person and jointly with close ties

> = Indicates the D developed out of the Events. COSO=Conflict over speaking out COSO; PITS=Powerless in the system as operationally defined (Baker et al., 2013)

To acknowledge the impact of the voice problem and the possible sense of loss

It is also during this very early exploratory stage of gathering information about incidents preceding the onset of the voice disorder that many individuals will begin to talk about the impact that the dysphonia has been having on their day-to-day communication with others, especially where their voice is their primary tool of trade. As emphasised by DiLollo (2014) in relation to counselling work for individuals with communication disorders, this enables the patient to consider the influence of the problem in their lives, with a shift from simply talking about the problem or themselves as the problem. The focus moves to '*the relationship between the person and their problem*' (p. 143). This is the foundation of the theoretical construct of *externalising the problem* as originally proposed by White and Epston (1990) and one of the cornerstone precepts underpinning narrative therapy.

For some patients, the emphasis of their distress may be expressed primarily in relation to auditory-perceptual-kinaesthetic symptoms such as: vocal fatigue, discomfort or pain in association with voice use; changes in the power of the voice and capacity for projection; alterations in vocal quality that make the voice unpleasant to their own or the ears of others; or in relation to embarrassing symptoms of alterations in pitch and quality that render the voice 'unreliable' under different circumstances.

Somewhat ironically, the impact of these changes as described by a patient is not always determined by the severity of the clinical signs as observed by others such as the otolaryngologist, SLP, or voice teacher. For example, the strong response of some patients to their voice changes can seem out of proportion to the very minimal clinical signs noted by others. However, such reactions should not be belittled or ignored. Teaching all day with a voice that feels tired and strained is extremely challenging both physically and emotionally. For the voice professional, where the demands for high levels of vocal control, flexibility, and projection are constant, it is far too easy to label the person as 'neurotic', 'overly anxious', or 'over sensitive'. On the contrary, performers are exquisitely sensitive to any suspected changes in their vocal health or vocal function and they are deserving of the closest professional attention and respect.

Alternatively, some patients with seriously dysphonic voices, or other individuals who possibly should be seeking help, may be strangely oblivious to their aberrant vocal function and appalling vocal quality. In Australia, one only has to listen to the gaggles of teenagers at the bus stop, to announcers on what are meant to be the top radio or television stations such as the Australian

Broadcasting Commission (ABC), or to the many well-educated and not-so-well-educated political leaders, to appreciate this anomaly. Grating glottal fry trundling along the moribund railway track is now the new normal.

Therefore, when the therapist endeavours to understand the impact of these changes, especially at this very early exploratory stage, some patients may only express a degree of annoyance or irritability. At the more conservative end of the counselling continuum this will generally require a supportive approach that lets the patient know they have been heard, with further educational explanations about how and why this might be happening.

Where other patients begin to express serious concerns about these changes to their voice, such as worry, sadness, or anger, a deeper supportive approach will be required. Here, it will be essential to convey to the patient that his or her feelings have been recognised, not just in the form of reflective listening or paraphrasing but rather 'the therapist making the most accurate possible statement he or she can about the client's emotional state' (Gibney, 2010) (p. 51). This can be integrated into educational counselling conversations about how various factors may have contributed to the onset of their particular vocal disorder, and the effects of stress on the physical and mental well-being of individuals in general, whilst also reassuring the person and alleviating their anxiety that these changes in the voice may well be amenable to intervention once therapy has started.

Sense of loss and early grieving conversations

'Grieving and the concomitant feelings are a normal response when a person is suddenly confronted with a life challenge for which there was not preparation; as a profession we need to give ourselves permission to do the necessary grief work' (Luterman, 2011) (p.3).

It is also a common phenomenon during this psychosocial interviewing stage that some patients will describe the impact of their vocal symptoms as extremely troubling, even devastating. As highlighted in Chapter 7, this may be expressed in terms of their voice no longer serving them during simple but important activities such as: reading aloud to their children; being heard on the telephone when speaking to close family members; or expressing their personality as they used to do in conversation with family or friends in social environments. This may carry over into the workplace where the voice problem has serious consequences for carrying out their job properly, whether this may be in fields of sales, classroom teaching, lecturing, or ministering to their religious community for example. For amateur singers or actors it may curtail their passionate involvement in the regular stage and musical events that have sustained and enriched their lives in the past. For professional performers, it may lead to the cancellation of a particular contract or completely threaten their ongoing performance career. Many of these individuals will describe the impact of their voice changes in compelling ways where they tearfully maintain "This is not my voice, this is not me, this is not who I am" (J. Miller, 2003; Rosen & Sataloff, 1997; Shewell, 2009).

When deeply felt statements like this are made, the patient is letting the therapist know that the impact of the voice disorder is challenging their sense-of-self, and their personal or professional identity. As emphasised by Luterman (2011), under these circumstances such a reaction is very natural, and he cautions therapists not to pathologise the patient's emotional responses to their communication or vocal problems. It is a fundamental aspect of the counselling work undertaken at this early phase to acknowledge the person's sense of loss and to let them know that it will be an important part of the therapeutic process to help them to resolve their grief (Baker, 1999, 2002; Bickford, Coveney, Baker, & Hersh, 2013; DiLollo & Neimeyer, 2014; Fourie, 2011a; Holland, 2007; Rosen & Sataloff, 1997). Further reference to ways of integrating deeper grief counselling work with voice therapy will be discussed in Chapter 12.

Coping

It is also during these processes of identifying the impact of the voice problem and sense of loss that the therapist will inquire about the patient's *coping strategies*. (Issues related to dispositional coping styles and coping in response to different kinds of voice disorders were discussed in Chapters 6 and 7.) Here, it is important to ask patients whether they feel they have been receiving adequate social support from those around them, and whether their current ways of coping are as effective as they were prior to this troubling period and if not, whether they have any ideas about what needs to change. This conversation may alert the therapist to any *major restraints to change* that are likely to influence the therapeutic process and that will need to be addressed during later stages of intervention. Some of these may be external constraints that seem to be outside of the patient's control. Others may be dispositional factors such as attitudes, beliefs, or entrenched patterns of operating that are likely to restrain the person from making the necessary changes to overcome their current vocal difficulties.

Alternatively, and of equal importance during this counselling conversation about coping, the patient may be invited to reflect upon their *strengths, resources,* and *powers of resilience* that have helped them to cope in the past (Oliveira,

Hirani, Epstein, Yazigi, & Belhau, 2012; Zambon, Moreti, & Behlau, 2014). They may be then asked to consider how these important motivational features can now be harnessed in the next phase of their voice therapy. It is essential for therapists to recognise the *role of hope* and *despair* in the therapeutic process, and one important component of hope is trusting that one has the inner resources to make the necessary changes to improve one's situation. A clinical vignette of a young man dealing with an OVD in association with severe recurring *vocal fold papillomata* highlights his sense of loss in relation to his vocal health, his longer term health, his sense of betrayal in his current relationship, and the importance of attending to his coping strategies in the future (Case 11.4).

Case 11.4 Issues revealed in the psychosocial interview related to sense of loss

A 29-year-old man (S) with recurring vocal fold papillomata and severe dysphonia was referred for 'straightforward assessment' of vocal quality pre- and post-surgical removal of the lesions. Medical history revealed changes to his voice were first noted 18 months ago.

Psychosocial issues related to aetiology

- Onset of a new sexual relationship had begun with this partner 2 years before
- Minor changes to his voice were noted shortly after, but were ignored initially since he was happily pre-occupied with his new relationship
- He had only learnt in retrospect that this sexual partner who had encouraged him to have oral sex, suffered from genital warts and had withheld this information
- He had previously been highly committed to this relationship that was now fraught with sense of betrayal and bitterness

Psychosocial issues related to the knowledge he had acquired about this condition and his current sense of loss, grief and coping

- The recurrence of the papillomata was possible and even likely
- Laryngeal examinations and surgical treatments would need to be repeated
- There was a risk of spread of the viral lesions into the trachea and vocal tract

- There was a possibility that papillomata may develop into cancer
- The hoarseness of his voice due to vocal fold scarring with repeated surgical interventions would be unlikely to improve
- Having been betrayed he was now withdrawing from close confiding relationships
- He was becoming super vigilant and anxious in relation to his vocal quality
- These factors had already started to have an impact on his current career prospects

To offer an assessment and diagnostic explanation that has meaning for the patient

'The purpose of taking a history is not just to obtain information – ideally, it also enables the patient to feel unburdened and to gain confidence in the doctor before the diagnosis has even been discussed' (Stone, 2016) (p. 7).

At the end of the initial consultation and psychosocial interview there is the expectation that the therapist will be able to offer feedback about the nature of the vocal problem in a way that makes sense to the patient. This explanation will take into account the findings from the otolaryngologist, the traditional case history and voice assessment, whether or not improved vocal function or normal phonation had been elicited during this preliminary session, and material emerging from a more comprehensive exploration of psychosocial issues where this had also been considered necessary. Such an explanation draws upon the considerable knowledge, skills, and experience of the therapist. While it is a relatively straightforward process with an OVD where observable lesions, vocal fold paralysis, damage to cartilaginous structures, or neurological disorder can clearly account for the nature and severity of a vocal problem, it may not seem such a clear cut process for the FVD group of disorders, especially those belonging to the PVD sub-group.

To some extent the inner conflict for the patient begins when the otolaryngologist reassuringly confirms "Your vocal folds are fine, the good news is there is nothing wrong with your larynx". However, by the time the patient comes to the SLP and has participated most co-operatively with an extensive initial assessment, there are a number of burning questions that are often asked of therapists, sometimes rather sheepishly and sometimes with a considerable degree of frustration or even anger: "Well if there is nothing wrong with my larynx or my vocal folds, why do I sound like this? If it's not in my larynx, is it all up in here, in my head? Is that what the specialist really thinks? Is that what you think too?" (Pain of death and I will be out the door if your answer to that one is a blunt "Yes".) They might even go on to say "I can't' really believe that it is normal. Do you think the doctor may have made a mistake?" "It's not in my head, it's in here, it hurts, and it doesn't feel right, this is not my voice, and I am not myself. I have taught for 20 years, so why now?" "I have sung this role 40 times before with no difficulties. It can' be my technique so what is going on?"

At this point we may be able to nod wisely and confirm with absolute integrity, "Well actually both are right. It is here (in your larynx), and it is in here (in your head, your brain)". However, what may be more difficult to explain is how it gets from the brain to larynx in a way that makes sense to the patient, that is meaningful in the context of their recent experience, and that is of therapeutic value, all at the same time.

This important explanatory process involves both *supportive* and *psycho-educational counselling conversations*. This will necessarily involve clarifying issues related to emotional, cognitive and behavioural aspects of the patient's history, with opportunities for dialogue about mind-body and functional-organic interactions, the effects of psychological stress on different systems in the body, and in particular, how this can impact upon our respiratory and vocal function. For some, it may involve suggesting possible associations between stressful incidents reported and whether they were deemed causally related or not. This comprehensive explanation will indicate the therapist's genuine respect for the patient's very reasonable questions "Why me, why this voice disorder, why now"?

In my clinical experience, the *diagnostic explanation* is integral to voice assessment and psychosocial interview, and rather than being tagged on the end, it is often interwoven or emerges in a dynamic way within these earlier conversations. When it is done well, it can substantially reduce the patient's anxiety, and can alleviate any self-consciousness where others may have implied that the symptoms were 'all in the mind' or being feigned. This then helps the person to feel empowered to take control of their situation. I have also found that when the therapist shares these findings, hypotheses, and formulations in a transparent manner, it strengthens the trust in the therapeutic alliance.

In some cases, for instance where a patient presents with a long-standing and severe PVD, it may mean having to admit that there are aspects that cannot yet be fully explained, and although no normal phonation has been elicited despite all best efforts on the part of the patient during the first session, there is every likelihood that it will be resolved in subsequent sessions. Such an explanation or admission can be a most powerful intervention in its own right. It can be so powerful, that for some patients, it triggers the resolution of their functional symptoms right there and then or shortly after, and in some cases, it may even obviate the need for further treatment. Essentially, a transparent diagnostic explanation along with acknowledgement that not everything is necessarily understood completely at this point, sets the scene for approaches to intervention that will take these 'functional' and psychosocial issues into account.

There have been a number of excellent papers devoted to this challenging issue of explaining the diagnosis by several teams of neurologists and psychiatrists seeing patients with complex 'functional' or 'psychogenic' neurologic disorders (Carson et al., 2016; Reuber, Mitchell, Howlett, Crimlisk, & Grunewald, 2005; Stone, 2016; Stone & Edwards, 2012). The conundrum over nomenclature and diagnostic terminology across disciplines remains problematic, but the primary focus of these discussions has been on how a neurologist or psychiatrist might communicate a diagnosis to a patient in such a way that it makes sense, and is also therapeutic. The suggestions made by these specialists reflect approaches that may well be integral to the clinical practice of many experienced otolaryngologists and voice therapists already. However, there is a refreshing transparency in some of the practical guidelines suggested by this team that are very helpful and entirely accessible to practitioners involved in voice care.

For instance, the neurologist Jon Stone (2016) argues convincingly that aspects of the diagnosis for various functional neurological conditions can be readily discussed during the actual assessment, and in such a way that it becomes a preliminary form of intervention. In a related paper, Carson and colleagues (2016) have presented a series of cartoon-like conversations to show how such a diagnostic explanation might be delivered by a neurologist to a patient presenting with a functional neurological leg weakness, and ending with a referral to psychiatry. They depict the scenario where it is not done very well at all, leaving the patient feeling frustrated and doubting that he has been taken seriously. In a second scenario, a clear diagnosis is delivered in a transparent manner with an explanation for how it is possible for this to have occurred and what can be done about it.

The authors recognise that this may seem an amusing way to highlight these serious issues, but these apt cartoon conversations offer a provocative challenge to practitioners to think about how such explanations might have deleterious or positive effects on both the patient and physician, with implications for later treatment outcomes. In my opinion, all of the issues are directly applicable to the way in which otolaryngologists or SLPs may give such explanations to patients with OVD and FVD, including those in the MTVD and PVD sub-group.

Some of the issues raised by these approaches will be discussed in further detail with respect to more complex voice disorders in Chapter 12. A brief summary of these key elements as highlighted by these authors is summarised in Box 11.6.

Box 11.6 Aspects of a diagnostic explanation for functional neurological disorders that are meaningful and therapeutic

- Indicate that the problem is being taken seriously
- Emphasise that the symptoms are genuine and common
- Explain that there is diagnosis that is both familiar and has a name
- Be prepared to offer a clear rationale for the diagnosis
- Explain the positive nature of the diagnosis
  - **Not a diagnosis of exclusion but based upon positive signs**
- There is an explanation of 'how' even if not 'why' at this point
- Reassurance that it is potentially reversible
- Simple advice in the form of:
  - Distraction techniques
  - Self-help techniques
  - Written sources of information
- Referral on to appropriate physiotherapy and or psychological services
- Offer follow up

(Extrapolated from Carson, Lehn, Ludwig, & Stone, 2016; Stone, 2016; Stone & Edwards, 2012).

To decide together whether therapy is warranted and formulate a contract for change

The final component to the initial consultation concludes with a discussion about whether or not therapy is warranted and if so, in what form it is likely to take. To a large extent this decision will emerge naturally from the earlier aspects of the initial consultation, where the therapist and patient collaborate to discuss the possible approaches to intervention, and the rationale for these options. It is helpful at this point to come to some form of *contractual agreement* where the therapist will undertake certain responsibilities for this process, but may also ask the patient to commit to aspects of the process as well. Reference will be made to a possible *time frame* so that the patient can anticipate how long the commitment to change may need to be, and it will be important for the therapist to recognise that the *priorities of the patient* may not necessarily be those that the therapist considers relevant.

For instance, where psychosocial issues have contributed to onset of a PVD, or where they are aggravating and perpetuating the symptoms, many therapists would anticipate working with the person to help them resolve these issues. They would consider this as their ethical responsibility, especially if they were seen as risk factors for relapse or recurrence. However, some patients with PVD seem to be totally satisfied once their voice is restored and they may well choose to walk very happily out of the door without looking back. This highlights some of the points raised earlier in this chapter where the perspectives of the patient and therapist may differ. In general, this last phase of the initial consultation is a most rewarding time in the therapeutic alliance, giving both therapist and patient an opportunity to outline their vision for the action phases that they are about to embark upon, and the optimism that is often felt at this stage. They will both need to recognise when they have achieved their goals, whether these are related to cognitive, affective, or behavioural changes, and how these impact on the person's voice. This final part of the conversation will also help the therapist to pre-empt some of the processes that will be involved in *ending therapy*, a stage that needs to be handled with sensitivity and one that can be as important as the very beginning. A summary of the counseling components involved in Stage 2 of the initial consultation is shown in Box 11.7.

Box 11.7 Stage 2: Gathering information and psychosocial interview

Main purposes

- To inquire about the nature of the problem as experienced by the person/others
- To conduct a psychosocial interview giving attention to the wider social context
- To acknowledge impact of the voice problem on the person and possible sense of loss
- To offer an assessment and diagnostic explanation that has meaning for the person
- To decide together if therapy is warranted and to formulate a contract for change

Levels of counselling

- Supportive counselling with empathic listening, seeking to understand
- Psycho-educational counselling offering information and advice where appropriate
- Preliminary grief counselling recognising sense of loss or altered sense of identity
- Explanatory counselling regarding differential diagnosis and approaches to therapy
- Early motivational counselling that seeks to harness motivation and foster resilience

Different intensities of therapeutic engagement

- Maintaining a holding environment during the process of systematic inquiry
- Strengthening the therapeutic alliance with transparency about systematic inquiry
- Exploring biographical details, current family constellation, stages in family life cycle
- Recognising the impact of the problem on the person and preferred coping style

Therapist skills, strategies, qualities and 'ways of being'

- Seeks to understand through listening, observing and being open to intuitive insights
- Empathises, affirms, reflects thoughts and feelings with sensitivity
- Clarifies attitudes, beliefs and concerns with different styles of questioning
- Reframes and externalises the problem where appropriate
- Inspires by giving authoritative and coherent explanation
- Pre-empts processes for ending therapy

References

American Psychiatric Association. (2013). *Diagnostic and statistical manual of mental disorders DSM-5* (5th ed.). Arlington: American Psychiatric Association. https://www.psychiatry.org/psychiatrists/practice/dsm [Accessed October 2016].

Amini, R. L., & Woolley, S. R. (2011). First-session competency: The Brief Strategic Therapy Scale-1. *Journal of Marital and Family Therapy, 37*(2), 209– 222.

Aronson, A. E. (1973). *Psychogenic voice disorders.* Philadelphia: Saunders.

Aronson, A. E. (1990). Importance of the psychosocial interview in the diagnosis and treatment of "functional" voice disorders. *Journal of Voice, 4*(4), 287– 289.

Aronson, A. E., & Bless, D. M. (2009). *Clinical voice disorders* (4th ed.). New York: Thieme.

Baker, J. (1999). Changes to women's voices following hormonal therapy. A report on alterations to the speaking and singing voices of four women. *Journal of Voice, 13*(4), 496– 507.

Baker, J. (2002). Persistent dysphonia in two performers affecting the singing and projected speaking voice: A report on a collaborative approach to management. *Logopedics, Phoniatrics, Vocology, 27*, 179– 187.

Baker, J. (2003). Psychogenic voice disorders and traumatic stress experience: A discussion paper with two case reports. *Journal of Voice, 17*(3), 308– 318.

Baker, J. (2012, 27 July). Workshop on Psychogenic voice disorders: Lost or mislaid, stolen or strayed: Perspectives on aetiology, assessment and intervention.

Baker, J., Ben-Tovim, D. I., Butcher, A., Esterman, A., & McLaughlin, K. (2007). Development of a modified diagnostic classification system for voice disorders with inter-rater reliability study. *Logopedics Phoniatrics Vocology, 32*, 99– 112.

Baker, J., Ben-Tovim, D. I., Butcher, A., Esterman, A., & McLaughlin, K. (2013). Psychosocial risk factors which may differentiate between women with Functional Voice Disorder, Organic Voice Disorder, and Control group. *International Journal of Speech-Language Pathology, 15*(6), 547– 563.

Baker, J., & Lane, R. D. (2009). Emotion processing deficits in functional voice disorders. In K. Izdebski (Ed.), *Emotions in the human voice* (Vol. 3, pp. 105– 136). San Diego: Plural Publishing.

Barnes, J. (Ed.). (1985). *The complete works of Aristotle* (Vol. Vol. 2). Princeton: Princeton University Press.

Bateson, G., & Bateson, M. (1987). *Angels fear: Towards an epistemology of the sacred.* New York: Macmillan Publishing.

Berne, E. (1977). *Intuition and ego states:* San Francisco: T.A. Press.

Bickford, J., Coveney, J., Baker, J., & Hersh, D. (2013). Living with the altered self. *International Journal of Speech-Language Pathology, 15*(3), 324– 333.

Bifulco, A., Moran, P., Ball, C., & Bernazzani, O. (2002). Adult attachment style I: Its relationship to clinical depression. *Social Psychiatry and Psychiatric Epidemiology, 37*, 50– 59.

Boeckx, C., & Longa, V. M. (2011). Lenneberg's views on language development and evolution and their relevance for modern biolinguistics. *Biolinguistics, 5*(3), 254– 273.

Bowling, A. (1995). *Measuring disease. A review of disease specific quality of life measurement scales.* Buckingham: Open University Press.

Brown, G. W., & Harris, T. O. (1978). *Social origins of depression.* London: Tavistock Publications.

Brown, G. W., & Harris, T. O. (1989b). *Life events and illness.* London: The Guilford Press.

Butcher, P., Elias, A., & Cavalli, L. (2007). *Understanding and treating psychogenic voice disorder: A CBT framework.* Chichester: Wiley.

Cade, B., & O'Hanlon, W. H. (1993). *A brief guide to brief therapy.* New York: W.W. Norton & Co.

Carr, A. (2012). *Family Therapy: Concepts, process and practice.* Chichester: Wiley-Blackwell.

Carroll, L. (1893). *Sylvie and Bruno concluded.* London: Macmillan & Co.

Carson, A., Lehn, A., Ludwig, L., & Stone, J. (2016). Explaining functional disorders in the neurology clinic: A photo story. *Practical Neurology, 16,* 56– 61. doi: 10.1136/practneurol-2015-001242

Cavalli, L., Butcher, A., & Elias, A. (2009). *Incorporating Cognitive Behaviour Therapy principles and skills into the clinical practice of SLT's working with Psychogenic Voice Disorders: A partnership approach* Paper presented at the RCSLT Scientific Conference, London.

Colton, R. H., Casper, J., & Leonard, R. (2006). *Understanding voice problems: A physiological perspective for diagnosis and treatment.* Philadelphia: Lippincott, Williams & Wilkins.

Crago, H., & Gardner, P. (2012). *A safe place for change. Skills and capacities for counselling and therapy.* Melbourne: IP Communications.

DiLollo, A. (2014). Constructivism and adaptive leadership: Framing an approach for clinicians to overcome barriers to counseling. In R. J. Fourie (Ed.), *Therapeutic processes for communcation disorders* (pp. 139–152). New York: Psychology Press.

DiLollo, A., & Neimeyer, R. A. (2014). *Counseling in Speech-language Pathology and Audiology.* San Diego: Plural Publishing.

Flasher, L. V., & Fogle, P. T. (2012). *Counseling skills for speech-language pathologists and audiologists* (2nd ed.). NY: Delmar, Cengage Learning.

Fourie, R. J. (2011a). From alienation to therapeutic dialogue. In R. J. Fourie (Ed.), *Therapeutic processes for communication disorders.* New York: Psycholgoy Press.

Fourie, R. J. (Ed.). (2011b). *Therapeutic processes for communication disorders.* New York: Psychology Press.

Geller, E. (2011). Using oneself as a vehicle for change in relational and reflective practice. In R. J. Fourie (Ed.), *Therapeutic processes for communcication diosrders* (pp. 195– 212). New York: Psychology Press.

Geller, E., & Foley, G. M. (2009). Expanding the "ports of entry" for speech-language pathologists: A relational and reflective model for clinical practice. *America Journal of Speech Language Pathology, 18*(1), 4– 21.

Gelso, C. J. (2009). The real relationship in a postmodern world: Theoretical and empirical explorations. *Psychotherapy Research, 19*(3), 253– 264.

Gibney, P. (2010). *The pragmatics of therapeutic practice*. Melbourne: Psychoz Publications

Hmelo-Silver, C., & Pfeffer, M. G. (2004). Comparing expert and novice understanding of complex systems from the perspectives of structures, behaviours and functions. *Cognitive Science, 28*, 127– 138.

Holland, A. L. (2007). *Counselling in communication disorders*. San Diego: Plural Publishing.

Hutchins, D. E., & Cole, C. G. (1992). *Helping relationships and strategies* (2nd ed.). Pacifc Grove. C.A.: Brooks/Cole.

Kollbrunner, J., & Seifert, E. (2015). Encouragement to increase the use of psychosocial skills in the diagnosis and therapy of patients with functional dysphonia. *Journal of Voice*. doi: doi:10.1016/l.jvoice.2015.11.021

Korzybski, A. (1933). *Science and sanity: An introduction to non-aristotlian systems and general semantics*. New York: Institute of General Semantics.

Lenneberg, E. H. (1967). *The biological foundations of language*. New York: Wiley.

Lindhe, C., & Hartelius, L. (2009). Speech-language pathology students' self-reports on voice training: Easier to understand than to to? *Logopedics Phoniatrics Vocology, 34*, 51– 59.

Luterman, D. (2011). Ruminations of an old man: A 50-year perspective on clinical practice. In R. J. Fourie (Ed.), *Therapeutic processes for communication disorders* (pp. 3– 8). NY: Psychology Press.

Mathieson, L. (2001). *Greene and Mathieson's: The voice and its disorders*. (6th ed.). London: Whurr Publishing.

McGilchrist, I. (2009). *The master and his emissary: The divided brain and the making of the western world*. New Haven: Yale University Press.

McLeod, J., & McLeod, J. (2015). Research on embedded counselling: An emerging topic of potential importance for the future of counselling psychology. *Counselling Psychology Quarterly, 28*(1), 27– 43.

Miller, J. (2003). The crashed voice – a potential for change: A psychotherapeutic view. *Logopedics Phoniatrics Vocology, 28*, 41– 45.

Miller, T., Deary, V., & Patterson, J. (2014). Improving asscess to psychological therapies in voice disorders: A cognitive behavioural therapy model. *Current Opinion in Otolaryngology and Head and Neck Surgery, 22*(3), 201– 205.

Morrison, M. D., & Rammage, L. (1994). *The management of voice disorders*. San Diego: Singular Publishing Group.

Muller, R., Ward, P. R., Winefield, T., Tsouros, G., & Lawn, S. (2009). The importance of resilience to primary care practitioners: an interactive psycho-social model. *Australasian Medical Journal, 1*(1), 1– 15.

Oliveira, G., Hirani, S. P., Epstein, R., Yazigi, L., & Belhau, M. (2012). Coping strategies in voice disorders of a Brazilian population. *Journal of Voice, 26*, 205– 213.

Pigliucci, M. (2012). *Answers for Aristotle*. NY: Basic Books.

Rammage, L., Morrison, M., & Nichol, H. (2001). *Management of the voice and its disorders*. San Diego: Singular Publishing Group.

Reuber, M., Mitchell, A. J., Howlett, S. J., Crimlisk, H. L., & Grunewald, R. A. (2005). Functional symptoms in neurology: Questions and answers. *Journal of Neurology, Neurosurgery and Psychiatry, 76*, 307– 314.

Rhodes, P., & Wallis, A. (Eds.). (2011). *A practical guide to family therapy*. Melbourne: IP Communications.

Rogers, C. R. (1951). *Client-Centered Therapy*. London: Constable.

Rosen, D. C., & Sataloff, R. T. (1997). *Psychology of voice disorders*. San Diego: Singular Publishing Group.

Schore, A. N. (2012). *The science of the art of psychotherapy*. New York: Norton.

Selvini Palazzoli, M., Boscolo, L., Cecchin, G., & Prata, G. (1980). Hypothesizing – circularity – neutrality: Three guidelines for the conductor of the session. *Family Process, 19*, 3– 12.

Shewell, C. (2009). *Voice work: Art and science in changing voices*. Chichester: Wiley-Blackwell.

Stemple, J. C., Roy, N., & Klaben, B. K. (2014). *Clinical voice pathology* (5th ed.). San Diego: Plural Publishing.

Stone, J. (2016). Functional neurological disorders: The neurological assessment as treatment. *Practical Neurology, 16*, 7– 17. doi: 10.1136/practneurol-2015-001241

Stone, J., & Edwards, M. (2012). Trick or treat? Showing patients with functional (psychogenic) motor symptoms their physical signs. *Neurology, 79*, 282– 284.

Stone, J., LaFrance, W. C., Brown, R., Spiegel, D., Levenson, J. L., & Sharpe, M. (2011). Conversion Disorder: Current problems and potential solutions for DSM-5. *Journal of Psychosomatic Research, 71*, 369– 376.

Sullivan, B. (2008). *Counsellors and counselling: A new conversation*. Sydney: Pearson Education Australia.

Talmon, M. (1990). *Single session therapy: Maximising the effect of the first (and often only) therapeutic encounter*. San Francisco: Jossey Bass.

Titze, I. R., & Verdolini Abbott, K. (2012). *Vocology. The science and practice of voice habilitation*. Salt Lake City: National Center for Voice and Speech.

Tomm, K. (1987a). Interventive Interviewing Part 1:Strategizing as a fourth gudeline for the therapist. *Family Process, 26*, 3– 13.

Tomm, K. (1987b). Interventive Interviewing: Part II. Reflexive questioning as a means to enable self-healing. *Family Process, 26*, 167– 183.

Tomm, K. (1988). Interventive interviewing Part III. Intending to ask lineal, circular, strategic, or reflexive questions? *Family Process, 27*(1), 1– 15.

Watzlawick, P., Weakland, J., & Fisch, R. (1974). *Change. Principles of problem formation and problem resolution*. New York: Norton.

White, M., & Epston, D. (1990). *Narrative means to therapeutic ends*. New York: WW Norton & Co.

Winnicott, D. (1982). *The Maturational Processes and the Facilitating Environment*. London: Hogarth Press.

Zambon, F., Moreti, F., & Behlau, M. (2014). Coping strategies in teachers with vocal complaints. *Journal of Voice, 28*(3), 341– 348.

12

Working through complex psychogenic and psychosocial issues during the action and closing phases of voice work

Introduction

'In many settings the psychotherapeutic practitioner applies his or her craft in addition to the tasks that are prescribed by their profession-of-origin, or if employed solely as a psychotherapist, it is often in a setting where psychotherapy is a secondary activity to the 'core business' (e.g. medicine, justice, education)' (Gibney, 2010) (p.4).

As mentioned in previous chapters, the degree to which counselling is integrated with direct behavioural approaches to voice therapy will depend upon the nature and severity of the voice disorder, and the extent to which psychosocial factors may have contributed to the clinical presentation or may be impacting upon the course of therapy. It will also be coloured by the preparedness of voice practitioners to engage in different levels of counselling depending upon their attitudes and beliefs about the place of counselling in relation to voice work. This in turn will be determined by what is considered to be the 'core business' of their work environment, and their respective levels of training and expertise in the different models of counselling and/or psychotherapy.

It is acknowledged by experienced voice therapists that in some cases relatively little counselling is necessary, and I would agree with this. However, generally speaking, *supportive, psycho-educational*, and *motivational counselling* by the speech-language pathologist (SLP) will be relevant across the full range of functional voice disorders (FVD) and organic voice disorders (OVD). For those patients with a psychogenic voice disorder (PVD), deeper psychological work with approaches such as *cognitive behavioural therapy (CBT)* or *relational therapy* is often the primary intervention. This is necessary both during efforts to facilitate and restore normal phonation for those who may be aphonic or severely dysphonic, and during the parallel processes of helping the person to make sense of their psychogenic symptoms.

For many individuals with disorders of the voice, *grief counselling* will be a significant component of the work, especially where the vocal problem challenges a person's sense-of-self or professional identity, or where different medical conditions such as endocrine dysfunction, traumatic brain injury, surgical mishap, total laryngectomy, or progressive neurological disorder lead to marked deterioration or loss of voice altogether. In those situations where change to an individual's *physiological voice* seems to represent a loss of his or her *metaphorical voice* in the context of family, occupation, and wider social networks, counselling where the *therapeutic relationship operates as the nexus of change* may be required. This may occur for instance in work settings or in personal relationships where a person is bullied or totally disempowered by others, and where ongoing uncertainties about the future remain a concern for the individual. These issues in relation to chronic stress, the ongoing anticipation of threat, and constant challenges to self-preservation were discussed in Chapter 3 and then highlighted in relation to different theoretical models accounting for FVD in Chapter 8.

In this chapter I suggest ways in which strategies from systemic and strategic family therapy along with other models of counselling may be combined with traditional voice therapy for both FVD and OVD. The discussion of these approaches is structured around the different levels of counselling that may be used during the third and fourth stages of intervention as described in Chapter 9. Stage 3: *The action phase*, involves finding ways to *restore phonation* for those with aphonia, or *facilitating improved phonation* for those with dysphonia. During this phase it is also important to help the person *gain further insights* into stressful situations that may have contributed to the onset of their vocal disorder, or those that may be operating to perpetuate their vocal symptoms. Stage 4: *The closing phase* entails *consolidating changes*, *weaning* from the therapeutic process and *ending therapy*.

Suggestions are made to help therapists recognise the more complex psychological issues that are often associated with particular voice disorders such as PVD, how to determine which levels of counselling may be appropriate during the different stages of intervention, and creative ways to go about this.

Guidelines are also proposed to assist therapists in recognising *restraints to change* that may impact upon the therapeutic process. These restraints might be related to external factors such as *stressful life events* or *conflict over speaking out (COSO)* situations impinging on the patient. Alternatively, they may be related to *personality traits* or *dispositional qualities* that affect the way in which individuals tend to cope in the face of stress or in relation to their particular vocal disorder. At the more serious end of the continuum, if these restraints to change are associated with more deeply suppressed or unconsciously repressed negative emotions, as seen in some cases of patients with conversion reaction aphonia, then interventions generally used by the SLP or even experienced clinical psychologists may not be effective in helping these patients to resolve their vocal disorder. Under these circumstances, referral to a psychiatrist or psychotherapist for more sophisticated levels of intervention would be more appropriate (Butcher, Elias, & Cavalli, 2007; Butcher, Elias, Raven, Yeatman, & Littlejohns, 1987). It is also the case, although not a very comfortable thought, that *one of the most powerful restraints to change is the therapist.*

For both patient and therapist this counselling work can be challenging and feel difficult at times, but it is also stimulating, thought provoking, and fun, always leaving both parties altered and changed as a result of the interaction (Holland, 2007; Sullivan, 2008). Once again, reference is made to the *main purpose* of the counselling work during Stages 3 and 4, the *specific skills* and *strategies* used by effective therapists during these activities, and particular *therapeutic qualities* and *ways of being* that enable this work to take place.

It is proposed that therapists who are recognised as being *master clinicians* in any therapeutic context openly admit to the limitations in their knowledge or experience with particular kinds of disorders or problems. They also remain vigilant to the nuances of *transference* and *counter-tranference* as this plays out in the dynamics of the therapeutic relationship. In the specialised field of *vocology*, therapists who may be identified as master clinicians, regardless of their preferred approaches to behavioural voice change or models of counselling and psychotherapy, are those who are open about their levels of expertise and are comfortable in declining to take on patients whose voice disorders lie well outside their levels of knowledge and competence. These are also the therapists who are willing: to *seek supervision*; *to work collaboratively* with more experienced therapists or other mental health professionals; to *refer on* to mental health professionals who are experienced in the clinical management of voice disorders; or to *undertake further training in appropriate models of counselling or psychotherapy* (Baker, 2010b; Butcher *et al.*, 2007; T. Miller, Deary, & Patterson, 2014; Nichol, Morrison, & Rammage, 1993).

Stage 3. The action phase, seeking solutions and gaining insights

'*..emotional growth does not readily lend itself to measurement, yet it is in the emotional realm where a great deal of the action takes place*' (Luterman, 2011) (p. 4).

The primary purpose of integrating counselling during this third phase is to support the medical and surgical aspects of intervention, and to enhance conventional behavioural voice therapies. For many patients with PVD, counselling will be the primary intervention. When this is done effectively it facilitates changes in thoughts, feelings, and behaviours and presents opportunities for the person to find both their physiological and metaphorical voice.

These processes may include *educational counselling* in order to clarify the diagnosis and rationale for recommended approaches to therapy, with important *direct advice* on ways to improve vocal health and hygiene (Pemberton, Oates, & Russell, 2009). Judicious suggestions and unobtrusive advice may also be offered throughout this action phase, where *psycho-educational counselling* conversations are focused on complex interpersonal issues or other psychosocial matters affecting the patient. It is my experience that student clinicians often come away from basic counselling topics in their training convinced that therapists should never give advice, and that giving advice will be frowned upon. This is one of the key tenets underpinning the non-directive supportive models of counselling where it is emphasised that each person has the potential and resources to find the answers within themselves, given the therapeutic climate to do so. These models of counselling maintain that it is not the role of the counsellor to give advice.

However, as highlighted by Paul Gibney (2010), while therapists should never force their recommendations or opinions on people, he has stressed that it is naïve for any therapist to think he can practise 'advice-free'. He reminds us too: '*In the same way that a therapist cannot be value-free, what she or he chooses to highlight by comment, or chooses to address by conversation, constitutes a reinforcement that has embedded in it advice as to a course of thought, reflection or action*' (p. 53). This reflects Karl Tomm's proposals (1988) as discussed in Chapter 11, that the type of questions we ask will determine the answers we want to hear.

In a most interesting discussion about the place or manner of giving advice in the context of family therapy, Couture and Sutherland (2006) challenge the notion that the giving of advice is always a one-way linear process from therapist to client, or that it is necessarily 'a form of social control with the locus of control for treatment lying in the expert hands of the counsellor' (p. 330). These authors suggest that it is not the advice in itself that is likely to hinder therapy or to diminish the capacity of the client to draw upon their own resources, but the manner in which it is offered. Using a detailed discourse analysis of therapy sessions with Karl Tomm and a family, they observe that moving into offering advice often occurs in a *stepwise progression*, with each party taking turns with responsive questions and answers, and with circular rather than linear interactions. Couture and Sutherland propose that if we think about *therapeutic advice* as the culmination of an *interactional process* evolving during the conversation between therapist and client, then the provision of advice can have 'a generative and healing potential' (p. 331). This perspective on the offering of advice in family therapy makes good sense in the context of voice therapy, and echoes the way in which I think about therapeutic conversations as resembling a dance. The notion of a 'stepwise progression' into the proffering of advice also supports the previous discussions in Chapters 10 and 11 advocating for a therapeutic relationship that is 'real'(Flaskas, 2011; Geller, 2011; Gelso, 2009).

Supportive counselling approaches will underpin all of the patients' efforts as they pursue both medical and practical solutions to their vocal problems, and as they strive to regain control over their voice (Egan, 2009; Flasher & Fogle, 2012; Holland, 2007; Riley, 2002). For some, a more energetic style of *motivational counselling* may be necessary as the person undertakes the practice of structured activities designed to regain improved perceptual-motor control over their respiration and vocal function (W. R. Miller & Rollnick, 2013; Moyns, 2015).

Throughout all of these activities the therapist needs to remain sensitive to the patient's feelings in relation to the nature of their vocal disorder and the adjunctive medical or surgical treatments that may be necessary, the meaning that their vocal symptoms have for them, and the impact of the vocal problem on the person (Aronson & Bless, 2009; Baker, 1998, 2002; Butcher & Cavalli, 1998; Butcher *et al.*, 2007; Elias, Raven, Butcher, & Littlejohns, 1989; Elkan, 1995; Geller & Foley, 2009; J. Miller, 2003; T. Miller *et al.*, 2014). This may entail creating psychological space for the expression of grief in relation to the vocal problem, a process that will be as important as the carefully structured and direct voice work. Attention to some of these issues may take place in brief, informal counselling moments but in other instances, time should be set aside for more formally structured *grief counselling* conversations (DiLollo & Neimeyer, 2014; Fourie, 2011a; Holland, 2007; Luterman, 2011; Rosen & Sataloff, 1997).

This counselling work will also allow therapists and patients to reflect upon the relative success or failure in achieving the changes that they have been seeking. It offers a platform for considering any persistent psychosocial factors that are blocking progress, or any positive features, such as the person's resilience, social support networks, or aspects of the therapy that have been particularly effective in achieving the mutually agreed goals.

It is during this reflective process that the attitudes, beliefs, life experience, and professional competence of the therapist should also be considered. For instance, in rare circumstances a therapist's lack of knowledge, biased perspectives, and personal baggage can operate as a negative influence that may limit or stultify a patient's progress even to the point of doing harm. (An example of this may be where a therapist insists that all patients with PVD have been sexually abused, and that resolution of the dysphonia will never be complete until this issue has been exposed and discussed.) On the other hand we should never underestimate the person of the therapist with his/her combined knowledge, empathy, and skills as being a positive force in facilitating change and healing (Sanders, 2012; Wendler, 2015). Pivotal to this effective process is the capacity of therapists to inspire their patients with hope and optimism for change (see Box 12.1).

Box 12.1 The role of inspiration in facilitating change and new insights

"It seems to me that we are all looking for inspiration from within and from those around us. I am very interested in what inspiration means, to appreciate the qualities of those who inspire us, and to understand what it is they do that is inspirational. It feels good to meet someone who is inspirational or to attend a function where we come away inspired, but what is it that happens that gives us this feeling, and why does it matter?

At a most basic level it seems to me to be inspired means to have taken something in and to be invigorated by it. This may be a wonderful view, someone's performance, or it might be the essence of what another does with a level of expression that gives meaning to thoughts, and feelings we've not been able to express ourselves. Whether through the spoken word, music, art, or sculpture, we often feel inspired when the expression of ideas or emotions affirms who we are and gives us hope. And I can think of no more important role for us as therapists, clinical educators, academics and researchers than to inspire our patients and our students to have hope, to find their own voice, and to fully realize who they are."

(Excerpt from the Elizabeth Usher Memorial Lecture as edited from Baker, 2010b).

To integrate counselling with creative and traditional approaches to restore phonation and improve vocal function

Another key purpose of undertaking counselling during this action phase is to support traditional and physiological approaches to restoring phonation and improving vocal function. This may involve integrating *top-down* approaches to counselling that capitalise on helping the person to modify ways of thinking and feeling in order to achieve changes in behaviour. Alternatively, it may involve *bottom-up* interventions that enable the recognition of more inhibited bodily reactions or more implicit emotional responses that can prevent a person from initiating voluntary phonation or modifying their voice. These approaches will require the therapist to join with the patient in a different way, drawing upon more intuitive, spontaneous, and creative strategies as a first step that later enables the top-down modulations to take place (Baker & Lane, 2009; Dietrich, Andreatta, Jiang, Joshi, & Stemple, 2012; Helou, 2014; Helou, Wang, Ashmore, Rosen, & Verdolini Abbott, 2013).

Many behavioural voice therapy techniques are used to facilitate improved vocal function for individuals across the full range of voice disorders, and in particular for those within the FVD sub-group of MTVD. These have been described and reviewed in a number of excellent publications including Eastwood, Madill, & McCabe, 2015; Ramig & Verdolini, 1998; Roy, 2008; Stemple, Roy, & Klaben, 2014; Titze & Verdolini Abbott, 2012. Although these direct vocal therapy techniques are not the primary focus of this text, it is important to recognise that well-developed skills in counselling are absolutely fundamental to these behavioural approaches. They apply to the micro-skills of teaching involved in modifying respiratory, extrinsic, and intrinsic laryngeal muscle tension patterns, to guiding patients with highly selective and supportive feedback in the shaping of the supraglottic structures (McDonald Klimek, Obert, & Steinhauer, 2005a, 2005b), and to sustaining the safety of a holding environment as patients both fail and succeed in their attempts to make such changes (Geller & Foley, 2009).

This counselling work requires the therapist to draw upon firm foundations of discipline-specific knowledge regarding normal and abnormal laryngeal function in combination with a strong sense of the psychosocial context for each person as gleaned from the initial consultation (Chapter 11). In setting about the task of helping patients to modify their vocal technique, or in the case of those with PVD to regain voluntary control over the initiation and maintenance of normal phonation, it is useful to reflect upon several factors that determine the complexities of laryngeal function. One of these relates to the structural positioning of the larynx in relation to other systems in the body. The other is linked to the more primitive role of the larynx in contributing to an individual's survival and the different forms of vocal communication (Sasaki, 2006).

Although these may seem so fundamental that they barely deserve mention, remaining alert to such factors can guide the voice practitioner to different ways of facilitating change, especially in those cases where complex psychogenic or psychosocial issues are operating. I suggest that holding onto these phylogenetic perspectives may also shed further light on the possible symbolic meaning of the 'non-organic' voice disorders, with implications for selecting *top-down* or *bottom-up* approaches to intervention. Some of these phylogenetically relevant features are discussed below.

The structural positioning of the larynx in relation to other systems within the body

Since the larynx is connected inferiorly to the respiratory system and superiorly to the supraglottic structures of the vocal tract and oral cavity, assessment, differential diagnosis, and approaches to therapy will need to take the interactions between these major components into account (Stemple *et al.*, 2014). Different behavioural approaches to direct voice work sometimes give precedence to strategies aimed primarily at respiratory control, some focus on modifying behavior at the level of the glottis, and others place emphasis on altering the shaping and configuration of the supraglottic structures and spaces. While there is a time and place to focus specifically on each of these major components, observations of experienced clinicians, and the finest vocal pedagogues working with actors, singers, and other professional voice users, suggest that the most effective behavioural approaches attend to interactions between all three components within the context of the body as a whole.

Other vital roles of the laryngeal valve

It is also essential to keep in mind that the laryngeal valve performs several other vital roles pertinent to survival, over and above those related to phonation (Aronson & Bless, 2009; Mathieson, 2001; Stemple *et al.*, 2014). These are achieved by interactions between the opening and closing of the three anatomical levels of the laryngeal valve comprising the aryepiglottic sphincter, ventricular folds, and supraglottic structures. The vital roles include: preservation of the airway during respiration; protection of the airway from foreign substances during breathing or swallowing; fixation of the thorax for effort closure during throat clearing, coughing, vomiting or sneezing; strong stabilisation of the thorax during weight bearing, lifting, pushing, defecation, or parturition; and significantly, as a stress response in preparing the body for *flight or fight*.

While these normal activities and functions contribute to survival, they may also occur in relation to phonation in everyday life. This may present as a marked constriction at any or all of these levels of the laryngeal valve, indicating abnormal levels of intrinsic muscular tension. During laryngoscopic examination, these involuntary postures are frequently observed in the form of excessive anterior-posterior constriction of the aryepiglottic folds, marked medial compression of the true vocal folds, or over-involvement of the false vocal folds. They may also be evident during voluntary efforts to phonate, during both quiet speaking and singing activities, and often during projection of the voice.

As discussed in other chapters, it is recognised that muscle tension patterns at the level of the true vocal folds and supralaryngeal structures may be evident to some degree in patients with OVD as well as FVD, and for these reasons they are not necessarily diagnostic (Behrman, Dahl, Abramson, & Schutte, 2003; Sama, Carding, Price, Kelly, & Wilson, 2001). However, in more severe presentations such as a PVD following a traumatic event, or in some cases of deeply entrenched mutational falsetto or puberphonia, marked constriction of the ventricular bands or tight anterior-posterior closure of the aryepiglottic sphincter may completely obliterate the view of the true vocal folds limiting phonation altogether (Baker, Ben-Tovim, Butcher, Esterman, & McLaughlin, 2013). This raises questions about the possible psychological significance of extreme degrees of inhibition from within, such as that which occurs in association with personality traits of introversion, perfectionism, and constraint (Dietrich & Verdolini Abbott, 2014; Helou, 2014; Roy & Bless, 2000b; van Mersbergen, 2011).

Alternatively, these extreme patterns of constriction may also reflect a bodily 'protectiveness', 'bracing of the self', or 'body armouring' against some form of insult from external factors such as highly threatening life events or conflicted interpersonal relationships (Baker, 2003; Baker & Lane, 2009; Butcher *et al.*, 2007; House & Andrews, 1988; Kollbrunner & Seifert, 2015). In some cases of severe PVD, the degrees of constriction may signal both elevated stress reactivity based on dispositional traits of introversion and as habituated patterns of behavioural inhibition in response to stressful incidents or longer-term difficulties.

The role of voice in non-verbal and verbal communication

Another primary function of the laryngeal valve is to produce phonation for different forms of communication. When this occurs at a non-verbal or pre-linguistic level, it is used for noise making to express the more primitive instinctive emotions such as groaning, crying, laughing, intimidating, and luring, with a gradual progression to the expression of the basic emotions of anger, sadness, fear, and joy. It is only through the engagement of the higher cortical levels of function in combination with further emotional development and socialisation, when the voice becomes integrated with the spoken or sung words, that we can communicate our thoughts more explicitly or express our emotions in the form of 'feelings' (Damasio, 2000, 2003; Lane, 2000). This more sophisticated use of spoken language enables us to express our more complex feelings of shame, humiliation, derision, uneasiness, affection, and humour. In various creative domains our voices may then be used to great effect in the expression of emotion through the more sophisticated avenues of poetry, acting, or oratory, and in the musical context of song. Ironically it is the voice, rather than the words alone, that conveys the extremes of passion or the meanings of these more nuanced emotions most effectively.

These sensitivities of the respiratory system and laryngeal valve in response to stress, and the different roles of preverbal and verbal vocal expression, render the laryngeal valve particularly vulnerable to the development of different kinds of voice disorders. As reflected in the closely co-ordinated links between the more primitive regions in the brain, via the limbic system, and then through to the central laryngeal control mechanisms of the cortex, I suggest that these sensitivities may also help to explain the different clinical manifestations of FVD such as MTVD or a PVD.

In an edited excerpt from a recent piece of work by Christina Shewell (2016), this distinguished SLP and voice teacher proposes how an understanding of these complex processes may influence a therapist's approaches to voice work (see Box 12.2).

Box 12.2 Speculative Model (Shewell 2016, In Progress)

Using Paul MacLean's model of three levels of the Triune brain (MacLean, 1990), I posit a speculative model as to the way that there may be a kind of 'pathway progression' in voice and communication between the lower instinctive levels of the brain to the higher cortical processes (see Fig. 12.1).

Area of brain	Main functions	Nature of voicing
Cortex	Conscious thought	Prose sentences Poetry Free voicing
Limbic structures	Emotions/images	Natural voicing
Reptilian structures	Strong sensations	Instinctual voicing
'Bottom-up connecting'		'Top-down connecting'

Fig. 12. 1 Speculative model illustrating pathway progression in voice and communication between the lower instinctive levels of the brain to the higher cortical processes

Reproduced with kind permission Christina Shewell (2016, In Progress) ©

At the lowest level of brain functioning that MacLean refers to as reptilian brain structures, the sounds that emerge are going to be primitive and *instinctual*, and linked to the basic business of survival, eating and mating, and their sensations. The snake hisses when under threat, and the lustful frog croaks. That kind of instinctual voicing is also heard in the noises mammals make – the yelp of the injured dog, or the growl of an attacking bear.

Human beings may yell in great pain, shriek in terror or moan with sensory pleasure. Even when unconscious, we may groan or cough. These sounds are not consciously controlled, but emerge from a physical state.

At the mid-level of brain function the limbic structures of the brain deal with basic emotional issues, core to which is recognition as to whether something is pleasant or unpleasant. Mammals and humans produce a range of non-verbal vocalisations reflecting different emotions.

I follow James D'Angelo's (2000) term, 'natural sounds' and use *natural voicing* for the non-verbal vocal expression of our emotional state. Unlike the more instinctual sounds, we can inhibit natural voicing if it is not socially appropriate to allow sound to emerge. These sounds include sighing, yawning, groaning, sobbing, wailing, laughing, yelling and humming. We can also make these sounds deliberately, extending and improvising with them in *free voicing* – no words but a wide range of vocal sound in a voiced improvisation.

Young children often enjoy playing with vocal sound, repeating sounds, syllables and sequences of sounds, and indeed the ability to babble is an important part of the development of language in the baby. And it is acceptable, when young, to be as loud as one wants. The voice of the thwarted two-year-old pulsates with energy, but as we grow more socially adapted, we have to learn to hide such 'sounded fire', even when we long to let it pour out in a stream of sound. It's the same with pleasure – cooing and swooping with the voice when happy is usually only socially acceptable when seen as singing – and even that has to be carefully rationed according to the context.

In *free voicing* a person allows himself to make any vocal sound that 'feels right'. He may start on a simple vowel sound and develop this into a voice improvisation with a spontaneous variety of intoned vowels, syllables, pitches, resonances and phonation qualities. It can be done alone or in a group, when wonderful choral harmonies and dissonances are woven into a creative cacophony. Such vocal improvisation is sometimes referred to as 'sounding' or 'toning'.

I see this kind of deliberate, exploratory, non-verbal vocal sounding as directly linking the lower levels of brain functioning and the higher. In a sound improvisation, we may start by making what seems like spontaneous, raw and undifferentiated sounds, but then move into repeated syllables that develop into particular words and phrases. These sounds and words may suddenly give us an insight into what we are feeling – a *bottom-up experience* where the hard-to-express, and the unspoken is given sound and then words, to lead to new understanding.

Parallel to this, we might enter the privacy of our home at the end of the day, aware that we feel furiously frustrated at something that has happened. We could take the time to lie on the floor (if in privacy, and where sound does not carry too far!) and allow our bodies and voices to go where they will, attending, trusting and responding to our feelings. We are then using a *top-down connection* – our cortex recognises we are stressed and tense, but the body and voice work connects us to the lower levels of brain, feeling and sound, and there is emotional and physical release.

Language is produced by a range of complex neuronal network functioning in the cortex. Here we think, plan, problem-solve, understand, negotiate and perform a multitude of other, high-level cognitive tasks. And we communicate our complex thoughts by speech or by writing. The model makes clear that both prose and poetry are predominantly functions of the cortex. However, I see *free voicing* as a kind of bridge between poetic language and the natural voicing sounds of the limbic system.

My contention is that poetry typically contains elements and aspects of what I would call natural or even instinctual voicing. It is produced from activity of the cortex, but its sounds and rhythms connect us to something more primitive – to those lower levels of deeper emotional or even instinctual feeling. This is why poetry – with its powerful use of sound, sensory words and metaphor – can express the inexpressible so effectively.

(Edited excerpt from paper by Christina Shewell (2016, in progress)
Reproduced with permission)

In translating these ideas into the practical context of voice work with actors, Shewell describes how combining improvised bodily movement with a range of exploratory voice sounds enables the voice to be produced freely 'without the pressure of text or meaning'. This is an example of *bottom-up* connecting. She also describes how performers may explore the text with *top-down* approaches. For example, an actor may speak the text, allowing the body to move or stretch in response to how the words 'feel', playing with them and improvising with words and free, non-verbal sounds. Shewell proposes that *'both of these processes enable an active exploration of the strength and flexibility in the voice, where a speaker may find a new feeling of a centered and embodied voice, where sound and word are 'organically' connected to emotional content'.*

Comment in relation to Shewell's (2016) model and implications for voice therapy

Reflections upon the vital functions of the laryngeal valve and differentiated roles of phonation within the context of Shewell's elegant model help to clarify why counselling or psychotherapeutic models that give precedence to *top-down* interventions may be entirely appropriate for many patients at various stages of voice therapy. These interventions will draw upon spoken language to clarify beliefs, attitudes, and feelings, and how these may work together to influence behaviours. As suggested in Chapter 9, such approaches will lie on the problem-solving or solution-focused end of the helping continuum, as exemplified in person-centered counselling and motivational interviewing, CBT, narrative therapy, and some models of family therapy (Crago & Gardner, 2012).

These reflections and Shewell's model also provide important clues as to the ways in which therapists may offer effective *bottom-up* interventions within the context of their counselling or direct voice work, with activities to help people access their more deeply felt but unexpressed emotions. It may be through free physical movement, play or other forms of intuitive and creative expression to facilitate *natural voicing* associated with basic emotions, or *free voicing* associated with improvisation. This may then transition to *top-down* strategies that draw upon metaphor, the language of poetry and song, and higher levels of verbal expression where thoughts and complex feelings may be put into words.

These different ways of intervening, as suggested by Shewell, lend further support to our theoretical model that seeks to explain the development of FVD (Baker & Lane, 2009). As described in detail in the publication cited above, and as discussed in Chapter 8 of this current text, we have proposed possible differences in emotion processing amongst patients with various voice disorders, and that individuals with FVD may have lower levels of emotional awareness in comparison to those with OVD or controls with normal voices. Our model proposes that therapists need to be able to join with patients at the emotional level at which they are currently functioning. For those patients operating at lower levels of emotional awareness, interventions will be required to help a patient to transition from poorly formulated or implicit levels of emotional awareness to more explicit emotional awareness where thoughts and feelings as mediated by language can then be expressed. This process will involve the *bottom-up* transfer of information from sub-cortical to cortical structures, which will then enable the appropriate *top-down* inhibition or modulation of sub-cortical activation, leading to better control over the voluntary and involuntary aspects of vocal function (Baker & Lane, 2009).

For instance, in the treatment of patients with PVD, this process might begin with the therapist stimulating involuntary vocalisations such a coughing, grunting, laughter or crying, which may be construed as intervening at the implicit level. It is only once these vocalisations have been shaped into syllables and meaningful words reflecting higher levels of emotional awareness, an understanding of the meaning behind the vocal symptoms, and the capacity to use the voice in speech with communicative intent, that true resolution of the voice disorder is possible. (Clinical examples to illustrate aspects of this process are given later in this chapter.)

As implied by Shewell's model and our model, to some extent the rationale for choosing to focus on *top-down* or *bottom-up* approaches may well depend upon the key purpose of the intervention (i.e., working creatively with actors or singers versus patients with voice disorders). In the specialised field of *vocology*, it will also depend upon the specific nature of the disorder, the personality of the patient, and, not to be forgotten, the training, experience, and personal inclination of the therapist. There needs to be 'a good fit' between both patient and therapist, and we need to keep in mind too that *it will be impossible for therapists to take their patients any further than they have been themselves.*

It is my firm conviction, that there is no one right way to go about helping our patients to achieve change, and it is so much more liberating if we are able to work in different ways. In order to do this, we need to recognise that our patients learn differently. Of equal importance, we need to know how *we* learn best, under what circumstances we are more likely to be influenced and to change, and to own that this will inevitably shape the ways in which we offer therapy to others. Such self-knowledge will not be found in lectures, on-line courses, books or journals. It will be gleaned through experiential activities to develop our own speaking and singing voice, and through training and participation as a patient or client in some form of counselling or psychotherapy.

As emphasised in Chapter 9, the most effective therapists are likely to be those who engage in both left and right hemisphere processing by integrating their academic and scientific knowledge with their 'embodied' vocal and/or counselling experiences. I suggest that when these higher levels of integration are mastered, therapists will be more adept at offering patients both *top-down* and *bottom-up* interventions. This in turn will place patients in a stronger position to achieve such levels of integration themselves.

Risky self-disclosure

Ironically, despite my lifelong quest for scientific, neurophysiological and psychological knowledge and an absolute commitment to using empirically based interventions, when it came to the very early development of my own speaking and singing voice, approaches that were more creative, playful, involving free movement, music, and drama always helped me to phonate more freely. This is a risky self-disclosure to make.

Two memorable experiences highlight why this was so and they also serve to illustrate Shewell's (2016) notion of 'pathway progression'. These experiences were deeply affecting at the time (many years ago now), but they imbued in me a deep understanding about why it is so helpful to be able to incorporate both *top-down* and *bottom-up* strategies into our counselling and behavioural approaches to voice therapy. Two voice-training experiences that fostered these approaches are described in Boxes 12.3 and 12.4.

Box 12.3 Possible approaches to facilitating development of the speaking voice

This first occurred during a one-month intensive workshop in the US with Shakespeare & Company, led by Kristin Linklater who is renowned for her book *Freeing the Natural Voice* (Linklater, 2006). All of the other participants were actors and directors, and the primary focus was on the further development of our speaking voices. After listening to 40 or so performers from both stage and film declaring their aspirations from the workshop in their deep and resonant voices across a huge room, it was my turn. In my very best "I-am-so-extremely-excited-to-be-here" and "I-am-here-to-help-you" therapist voice (all rather high-pitched, breathy and ineffectual at the time), I explained how I specialise in the treatment of voice disorders and like the others, wanted to explore and develop my own voice. At this point I saw the raised eyebrows of one of Kristin's colleagues and lip-read her muttering to Kristin, *"She's not going to know what's hit her when she has been here for a month!"* Kristin smiled a Mona Lisa smile, and I felt suitably terrified!

The approach to voice work included an intense and wonderfully structured 12–14 hour day with an inspiring programme. Some of the activities were *top-down* approaches that were strongly text driven and focused upon the iambic pentameter of Shakespeare's sonnets and plays, many of which I knew and loved already. These were integrated with many other activities that I now recognise as *bottom-up* strategies involving movement, music, and all different modes of vocal and dramatic performance. Indeed, it was only when I escaped behind a dramatic Greek Tragedy mask, or when cavorting as a comical clown, wickedly outrageous at one minute or perversely provocative in the next, that my voice began to emerge.

I still recall the day, when after euphoric moments of improvising with dancing and voice around the massive Wellesley College ballroom to the strains of Pachebel's Canon in D major, my voice totally flourished. It seemed to grow into gargantuan sounds, projected freely onto the floorboards, as if from some other place or person. The only time I have ever felt or heard it again with that incredible intensity or degree of freedom has been when singing lieder and oratorio, where the beauty of the music has transported technique to another plane.

Comment: In these activities where I had to decommission my thinking, let go of my critical parent, abandon the running commentary about what was happening physiologically, I discovered what it felt like to have a free voice. For someone aspiring to be an exemplary clinician scientist, this was and has continued to be a rather confronting revelation.

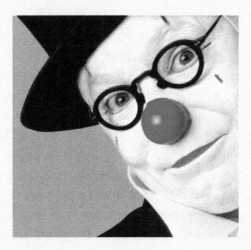

Fig 12.2 Land of Clowns
Courtesy Open Eye Figure Theatre, Minnesota

Box 12. 4 Possible approaches to facilitating exploration of the singing voice

The other experience occurred in a voice workshop with singer/song writer/ social worker Frankie Armstrong, where many cognitively high-powered professionals from medicine, psychology, psychotherapy, law, or accountancy came to explore their singing voices. The odd speech pathologist was allowed in too.

Many of the participants wanted to improve their singing voices, while others admitted to a lifelong yearning to be able to sing at all. A surprising number explained how their decision never to sing dated back to the age of 5 or 6 years old during singing activities in Grade 1:

"No, not such a good idea Johnny, not in the front row for you today dear – stand on the plank in the back row with Mildred. Don't bother to sing, just mouth the words."

Frankie Armstrong played examples of singing and vocalising that she had tape recorded during her travels all around the world. She then briefly demonstrated the different ways of singing with related actions that brought these activities to life. We joined in singing as a group, with the occasional foray into personal improvisation for those who wanted to try. The modelling with the tape recording and then demonstrating with her own voice helped to create a *holding environment* that felt safe, while also creating the space to play more creatively with our voices if we wished.

We were all rather trussed up and awkward at the start, but by the end of the day the energy in the room was totally transformed. Even the most inhibited were singing with total commitment as we incorporated the movements for scything of the wheat in the fields in Hardy's England, calling in the goats across the craggy hilltops of Cyprus, weaving and spinning the wool in the cottages of Scotland, yodelling from one snowy mountain top to another in Switzerland, or keening with mournful anguish over the death of a tiny infant in Iran. With all of these activities we envisaged ourselves in a different time, place or emotional state, finding ways to use our voices that we had never tried before.

Comment: I learned a great deal from this experience about how to support patients as we encourage them to use their voices differently, and how it helps to hear someone model the sounds first, making first attempts to produce these sounds with the safety of the therapist joining in at first to effectively create a Lombard effect (Lombard, 1911; Zollinger & Brumm, 2011), and then experimenting with vocalising in different ways independently without fear of making mistakes or ridicule.

It is terrible to be relegated, like Johnny, to a plank in the back row. It is also uncomfortable to be asked to perform on the spot. In moments like these we may react with a pre-emptive shutting down of our three-tiered laryngeal valve, or lose our feathers like this unfortunate cockatoo in the theatre production '*Fright or Flight*' (Fig. 12.3).

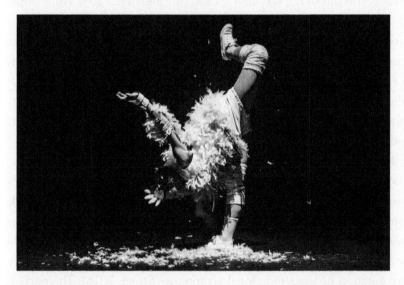

Fig. 12.3 Cockatoo in a state of Fright or Flight – Photographer Sean Young
Performer: Bianca Mackail Theatre Production Fright or Flight by 3's a Crowd

To prepare the person for strategies designed to facilitate improved phonation

As emphasised above, counselling skills will be integral in helping patients to improve their vocal function with physiological and behavioural approaches across the full range of voice disorders. However, more sophisticated counselling skills are often needed in helping patients to restore voluntary control over the initiation of phonation where they present with a PVD.

Although many patients with a psychogenic aphonia or dysphonia achieve normal phonation in the first session, others may take many weeks, even months.

Moreover, while we might think of total loss of voice in the form of an *aphonia* as being a more severe psychogenic or conversion reaction symptom, sometimes a *psychogenic dysphonia* can be the more difficult to resolve. The preparatory counselling that will be important prior to introducing strategies to facilitate normal phonation for patients with PVD is the focus of this first part of the discussion.

Subtle counselling work helps to set the scene for introducing a range of strategies that will help the patient to reclaim their voice. This may be offered in the context of the psychosocial interview, during activities to demonstrate symptom reversibility, or just prior to attempts to facilitate normal phonation. Many therapists do this in the very first session (my preference too), while others wait until the more direct action phase.

Students and experienced therapists often ask questions about what to do first with patients with PVD. Is it better to introduce strategies that clearly reaffirm symptom reversibility, and then move into offering strategies to help the person regain voluntary control over the initiation of phonation? Or, as a first priority, is it preferable to focus on the psychosocial issues in the anticipation that with insight and understanding the dysphonia will resolve spontaneously?

While there is no rigid rule about this, once the assessment and psychosocial history have been undertaken, I like to begin by talking together in very general terms about what we know about functional symptoms and the possible links between stress, strong emotions, and our voices. At the same time, it is important to acknowledge that even if there have been psychosocial issues impinging on the person, or if they are still operating, they may not necessarily be relevant to the current presentation of their functional symptoms (Stone, 2016). The purpose of this *double-bind message* is to reduce the anxiety and threat for those who may feel very self-conscious or defensive about the possibility that psychological issues may underpin the development of their symptoms, while simultaneously unlocking the door and leaving it open for deeper conversations about such issues at another time. I then explain that we are going to work together 'to find their normal voice again' using a range of strategies that are known to be effective in giving people mastery and control over initiating phonation and using their voice normally. I then suggest that once their voice has returned, we will be in a much stronger position to explore any issues that may have contributed to the development of the vocal problem, and to gain further insights into the meaning of their vocal symptoms.

Counselling prior to manipulation of the larynx

Some interventions that are very effective in triggering symptom reversibility and that enable the more conscious control over initiating voice involve repositioning or manipulation of the larynx in order to increase the thyrohyoid space (Aronson & Bless, 2009; Rammage, Morrison, & Nichol, 2001; Roy, 2008). Prior to palpation of the thyrohyoid laminae to assess any acute sensitivity, or any manoevering and manipulation of the larynx, the therapist needs to ask the patient's permission to touch their larynx and neck and to explain why this is going to be important. While most patients would expect this to be part of any assessment from a laryngologist or SLP, for some patients to be touched around the neck and throat can provoke extreme anxiety. This may occur if they have had prior experience of violence or strangulation, or if they have had any medical condition causing pain and marked discomfort in the laryngeal area. It is important to speak with the patient about why we are doing this, and what is being noticed as we undertake this procedure.

Counselling about 'pathway progression' to normal phonation

Other interventions are used to trigger the more primitive or *involuntary sounds* such as coughing, grunting, the *natural sounds* that accompany sighing, yawning, wailing or laughing, or the *free sounds* such as vocal improvisation that may be referred to as 'young' or 'playful' sounds. It works more effectively if these young, playful or expressive sounds are produced 'as if' with a particular emotion. These are then shaped into syllables, automatic and familiar utterances, and communicative speech.

Educational counselling will be an important part of this whole process because coughing and grunting, or the vocal sounds that we associate with communicating affectionately with a baby or small child, or the playful sounds that we recall from childhood, may seem totally unrelated to normal use of the voice for our adult patients. Being asked to make these sounds may even spark some indignation where the patient wonders "Why is the therapist treating me like a child?" Here it is essential to give a very clear explanation for eliciting these 'earlier' vocal sounds based on the neuroscience above, and why they are more likely to trigger free phonation if imbued with different emotions. Without the emotion they are just exercises. A selection of strategies that may be used to affirm symptom reversibility or trigger normal phonation is shown in Box 12.5.

Box 12.5 Strategies to demonstrate symptom reversibility or to facilitate healthy phonation in patients with PVD

Vegetative, reflexive or instinctive behaviours accompanied by sound

- Cough and clear the throat (allowing voice to be present if possible)
- Yawn followed by a sigh (as if with genuine relief)
- Whimper sounds (as if a small distressed animal such as a kitten)
- Grunt or groan (as if in pain, shifting posture, reflecting effort in lifting heavy item)
- Comfort moaning sounds (associated with pleasure, eating something delicious)

Playful pre-linguistic vocal sounds that we might enjoy with an infant or young child

- Blow raspberries while voicing
- Phonate with a rising and falling scale blowing the lips like a horse
- Move finger rapidly in between the lips shaped for 'ooh' with a falling inflection from high to low (you are so cute)
- Pat the lips with hand while phonating (gentle affectionate tone as if to infant)
- Gently pat the patient's back while they sigh out 'ah' (as if with comfort)
- Patient pats own chest firmly while sighing 'ah' (with a sense of comfort or relief)
- Siren quietly down the scale using nasal sounds such as /m/ /n/ or /ng/
- Produce a low-pitched glottal fry at the very bottom of the vocal range
- Giggle or laugh (as if in absolute delight)
- Gargle with a firm sound (firstly with water then simulated without water)
- Hold a tube of paper to the lips, phonate 'ooh' and notice sensation of lips vibrating
- Sing a rising and falling scale on tongue trill with a firmly voiced consonant, e.g. 'drr'

Automatic phrases and utterances with minimal communicative responsibility

- Respond with short "Mm" "Okay" "Uh huh " (as in response to question)
- Count and recite the days of the week, or sing "Happy Birthday" or favorite song

(Compiled for a workshop for Speech Pathologists, Adelaide, Australia (Baker, 2015))

Challenges for patients and therapists during this 'pathway progression'

A deeper level of *supportive counselling* may then be required as patients attempt the various strategies to elicit phonation. It is important to warn patients that there may be a degree of trial and error and that their voice may go through different stages as the dysphonia resolves. This may be experienced as occasional glimpses of normal voice that 'leak through' suddenly, with equally sudden loss of voice again, moments of coughing or choking noises, or changes in vocal quality that make the voice sound worse than their original a/dysphonia. Some patients begin to use involuntary *struggle behaviours* that manifest as exaggerated lip, tongue, and respiratory movements that are out of proportion to the actual physical effort required to phonate normally. These *struggle behaviours* may resemble those seen in association with articulatory or phonatory apraxia of neurogenic origin (Baker, 2016). These changes can be alarming to patients and it is important to reassure them that they often occur as a voice returns to normal function.

These transitional phenomena can also be quite disturbing for student clinicians and even experienced therapists, to the extent that they may retreat and quickly abandon their chosen interventions. There is the natural fear that they may have done something wrong or that they may be making matters worse. In these situations it is really important that therapists can 'hold their line with conviction' as long as they can justify their rationale for what they are doing, but also have the presence of mind to shift the focus or attempt another strategy that will achieve exactly the same outcome. I have described this to therapists as knocking on the front door and there if no answer, trying the side door, and again if no one answers but we know they are home, going around to the back door to give that a friendly knock. I also caution firmly that we must never 'break in'. The way in which I may have offered counselling during this process to a young person with PVD where it proceeded smoothly is illustrated in Case Example 12.1.

Case example 12.1 Preparatory counselling prior to laryngeal manipulation and making unusual sounds

A 15-year-old boy, S, presented with PVD in the form of a *mutational falsetto*. His parents instigated the referral and in addition to concerns about his voice, they wondered whether their son was struggling with concerns about his sexuality. Although popular at school, S told his mother that he was very embarrassed about his voice, especially as it alternated between a high-pitched falsetto and a rough, harsh, unpredictable pitch with phonation breaks. He understood that this was probably related to other normal maturational changes, but his voice was not breaking in the same way as that of his friends. At first, S was predictably shy and awkward, tending to wriggle in the chair and to giggle in a self-conscious manner as we talked about his voice. However, when asked about how much his voice was troubling him and if he was really motivated to do something about it, he became serious, his eyes filled with tears and he said "I really want it fixed". After a preliminary case history, which on this occasion did not involve an extensive psychosocial interview as his mother was present, I explained to them both what a mutational falsetto voice or puberphonic voice problem is, asked his permission to move his larynx in order to alter its position slightly, and warned him that together we were going to make some sounds that may seem a bit unusual. I explained that the reason for the *laryngeal manipulation* and making different sounds was to help me to determine how low his voice might be able to go, and to experiment with how his voice would work best. Since I had already heard inadvertent 'leaks' of normal, low-pitched phonation during our conversation, I was reasonably confident he would be able to achieve normal voice in this first session. For some patients, this can be a profound shock, even more embarrassing than their former dysphonia. So I spent some time pre-empting how loud and strong his healthy, low-pitched voice may sound, but that it would be entirely appropriate to his age and maturity and surprisingly effortless to produce..

Here, there were embedded hypnotic suggestions that his new voice would be *normal*, it would feel *relatively effortless*, it would be *age-appropriate* and fitting his *psychosexual maturity*. I also warned him that when I lowered the larynx, and as he imitated some of my sounds, his voice might seem momentarily worse (i.e., more roughness in quality as he transitioned from high-pitched breathy falsetto to a low-pitched modal voice), but not to be

400

alarmed by this transitory roughness or unusual strength and difference in volume. I reiterated and questioned him several times in a slightly cajoling and challenging way that seemed to fit with his joking personality and humour: "This will sound different". "Are you sure you are ready for this new, normal, healthy voice that will feel and sound just right for your age, your height, your build – low, strong, and easy to project?" He joined in with this sense of fun and challenging restraint by looking sideways with a playful grin at his mother who was smiling encouragingly and he said, "Let's go for it"!

I then gently but firmly lowered his larynx according to currently advocated methods (Aronson & Bless, 2009; Roy, 2008) and asked him to join me in making an exaggerated, low-pitched "ooh" sound. With this simultaneous intervention he produced a strong, low-pitched modal voice a full octave below his former falsetto voice. He was visibly shocked, looked sheepishly at his mother who also looked with genuine surprise and delight, and together they burst out laughing. With a sense of excitement and happy anticipation we set about more playful activities to facilitate shaping his low voice. Apart from occasional lapses into pitch breaks and harshness in vocal quality, he quickly mastered lowering his larynx himself with no need for external manipulation and gained voluntary control over initiating normal phonation. Within two subsequent sessions he was maintaining his normal voice and could no longer revert to his puberphonic voice, a phenomenon that fascinated him. In subsequent sessions in my capacity as a family therapist, we addressed the more sensitive issues related to his psychosexual development and concerns about his sexuality.

Restraints to change requiring more creativity and deeper levels of counselling

When facilitation of normal phonation in patients with PVD can be achieved quickly as in the example above, it enables the deeper counselling work to take place much more easily. However, as mentioned above, recovery of normal phonation in patients with PVD does not always proceed smoothly and it does not always occur quickly.

For instance, in rare cases, virtually no normal voice can be elicited at all. In other situations a person may be able to achieve a clear voice during facilitating activities but be unable to sustain it beyond the vegetative noises, playful sounds or automatic utterances. These patients might reach a point where they can sustain their voice in conversation with the therapist with non-threatening topics but as soon as it becomes more emotionally charged their voice begins to deteriorate, or once they leave the safety of the therapeutic relationship and return to their family or work settings where nothing may have changed, their aphonia or dysphonia returns. In any or all of these scenarios, as outlined above, it can become a significant intellectual, psychological, and emotional challenge for both parties and raises a number of important questions.

Does the patient really want to change?

First, some therapists may begin to wonder whether or not the patient really wants to get their voice back. I admit, with some discomfort now, that in my very early years of practice I might have held a rather sanctimonious and all-knowing view that "He is clearly not ready to change" or "She seems very highly defensive". However, after many more years of working with children, adolescents, and adults with PVD, I see things differently. It is my impression that most patients really do want to get their voice back, at least at a conscious level. That is why they are there in the first place. It is also reflected in the way patients describe how "having no voice" or "having this strange voice" is seriously compromising both for them and for those around them. In the short-term they describe it as puzzling, embarrassing, humiliating, and even rather frightening. In the longer-term they may admit to becoming increasingly affected and troubled by it, more constrained in their family and interpersonal relationships, having doubts about future studies or career paths that may be open or closed to them, or considering changes of employment.

For those experiencing these disorders over months and years, and admittedly these are rare, they often reflect upon how this has acted as a restraint to change with its subtle impact upon their personality, their gradual but strategic withdrawal from social settings, and tendency to anxiety and low mood. Sometimes this leads to a clinical depression. Despite the possibility that for some there are real secondary gains, generally speaking the sense of loss from having no voice or a severe dysphonia is genuinely troubling with significant implications.

Similar issues have recently been emphasised by Jane Bickford and colleagues (Bickford, Coveney, Baker, & Hersh, 2013), where men and women described the challenges of communicating after total laryngectomy. They have recounted how difficult it can be to express their emotions in such a manner so that others will take them seriously, and the marked limitations to the pragmatics of communication such as loss of spontaneity, being unable to interject, to be humorous, or to be heard in a noisy environment. These constraints often lead them to develop non-verbal strategies of communicating politely but briefly, limiting their verbal interaction with strangers or even family and friends, and avoiding face-to-face contact or conversations over the phone.

Therapist approaches as a possible restraint to change

Rather than suggesting that a failure to change reflects a patient's ambivalence in wanting to get their voice back, we might approach this differently. Alternative questions might be: "Was the therapist's decision to focus on restoration of phonation as a first priority the best choice?"; "Would it have been better to undertake the deeper counselling work aimed at understanding and insight first?"; "Was something missed in the psychosocial interview that might still be operating as a restraint to change?"

Certainly, one answer might be that issues raised during the psychosocial interview have not yet been fully explored and that for full resolution of the voice disorder, these issues do need to be formulated and understood. However, as emphasised above, it can be very difficult to talk about and give full expression to deeply troubling issues without a voice and therefore, it is not necessarily a mistake to try to elicit phonation first. Alternatively, in cases where the tight locking of the laryngeal sphincter is so severe that no voice can be achieved at all, this would suggest that more deeply suppressed or repressed emotional responses to stressful issues are operating. Under these circumstances, it could be argued that persisting with efforts to elicit phonation is not appropriate unless combined with deeper levels of counselling than are offered in traditional speech pathology practice. Another equally valid answer might be that despite the fact that there were some psychosocial issues that appeared to have contributed to the onset, these are no longer operating. Rather, the perpetuation of the symptoms is linked to deeply habituated extreme patterns of laryngeal muscular tension, and that modifying such a dysfunctional pattern takes time (Rammage *et al.*, 2001).

For how long should therapists keep trying to elicit phonation in patients with PVD?

In addition to the questions above, it is relevant to press for some other answers related to basic procedural issues. Many clinicians will ask: "Well, for how long should we keep trying?"; "Should we have offered more strategies or different kinds of interventions?"; "Would it have worked better with more intensive therapy rather than only once a fortnight or a month?"; "Is a failure to elicit normal phonation an important sign that we should *not* persevere and that we need to seek supervision, to work in collaboration with a more experienced therapist or refer on to a mental health professional?"

Transparency in reflecting upon the therapeutic process

These are all questions that need to be asked both during and after the more challenging therapeutic encounters. They serve to highlight the fact that in clinical practice it is never black and white, and that there will be times when work with our patients entails a degree of uncertainty and admitting to 'not knowing'.

As implied by the wording of many of these questions, they have all been generated and considered in the mind of the therapist. Certainly in the earlier days of my clinical training and practice, this is how it might have been. These private thoughts would have been accompanied by negative self-talk about a lack of competence, with further misgivings about facing another harrowing session where whatever we were about to do was probably not likely to succeed. While not at all ideal, in the early days of my striving to be independent and seeming to cope, it often happened in this way.

However, with much more experience and with further advanced training in the different domains of vocology, counselling, and psychotherapy, I prefer to be more open and transparent with patients about what is happening. This includes those occasions when everything is going well, but much more importantly, when they are not. I now raise these confronting questions or misgivings with my patients and invite them to share their perceptions and feedback too. This transparency shows more genuine respect for the patient and diminishes any sense that the therapist is the one who really knows what is going on. Admittedly, being all-knowing may well have been a defensive position in the heady days of early career omnipotence, but it is no longer the case.

Courage, creativity and responsive persistence in the face of restraints to change

Such a protracted and complex process draws upon the considerable trust, motivation, and determination of the patient. Even for clinicians with years of experience and expertise in the area, it takes additional creativity, courage, and tenacity to continue offering a *safe holding environment* while the patient struggles through this process. In reflecting on my own practice, I have sometimes described this tenacity as sheer pig-headedness or like 'a dog with a bone who refuses to give up'. A *positive reframe* of this might be *responsive persistence* (Sutherland, Dienhart, & Turner, 2013; Sutherland, Turner, & Dienhart, 2013). This is a far more tolerable description.

I now present a case that illustrates a much more complex journey in helping another 15 year-old boy diagnosed with a severe long-standing puberphonia. The aims of describing the challenging processes involved in helping this young man 'to find his voice' are:

1. To support the proposal that we need to be able to join with the patient at the emotional level at which he or she is operating (Baker & Lane, 2009)
2. To demonstrate how the interventions that assisted in triggering normal phonation validate the *'pathway progression in voice and communication from the lower instinctive levels of the brain to the higher cortical processes'* (Shewell, 2016)
3. To highlight several principles of systems theory and family therapy that helped to overcome some restraints to change, but not all.
4. To encourage therapists to be brave, creative, and persistent while also recognising when to seek help, to work collaboratively, or to refer on (See case example 12.2).

Case example 12.2 Complex challenges requiring more creativity & counselling

A 15 year-old boy presented with a severe PVD in the form of a severe puberphonia. S was in year 10 at school, he had a sister aged 12 years, and his parents worked professionally. He recalled his voice beginning to change, with other signs of physical maturation, at the age of 11, and that he sounded as if he had a cold. This became firmly entrenched as a tight, high-pitched falsetto voice sometimes deteriorating with pitch breaks into a rough and harsh dysphonia that would then shift back to the high falsetto phonation. He admitted that on occasions when he heard his lower voice breaking through he did not like the sound of it at all. At no time had he been able to use a normal low-pitched voice befitting his maturity.

History of previous interventions

A detailed case history and review of laryngoscopy reports revealed that S and his family had been seeking help for over 4 years. This had involved three consultations with otolaryngologists, each confirming a diagnosis of a puberphonia with no medical or structural abnormalities sufficient to explain the severity of his voice disorder. On one of these visits, a Botox injection was administered into his tightly constricted false folds that were completely obliterating the view and interfering with the function of the true folds. It was hoped that this temporary intervention would enable the SLP's facilitating techniques to elicit phonation more readily. This is a procedure that has been shown to be effective, but on this occasion it was not successful in facilitating change.

S had attended 40 consultations with four different SLPs during this 4 year period, some in the public sector, some in the private, but with little or negligible success in achieving normal phonation. Due to the constraints of distance, school commitments, and reported upper respiratory tract infections there was a pattern of missed appointments or therapy sessions taking place on an irregular basis, sometimes weeks or even months apart. In view of the poor progress in eliciting phonation, and concerns that psychological issues may have been underpinning this ongoing lack of progress, one SLP recommended referral to a clinical psychologist to be offered concurrently with the ongoing voice therapy.

S attended 10 sessions with the clinical psychologist on his own with no parental involvement. It was difficult to establish with either S or his parents what had happened during these sessions, but his main recollection of the process was being advised 'to go somewhere and shout loudly'.

Initial consultation

S's parents accompanied him to our initial session, having driven for an hour from the country. They were not emotionally effusive about all that had transpired but they were worried about the fact that S had reached a stage at school where tertiary studies and career choices were being discussed, and that his severely dysphonic voice could limit these choices. S was concerned about this too and said he felt rather disheartened and desperate. While he mentioned possible courses and careers based on maths and science, he later admitted that his main ambition was to sell cars. I must have looked surprised at the thought of his wanting to be 'a used car salesman', but he was quick to clarify that these would be *seriously expensive cars*. I was put firmly in my place.

Psychosocial interview

A review of laryngology reports, the detailed case history with S and a comprehensive psychosocial interview with S, and later with his mother, failed to reveal any obvious stressful events that may have precipitated the onset of his symptoms, or that might be contributing to the perpetuation of his voice disorder. There was mention of changing schools and some teasing, but nothing stood out as being highly significant. The parents described their son as enjoying school, having good times with friends, and home life as being contented. I noted that his mother seemed more in touch with various aspects of his everyday life, and that S described his relationship with his father as being more distant. S's parents were very quietly spoken, especially his father, however, they were both most supportive and cooperative throughout the whole process.

S was immaculately groomed and polite at all times. He answered questions with one-word answers but never generated any conversation and did not raise any concerns about family or interpersonal relationships. His overall posture as reflected in raised shoulders, high clavicular breathing, tight jaw and uneasy stance suggested extreme anxiety and tension. He seemed to be inexorably shy and self-conscious.

S commented that he appreciated the efforts that his previous therapists had made and respected his last therapist who had quickly referred him on rather than persevering with therapy where no voice could be elicited. He admitted to thinking at this point "Things must be pretty serious – what's wrong with me – and if this new lady can't help me, well what then?"

I had some misgivings too, with a heightened sense of responsibility and a powerful imperative to succeed. To some extent, this started with the referral coming from two highly respected colleagues. The misgivings were also reinforced, having heard about the long quest for help from multiple practitioners and then on meeting S, who seemed so highly anxious and inhibited. Further, this family had very high hopes and expectations, but they also emanated a real sense of resignation, suggesting concerns that this might be yet another disheartening experience with another health professional offering more of the same.

Restraints to change

There were a number of restraints to change operating. One was the obvious possibility of both primary and secondary gains associated with this ongoing puberphonia. Another was the enormous commitment that S and his family had already made and were about to make again, both in terms of time and money. They would have to drive an hour each way to attend sessions; S would need to take time from school and one or other of his parents would have to take time from work; and there were fees to be paid too. Further, since S had received 40 sessions of therapy from several experienced and competent therapists specialising in voice, and 10 sessions from a clinical psychologist, the risk was that 'succeeding' might matter more to me than to my patient.

I may be tempted to try too hard, even harder than my patient. In view of the long-term nature of his dysphonia I warned the family that it would take time, but that I would persevere with S for as long as it took. I also undertook to seek review laryngoscopy and referral for a psychiatric opinion if no progress was made. I was under no illusion that I would do any better.

Course of therapy

The therapy process involved a concerted effort over many months with a number of interruptions to the time line. We worked intensively on trying to elicit normal phonation with the facilitating strategies shown in Box 12.5. Excerpts of teaching videos were shown to S and his parents so that they could see how these different strategies might work, and I gave S published case reports that highlighted different presentations of puberphonia with alternative theories about causality. Some of these referred to *habituated mutational falsetto* as the main aetiologic explanation; others detailed different forms of *stressful life events* and *difficulties* or issues related to *psychosexual immaturity*. Notions related to events or difficulties characterised by *conflict over speaking out (COSO)* or *powerlessness in the system (PITS)* were included in these discussions, with careful emphasis on the theoretical notion that in any COSO situation it is not merely a matter of feeling some ambivalence about speaking out. Rather, that if one chooses to speak out about some sensitive issue it might make matters worse, and if one chose *not* to speak out, that this too will have negative consequences. S found this all very interesting and decided that his disorder was more typical of a *habituated mutational falsetto*.

Rationale for psycho-educational counselling

The aim in sharing videos and written materials was to shift the dynamics in the relationship from one where S and his parents had felt like passive recipients of a complex process but not really knowing what was going on, to one of mutual participation. In presenting S with a number of options about possible psychological issues that might be operating, it was hoped that when he felt safe enough to raise these more sensitive issues, he would be sufficiently empowered to do so.

Integrating direct voice work with person-centered counselling

The direct voice work was interspersed with counselling conversations where possible associations between stress, COSO, or feelings of PITS in any aspects of his life were explored. Any concerns with respect to his sexuality, or troubling aspects to relationships such as those in the family, school or wider social network, were also raised, but nothing emerged as being troubling to S at this point. At one level, this was rather perplexing in the light of my strong intuitive sense that something was troubling this boy very deeply but, given how very anxious and inhibited he appeared to be, it was decided that delving too deeply or too quickly would not be appropriate at this time. It was also a possibility that S was right in his assessment that his dysphonia was simply a deeply habituated dysfunctional pattern, and that there were no significant psychosocial factors to explain the onset or perpetuation of his dysphonia. This was not my position, but it was possible.

New revelation

Prior to leaving for a family holiday S mentioned that he sometimes noticed unnerving feelings of light-headedness when people were behind him in places like churches or shopping centres. This was not a good sign. Was this related to the limited progress in obtaining clear modal voice at an appropriate pitch level during any facilitation activities? Had we missed something in the psychosocial history that had been re-awakened for some reason? There had been intense media coverage exposing rampant sexual abuse of boys in the Catholic Church and other respected institutions at the time. It was relevant to consider this, given that conversion reaction symptoms or other symptoms related to anxiety often follow such incidents. While there was no indication from S that anything like this had occurred, it was suggested he see his GP to exclude any other medical explanation for this new symptom. S did not feel that it was all that serious and never raised the issue again in therapy. It stayed in my mind.

Time for serious reflection

On his return, and recognising that there had continued to be been very little progress with the additional knowledge that I was going to be away for several weeks, this was a time for serious reflection. Therapy had become too drawn out, there was a risk that I was falling into the same pattern of offering more of the same, and whatever we were doing was not allowing new information into the system – certainly not enough to make a difference. In thinking about possible restraints to change, where of course the therapist can be at the top of the pile, several key issues stood out.

Different restraints to change

Our counselling conversations had not revealed any factors sufficient to explain this difficulty in moving forward. It did not mean there were none, but they had not been revealed or made explicit. Further, the interventions that we were using to elicit normal phonation were not triggering any *instinctual*, *natural* or *free voicing* at all. If anything, they seemed to be causing more *anticipatory stress* (as discussed in Chapter 3) and stronger inhibition at the level of the laryngeal valve. ***Perhaps this was the crux of the issue.***

As previously mentioned, eliciting and gaining voluntary control over these non-verbal but vocal sounds works better if a person can produce them when imbued with various emotions. However, if a person is intrinsically introverted, or at a stage in their maturity where they are extremely inhibited and operating at a low level of emotional awareness, it will be much harder to engage in these extrovert activities which require considerable empathy or at least a degree of playfulness. If these aspects of the self cannot be readily accessed, it is difficult to improvise with sounds 'as if being affectionate to a young child', 'as if feeling sad', 'as if sighing with relief', or 'as if chuckling behind the teacher's back'. Clearly we needed to be triggering responses from even lower down, either by tapping into the more basic sounds that we associate with survival, or by facilitating the more spontaneous expression of emotion linked to limbic system functioning without any moderation from by *top-down* processing.

News of difference

With these reflections in mind, I asked the family if they were absolutely sure they had never heard any normal voice under any circumstances. S's younger sister then recalled that she had heard him laughing out loud when watching television 'behind closed doors in his bedroom'. S had not noticed this and his parents had never mentioned it either. I had never heard this serious young boy laugh at all.

This was important new information that could be perceived as *a difference that makes a difference* (See Chapter 10). It opened up new conversations about what S liked watching on television, but in particular any programmes that made him laugh. He said he always found any films starring John Cleese very funny and especially *Monty Python*. This was such a fascinating revelation, because to laugh at Monty Python shows a rather black and irreverent sense of humour, especially for a young person who was so emotionally and behaviourally constrained. Somehow, we needed to capitalise on this new information. We also needed to use the knowledge that this loud, spontaneous laughter only ever occurred in the privacy of his room (see Fig. 12.4).

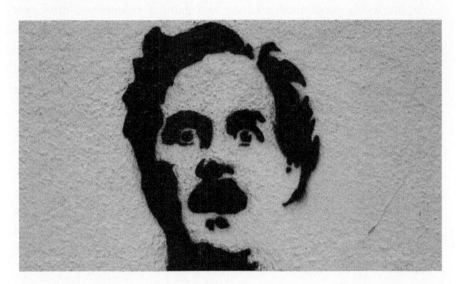

Fig. 12.4 John Cleese 'a la graffiti', artist unknown

Extending the news of difference and more creative interventions needed

As I was about to go away at what seemed like a crucial time in therapy, there was only one way to manage this. S was asked to keep his recording device on while he was watching his next Monty Python film, so that if any laughter occurred, it would be recorded without his thinking about it. He agreed to send through any brief moments of laughter, and in collaboration with his parents, I agreed to offer a series of brief but frequent Skype sessions to give feedback about the pitch and quality of his voice during spontaneous laughter. It was important to ensure that if he could produce any low-pitched phonation, the new voice was of good quality and free of any undue strain. (There was a risk he could shift into a very harsh low-pitched ventricular phonation.) It was also necessary to be prepared for S to experience a *flight or fright* reaction to his new voice, with a metaphorical loss of all his feathers, or a further closing down of his laryngeal sphincter.

Success at last

This approach worked. Within the safety of his familiar private space, and knowing that despite the distance, the therapist was not going to abandon him but would continue to offer a holding environment, something had changed. Once he had sent through one voice sample taken from spontaneous laughter, he gradually mastered voluntary initiation of normal phonation, and sent through excellent samples of his new, very deep voice. The technology side was easy and exciting for S, as one might expect for a boy of this age, and there was no hiding the fact that when I received the first recording of an extremely short but low pitched "Hi" that sounded like Morgan Freeman, I was extremely delighted.

Adjusting to his new voice

In response to his anticipated concerns that maybe his new voice did not sound very good, I sent emails embellished with photos of 'seriously expensive cars' to give him careful feedback about his voice (see Figs 12.5a and 12.5b).

HEADLINES IN DAILY NEWS

VOICE EXPERT WITH SOPHISTICATED KNOWLEDGE OF HIGH-END CARS

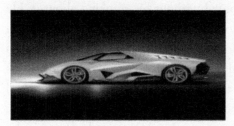

Voice like an Alpha Romeo

"Smooth, sleek, effortless, excellent colour, lots of power and substance.

All the things your voice is fast becoming"

To some extent, these messages represented a 'playful' joining with S and his passion for seriously expensive cars, while also joking at my own expense because S knew full well I knew nothing whatsoever about cars. The messages were also entirely serious in their intent, with gently embedded constructs within the metaphors designed to motivate and support S in his courageous efforts to make these behavioural and psychological changes.

HEADLINE IN AUTO MONTHLY

Voice that befits the owner of a Lamborghini

"Deep powerful motor with 10-gig horsepower, synchromesh & capacity to double-declutch with smooth easy confidence. A reliable voice that holds the road with assurance"

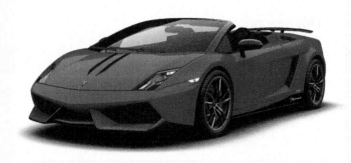

Generalising his new voice

Once he could reliably initiate voice with the anonymity of audio-recordings, we then scheduled short but frequent Skype sessions over a period of 2 weeks, where he began to generalise into brief moments of speech. Subsequent face-to-face therapy sessions were then devoted to activities to stabilise his voice beyond the clinical setting that involved walking energetically outside in the park while talking, inviting a close friend into therapy so that S could show him how his voice was changing, ringing the school for support when S was due to attend using his new deep voice, and a Skype session from his home where he invited different family members to come in and join our conversation. Again, I attempted further exploration of any possible psychosocial issues and again, nothing emerged.

Consolidating his new voice

This entire process took 7 months, but it required 3 of those months for S to consolidate his voice so that he could use it reliably, and in company with others. It was notable that S was the most severely inhibited in using his normal low-pitched phonation with his parents, and in particular his father. Even when S's voice had become entirely normal, his father never commented in my presence about being relieved or pleased for his son.

Maybe he *was* relieved but also holding some ambivalence about how much time this had taken and how much effort had been required from all concerned. Possibly, expressing feelings was not something that came easily to him. This was an observation made frequently by S. I wondered, too, if his father might have been harboring some deep concerns that his son's particular voice disorder reflected a psychological problem related to a degree of psychosexual immaturity, or some anxiety about his emerging sexual orientation that was too difficult to talk about together.

Ending therapy

It would have been my preference to keep working with this young man on aspects related to his extreme levels of emotional constraint and shyness, and his apparent levels of anxiety that I felt were probably related to his psychosexual development. However, he was very happy indeed with his voice, and relayed with some jubilation how his life had begun to change.

School was going really well, his friends and staff responded very positively to his 'normal' voice, and he had a renewed confidence in himself. S and his family ended therapy on a very happy note. I was delighted that S and his family felt this way, but I had serious reservations that all had not been resolved. Many clinicians would admit this is often the case.

Resurgence of anxiety

Six months later, I heard from his mother that S had started to show serious signs of anxiety and refusing to attend school. Some of his symptoms suggested panic attacks, and he was becoming abnormally obsessional about tidiness and cleanliness. S and his parents wanted to know if I would be in a position to help him again, but on this occasion I felt that he needed more highly specialised care of a clinical psychologist or psychiatrist experienced in working with adolescents with more serious psychological problems. I suggested they seek referral to a male therapist, and over the following months S was offered CBT with a clinical psychologist to help manage his anxiety with support from a psychiatrist when symptoms became more extreme.

Final revelations about the key conflict over speaking out issue

Over the next 2 years, S occasionally sent a short email letting me know how he was going in therapy and with his job. Progress with the psychologist had also been slow, with S sometimes feeling things were getting better and at other times feeling very rather disillusioned. Then one day he rang and casually asked for my advice on a practical matter. Even though therapy had finished well over 2 years before, I always keep the door open based upon my fundamental tenet that '*the therapeutic relationship once established need never be broken*' (Baker, 2010a).

He set up a session and in rather a roundabout way, referred to a recent friendship, and wondered how best to let his parents know about this person. When I asked gently if his special new friend was a male, he hesitated slightly as if surprised that I might know this and said "Yes, he is, and I'm gay". At last! He then explained how this secret had been taunting him since the age of 11, directly coinciding with the changes to his voice. He reported feeling totally preoccupied with conflicted emotions about his sexual orientation at the time.

On the one hand he desperately needed to tell someone, but on the other hand he was concerned about the consequences of his doing so – especially with his parents and, in particular, his father. This inner conflict over speaking out (COSO) turmoil had plagued him for the entire time that his dysphonia persisted, and in my opinion, it was still playing heavily on his mind while he was seeing his other therapist for 'anxiety-related symptoms'. As proposed so eloquently in the *cascade model of coping* that explains the persistence of voice disorders for some individuals (de Jong *et al.*, 2003), it was as if he had become 'deadlocked' in a coping pattern of denial, dilemmas over confiding, and withdrawal.

After declaring himself in this way and talking about it briefly together, he spoke with his mother, consulted his GP and once again, sought further appointments with his psychologist. He was now feeling able to 'come out' and he felt ready to begin to reconcile this part of himself in a way that would no longer constrain and hold him back. He had found his true voice. A short time later when he sought a follow-up review appointment, he came with a friend and was driving himself – his car – a second hand, but genuine Alpha Romeo!

To gain further insights into precipitating or perpetuating psychosocial factors

Another key purpose of integrating counselling with direct voice work during this action phase is to help the patient to gain a genuine understanding of the essential nature of their voice disorder and the meaning behind their symptoms. This then helps the person to appreciate why some interventions rather than others will be recommended.

Within the context of the early educational counselling conversations for a FVD (MTVD or PVD), a therapist may map out a range of aetiological possibilities that are often associated with onset or perpetuation of symptoms. These factors do not all need to be laid out at once. Rather, they can be presented gradually as options during the psychosocial interview and then be interspersed during the practical interventions to elicit initiation of normal or improved phonation.

As highlighted in Chapter 5, these may include factors related to a person's general health, especially URTI, the vocal demands on them in their work and family life, or in relation to advanced levels of vocal performance. It might also be suggested that these disorders develop suddenly in close association with acutely stressful situations, some time after a traumatic event or later where a memory of that trauma has been triggered by some incident, or gradually in response to chronic difficulties that have had an impact on the person's overall sense of physical and psychological well-being. In some cases, the difficulties may be associated with issues related to maturity, changes in the context of the family life cycle, or arising directly from a severe event (e.g., learning of a spouse being diagnosed with a progressive neurological disease and the ensuing efforts in adjusting home and work life to accommodate to this). In addition to the more severe events and difficulties, others are characterised by conflict over speaking out (COSO), or feeling powerless in the system (PITS) to which they belong (Baker, 1998, 2003; Baker *et al.*, 2013; Butcher & Cavalli, 1998; Butcher *et al.*, 2007; House & Andrews, 1988)

In Case Examples 12.1 and 12.2, having alerted these young boys and their families to a range of factors that may contribute to the onset or aggravation of puberphonia, the first priority was given to eliciting normal phonation. We then explored relevant psychosocial issues while reflecting on the meaning of the symptoms and the impact that their dysphonia had been having on them. It was a clinical judgment, rightly or wrongly, that these conversations would work better if they could use their voices normally.

In other cases of MTVD and PVD, clues to possible precipitating factors are revealed early on in the case history and psychosocial interview. They may not necessarily be considered pertinent by the patient, but they may suggest to the therapist that this is an area to pursue later. It is not a matter of the therapist rapidly leaping in to make causal links between the vocal symptoms and every adverse situation that a person may talk about. Rather, it is important to provide the time and space for both parties to think about what had transpired immediately prior to, or in the months preceding onset, and to reflect on how the person responded at the time, or how they are coping now. While telling their story there may be something about the demeanour of the patient that intuitively alerts the therapist, with a kind of 'knowing without knowing how she knows', to explore aspects of this account for more detail (see Chapter 11 for discussion about intuition).

Sometimes it is in this active phase of following up and asking more searching questions that patients make their own conscious connections between what has been happening to them and how this may have precipitated changes to their voices. During these transformative 'ah ha' moments, the person may begin to cry quietly or to express a strong sense of relief with a big smile. When this occurs, it seems to trigger a *top-down* modulation of the extreme levels of extrinsic and intrinsic laryngeal muscle tension, making the task of eliciting voluntary control over the initiation of phonation or improved vocal function so much easier (Case example 12.3).

Case example 12.3 Insights that enable resolution of the vocal symptoms

Transparency about a psychogenic aetiology

The 72 year-old woman previously mentioned in Chapter 11 (Case example 11.3) had been diagnosed with a sudden onset MTVD thought to be the result of vocal strain in association with an URTI and a heavy singing load in her local choir. The clinical presentation was not in keeping with a hyperfunctional dysphonia typically seen in association with heavy voice use or strain. Her high-pitched falsetto phonation with squeaks and occasional pitch breaks into normal phonation, and her inability to voluntarily initiate any modal voice, suggested a PVD. She had been aphonic and dysphonic for 6 weeks before being referred for SLP assessment. Having let S know that this was a PVD rather than related to over use of her voice in singing, she then nodded knowingly, settled comfortably into the chair, and stated firmly "I think it might have been something to do with stress". Such openness was a gift.

The power of insight and putting words to feelings

S was then invited to talk about what had been happening in the period prior to the onset of her aphonia. She recalled receiving a phone call from her daughter, informing her that she had just been diagnosed with a severe form of cancer, requiring immediate surgery. S described how on one hand she felt *frightened and absolutely devastated* by this news for her daughter; on the other hand, she felt a strong imperative to *hold herself together* and *to be strong and brave* so that she could comfort her daughter in a way that would give her strength and hope. It was later that evening as she wrestled with these conflicting feelings that her voice began to disappear. At the point that she divulged this information to me, she began to cry and then revealed that this was the first time she had told anyone else about it (other than her husband). It was also the first time she had been able to cry. This issue was discussed quietly and gently for some time until S wiped her eyes, smiled bravely and said 'I think I can start to get my voice back now'.

Intuition about other possible issues

In setting out to do this, while palpating her larynx, moving it gently from side to side and reassuring her quietly that there was no undue tension that would get in the way of our restoring her voice, I noticed that this lady was very thin. As with all functional symptoms, however positive they may be, there is always the other consideration that something organic may have been missed, and the inevitable thought was, could there be anything affecting her thyroid, anything impinging on her recurrent laryngeal nerve, anything affecting her overall health that might also account for her vocal symptoms and her physical fragility. Without quite knowing why, I began to explore this further and asked her gently if she had lost weight for any reason in recent months. She then revealed that she had suffered from breast cancer and had had a mastectomy some years before. She began to weep more profusely at this point, and admitted that her *deep unspoken fear throughout the last 6 weeks* was that there may have been a recurrence of some kind, or that she might have a new primary in the larynx. This revelation was equally important to the conflicting situation with her daughter, and one that had obviously been troubling her in a profound way.

Top-down modulation of fear

Here, the counselling was devoted to clarifying the ENT examination findings for an entirely normal larynx, and at the same time acknowledging that this would naturally have been a fear, especially given her daughter's diagnosis of a life threatening illness, and then her powerful recollections of her own vulnerability with cancer. After we had talked about this she became calm, and together we set about finding ways to trigger elicited normal phonation (see Box 12.5). S had achieved a perfectly normal voice by the end of this first session and with some trepidation and celebration, enjoyed my challenge of asking her to pick up the phone to ring her husband to say "Guess who this is – you can come and get me now!" Follow up sessions were offered to ensure stabilisation of her voice and to continue conversations about how best to support her daughter and her young family through this trying time.

Insights to enable resolution, transformation and reconstitution of the self

'If you don't consider the song of yourself, you become lost, and when you are lost you do lost things, and if you're lost for long enough you stop looking to be found' Wynton Marsalis (Personal communication, March 30, 2009).

Deeper levels of counselling may be a vital component in helping individuals to recognise how a long-standing dysphonia (now resolved) may have shaped their personality as they adapted and learned to cope with it over time (Epstein, Hirani, Stygall, & Newman, 2009; Oliveira, Hirani, Epstein, Yazigi, & Belhau, 2012). This counselling work will encourage the continuity of a person's *'core essence'* and 'private aspects of the self' (Gelech & Desjardins, 2011), while making adjustments to their public persona that is no longer characterised by an unusual voice. This may involve recognising that *avoidant coping patterns*, while appropriate at the time, are no longer necessary (McLeod & Clarke, 2007).

This process will require deeper levels of *person-centered counselling* by the SLP, or even *relational counselling* by a psychotherapist, where the therapeutic relationship is the nexus of change. In the safety of this holding environment the person can begin to envisage how life might change now if they see and hear themselves differently and if others are likely to view them differently too. The psychological work involved in the *reconstitution of the self* may be confronting or painful, but not necessarily so. It can evolve with an exciting momentum driven by the psychological mindedness, resilience, and renewed optimism of the patient (Ward *et al.*, 2011). As highlighted in Chapter 9 and emphasised by Paul Gibney (2010), on those rare occasions when patients create their own transformation and healing before our eyes, being a witness to this memorable experience promotes the growth of both the patient and the therapist (Case example 12.4).

Case example 12.4 Insights to enable resolution and reconstitution of the self

Speaking voice

A 21 year-old male student of drama and classical singing (S) was referred for assessment by his drama teachers who noted his unusually high pitched and ineffectual falsetto speaking voice during performance classes. When S made efforts to project with greater volume or emotional intensity, his voice would crack and break. His speaking voice was being consistently produced well within the female range, placing restrictions on parts that he might be offered, such as humorous, buffoon, or character roles. While these were considered well within his acting range, there were concerns from his drama teacher that in the long term this would lead to stereotyped casting. In addition, he noted that considerable co-operation was being required on the part of his fellow actors and audience to reconcile the incongruity of his feminine voice against his masculine role, dress, and appearance. S was not so concerned about this, having come to accept that *this was his voice, this was who he was.*

Singing voice

S was also undertaking singing lessons for classical voice. His current teacher, and several of those before him, had never queried his high falsetto speaking voice because this was all that he had ever heard. S was regarded as having a most rare and exceptionally beautiful singing voice and it was hoped that he might be developing into a rare male alto or counter-tenor. Training had been focused on the further development of his high falsetto range with repertoire traditionally sung by mezzos and contraltos. Simultaneously with the trouble that S was having with his speaking voice, he began to experience what appeared to be frequent sore throats or colds, difficulty in sustaining the strength in his projected falsetto singing voice, and involuntary cracking or breaking in the lower part of his alto range. He attributed this *increasing instability of his singing voice* to nervousness, mucous on the vocal folds or poor vocal technique. His singing teacher was fully supportive of his seeking assessment and chose to accompany him to the assessment session.

Clinical management

ENT, endocrinologist and SLP assessments confirmed a diagnosis of PVD in the form of puberphonia, and diagnostic probes by the therapist revealed that normal modal voice an octave below his falsetto phonation could be readily elicited. Considerable time was spent in explaining to S and his singing teacher that subsequent strategies might bring some exciting as well as somewhat confronting consequences. They were warned that it was likely that a normal low-pitched voice appropriate to S's size, gender and maturity would be elicited, and that this would have implications for them both. It would throw up some very real dilemmas for the young man and for his teacher, who may well face the prospect of working with a student who was not only a counter-tenor but a singer with the potential to become a baritone. This information was met with scepticism, but it was considered very important to prepare both of them for these impending changes.

Resolution of a dysphonia that may challenge a person's identity

In the therapist's opinion this was not just about this young man finding his normal voice for the first time. It was also about challenges to his personal identity that had been formed on the basis of his especially beautiful singing voice as a little boy that continued to shape his identity as he transitioned into adolescence and adulthood, with his unusually high singing and speaking voice. It was not my fear that he would no longer be able to sing beautifully; rather, that so much of his persona and reputation, that were loved and admired by family, friends, and teachers, were attached to his different singing and speaking voice. Therefore, once we had established his normal low-pitched voice and he was able to use it comfortably with family, friends, and during drama and singing activities, further counselling was recommended. Here, we explored a number of issues that had been raised in the psychosocial history that related directly to the way in which his special gift (his singing voice) and the perpetuation of his abnormally high speaking voice had influenced the development of his personality and ways of coping.

Relevant personal and vocal history that shaped his personality

S recalled being a chubby child with a beautiful singing voice who failed to fit in at primary school. At the age of 12 he recalled going through the normal pubertal changes but at not time was aware of his voice breaking. As he grew older, he became the butt of much teasing and harassment primarily about this weight and physical awkwardness and because his voice set him apart from others. He felt unable to defend himself in the schoolyard and would rather have been anywhere but at school. Although he was seen on a number of occasions by a school counsellor in relation to his adjustment problems he was never advised to seek a medical opinion in relation to his immature voice or excessive weight.

Relevant person and vocal history that helped to shape who he had become

S recalled being a chubby child, with a beautiful singing voice, who had failed to fit in at primary school. From early school days he was selected as a soloist in the local church choirs or for special functions at school. At the age of 12, he went through the normal pubertal changes but at no time was he aware of his voice breaking. He continued to sing and to be selected for solo work, and came to accept that his unusually high speaking voice was part of the special gift that he had been given with his singing voice. As he grew older, he became the butt of much teasing and harassment, primarily because of his weight and physical awkwardness and also because his voice set him apart from others. The mockery and rejection from boys in particular continued, and he privately resolved that all of this was *a test or hurdle that God had sent me to surmount over my lifetime*. He felt unable to defend himself in the schoolyard and would rather have been anywhere else but at school. He was seen on a number of occasions by the school counsellor about his 'adjustment problems' but was never advised to seek a medical opinion in relation to his immature voice or excessive weight.

Emotion focused coping in order to adapt

S recalled these transitional years as being very difficult until year 11 when he discovered *The Greek Girls*, a group who really liked him and enjoyed his company. He found it easier to be with girls and, having a voice like theirs, fashioned his intonation, linguistic, and paralinguistic features on these female friends. He found it easy to listen to their interests and attitudes and began to identify strongly with their thoughtful and sensitive ways of approaching and exploring personal problems. In order to cope with the alienation from the more masculine side of himself, he unconsciously developed '*a clown personality, somewhat larger than life, witty, dramatic, over the top, even camp. It all fitted with the mask, the armour and the image*'. Underneath all the jollity and hype, he felt he was an unusually sensitive and reflective young boy for his age, and that now as a young man, this was also how he regarded himself. I totally agreed.

Insights leading to transformation and reconstitution of the self

During these further counselling sessions we contracted to explore possible psychosocial factors that may have contributed to the onset of maintenance of his dysphonia and obesity beyond puberty. We also discussed how he thought his remarkable singing voice and unusual speaking voice had influenced who he was then and who he had become. In addition, he was strongly motivated to think about how his new voice might open up some new ways of being.

S described himself as coming from a loving and secure family home with one younger sister. As a family they were not inclined to be articulate about many things, certainly not about feelings. However, in keeping with their faith and family ways '*it was a given that we were loved and cherished by one another*'. His parents never criticised his appearance or his voice and simply accepted that 'this was who I was'. There did not seem to be anything of obvious significance in his family life that might have accounted for his psychosexual immaturity, but it was acknowledged that at some stage issues related to sexual preference might be raised by this young man for discussion.

What emerged most strongly with these deeper counselling sessions was the powerful impact that his remarkable talent had on his life from an early age. For many mates at school his singing was a point of ridicule but for others, and for the adults in his life, it was a source of considerable wonder and positive affirmation. As S explained '*I was known for my voice, through my voice, because of my voice: it was a gift, which both confined and defined who I was.*' This young man, who had come from a family unaccustomed to putting things into words or expressing feelings, was now articulating with remarkable insight one of the most crucial issues that may have contributed to the perpetuation of his dysphonia. Part of this ongoing psychotherapeutic work then involved discussing ways in which he might have unconsciously held onto young behaviours that brought both primary and secondary gains.

This led to his exploration of issues in relation to gender, in particular his highly feminised persona and apparent alienation from his more masculine self. He felt that this part of his self had remained quiescent and repressed under the flamboyant guise of his *'jolly androgenous clown mask'*, and in the final sessions he began to discuss his obesity and underdeveloped psychosexual maturity. He saw both of these phenomena as directly linked to his dysphonia and distorted vocal image that he now quite spontaneously referred to as *'false – it's so false'*. How amazing for a young man with puberphonia to choose use language like this.

Finally, and perhaps most significantly of all, he began to explore his thwarted capacity for intimate relationships. This had given him the greatest pain of all as he realised how rarely he had experienced *'things from the inside'*. He sensed instead that intimate relationships had been sacrificed while he had provided the understanding and confidential ear to others: *'always the witness, the observer, the spectator to the legitimate and inevitable intimacy of others'*.

I now understand what Paul Gibney (2010) meant when he referred to those extremely rare moments in a therapist's lifetime when we might witness the transformation of a person driven by their own insights. Such moments are never forgotten and as emphasised in Chapter 9, they serve to remind us about the difference between treatment and the removal of symptoms as opposed to therapy that heals.

(Edited and expanded excerpt from Baker, 2002)

To recognise the impact of the vocal problem and grieve different forms of loss

Grieving and concomitant feelings are a normal response when a person is suddenly confronted with a life challenge for which there was no preparation; as a profession we need to give ourselves permission to do the necessary grief work' (Luterman, 2011) (p. 3).

It is notable that in all of the excellent texts devoted to counselling for a broad range of communication disorders, a strong emphasis is given to the role of the

SLP in offering grief counselling to patients and their families in relation to their communication problems (see Chapter 9, Text Box 9.6 for a list of these texts). These different authors suggest that in most cases we are dealing with people who are in transition, and that as a result of their communication disorder these individuals 'are emotionally upset but not emotionally disturbed'(Luterman, 2011) (p. 3).

Notions with respect to grief and loss and mental illness

In a most moving editorial article, Arthur Kleinman (2012) also highlights recent controversies over listing *grief as a mental illness* in the *Diagnostic and Statistical Manual of Mental Disorders (DSM-V)* (American Psychiatric Association, 2013). He writes this critique from the dual perspectives of one who had recently suffered the loss of his wife after 46 years of marriage and in his capacity as Professor of Psychiatry and Medical Anthropology, Harvard Medical School. His concerns are related to the way in which the APA has determined that if a person is still experiencing feelings of grief characterised by 'sadness, disturbed sleep, loss of appetite and energy, agitation, difficulty concentrating, and other psychological and physiological sequelae of such profound loss' for more than 1 year (DSM-III), or for more than 2 months after the death of a close relation (DSM-IV), then this warrants a diagnosis of depression and 'treating it with pharmacological agents and psychotherapy' (p. 608). He proposes that the APA experts have shown little or no regard for different cultural attitudes, beliefs and practices around sense of loss, grief or bereavement, and challenges the shocking assumption that anyone from any society or religion has a right to determine that if someone is still grieving 2 months after a profound loss, then they must be depressed and in need of medical treatment.

Kleinman also points out that '*the experience of loss is never neat: that is, out of context. It is always framed by meanings and values, which themselves are affected by all sorts of things like one's age, health, financial and work conditions, and what is happening in one's life and in the wider world*' (p. 608). He finds it disturbing that the normal and inevitable process of grieving is becoming increasingly medicalised with the implicit message that grief should not be tolerated, certainly not for too long. He wonders if the new generation, in this day and age of the internet with all its technological advances, '*may no longer want or need the suffering of grief to affirm its humanity, redeem its deepest values, and frame its collective and personal experience of loss*' (p. 609). He goes on to propose that if and when this happens, we will lose what it is to be human.

Grief and loss in relation to the voice disorder

In the field of voice disorders, these same sentiments also hold . The person grieving changes to, or loss of their voice is not generally suffering a psychological disorder or psychiatric illness, rather a normal reaction to a discomforting and affecting situation that is sometimes experienced as being dreadful. In many instances it may be quite sufficient to listen gently and empathically to this, and to try to appreciate how the person is feeling before moving into any form of intervention. In other cases, it will be important to offer deeper supportive counselling that takes their more profound grief reaction into account. This does not mean that the therapist views this grief reaction as pathological. Rather, it reflects the therapist's recognition that the patient's feelings of grief may be so painful that they may be temporarily restrained from committing to more practical activities intended to facilitate improvements to their voice.

Grief in relation to diagnosis and stressful incidents preceding onset

Initially, the grief may arise in response to the diagnosis and all that the person has gone through to reach this point, as described in the examples below.

- Administration of testosterone implants originally intended to boost the libido of a professional female singer led to permanent changes to the pitch, stability and control over her speaking and singing voice. She lost an international singing contract and her voice was never the same again (Baker, 1999).
- Severe problems were experienced by a 34 year-old singer who struggled with difficulties to her speaking and singing voice over a period of 19 years as she sought to overcome what were labelled as 'problems with poor breath support', 'unreliable vocal technique', and her 'somewhat hostile and belligerent attitude to vocal teachers'. Early recordings showed that she had an extraordinarily beautiful contralto voice. A continued search for a more satisfactory explanation eventually led to a diagnosis of 'focal dystonia of the larynx of neurologic origin'. Her sense of loss was related to the 19 years of struggling to control her voice and feeling both misunderstood and stigmatised. Although she was grateful and relieved with a more accurate diagnosis, this new knowledge marked the end of hope for ever recovering her former beautiful voice again (Baker, 2002).

Grief and loss in relation to stressful incidents preceding onset

Other grief work will be devoted to helping patients deal with emotional responses to stressful life events or difficulties that preceded the voice disorder, and that may have contributed to its onset (Aronson & Bless, 2009; Baker, 1998, 2003; Baker & Lane, 2009). As highlighted in Chapter 5, and as originally described by Brown *et al.* (1987; 1978), severe life events and difficulties may be a threat to the self or close others, resulting in different forms of loss. These may include loss of health, loss of a partner or close family member through illness or death, loss of one's job, property or financial security, loss of confidence in important personal relationships through rejection, separation or divorce, humiliation, entrapment, or disempowerment, or loss of a trust and cherished beliefs through betrayal by a respected institution such as a religious or government body. Other researchers have highlighted that these events and difficulties may be characterised by conflict over speaking out (COSO) or dilemma, and more recently by powerlessness in the system (PITS) (Baker *et al.*, 2013; Hatcher & House, 2003; House & Andrews, 1988).

Grief and loss in relation to the impact of the voice disorder

Grief work often focuses on helping a person to come to terms with the immediate impact of a vocal problem on their lives, and the many adjustments that need to made, at least in the short term. For professional voice users such as teachers, where the severity of their voice problem may lead to worker's compensation, taking time out from classroom work, and even retraining in another field of work, or for performers who have to cancel performance engagements, the sense of loss can be traumatic. Possibly some of the saddest and most troubling grief work for patients, their family and the therapist, will be in cases of traumatic brain injury where prognosis for improvement or resolution of the voice problem and other aspects of communication remains uncertain. Equally challenging grief work will be integral to the therapy for patients with a progressive neurological disorder where the therapist works alongside the patient and family as they face a gradual deterioration in the voice, speech, and swallowing, or where total loss of verbal communication is imminent. Under both of these circumstances, the therapeutic task for all concerned will be to tolerate a more ambiguous or open-ended type of loss, with a concerted *search for meaning* (Boss & Carnes, 2012).

Grief and loss in relation to one's personal identity, public and private

As a person with a voice problem goes through the various processes of assessment, diagnosis and interventions to promote change, or faces incomplete resolution and possible further deterioration, the grief process changes too. In some cases it may be relatively short-lived, while at other times it may be prolonged and intense as the person deals with mixed feelings of anger, sadness, and even disillusionment.

A constant undercurrent that often runs throughout this therapeutic process is the patient's sense of being 'alienated' from their physiological voice and, of equal significance, the feelings of loss with respect to their *'compromised self'* or *'altered self'* that can be experienced as a threat to personal identity, both public and private (Bickford *et al.*, 2013; Fourie, 2011a; Jacobs & van Biene, 2015; Rosen & Sataloff, 1997).

As highlighted in Chapter 7, there is no way of predicting how profound the sense of loss may be for a patient on the basis of symptom severity alone. What seems to matter most is how the person sees, hears, and experiences themselves in relation to their voice and how others may perceive them. When the young man with puberphonia and the counter-tenor singing voice said *"I was known for my voice, through my voice, because of my voice: it was a gift that both defined and confined who I was"*, this was not inflated ego or arrogance. This was his reality, and for other individuals for whom the voice is the primary tool of trade, such as actors, teachers, radio announcers, auctioneers, and parents, the threat to their sense-of-self can be equally troubling. For many who value singing as an essential and integral part of their lives, a loss of voice can deeply affect their overall sense of well-being but for professional singers, a threat to their singing voice often feels like a threat to their very existence. This is not just a threat to their next singing engagement or their career. It is a threat to their essential core (Baker, 1999, 2002; J. Miller, 2003; Rosen & Sataloff, 1997; Sataloff, 1991; Shewell, 2009).

These sensitive issues related to a sense of loss and personal identity are captured most wonderfully in David Bromley's painting *'The Heavy Crown II'* (also referred to as *'The King of Suburbia has Lost his Crown'*). What is so special about the painting in this context is that it evokes the notion that whoever we are and wherever we come from, whether La Scala or 'La Suburbs', our voice may feel like our crowning glory. When the crown becomes too heavy, or if we lose our voice, our world can be turned upside down (see Fig. 12.6).

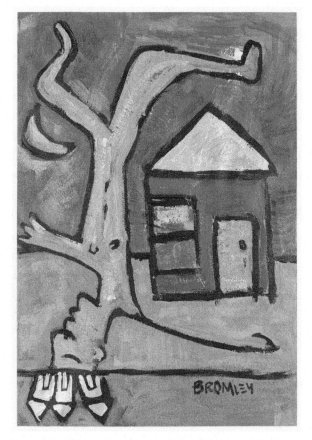

Fig. 12.6 "The Heavy Crown II" or "The King of Suburbia has Lost his Crown" David Bromley (1990)

Courtesy Bromley & Co.

Integrating grief counselling with traditional voice work

David Luterman (2011) strongly advocates that therapists should undertake grief work with their patients, but cautions against trying too hard to make them feel better. He notes that student clinicians often strive to alleviate the person's pain by doing more, talking more, trying to instil hope with optimistic comparisons, or by rescuing too soon. He reminds us that many communication disorders represent a temporary loss, but in the case of a disability, the loss will always be there regardless of what we may say or do. Therefore, when we create the time and space for grief that involves giving the person permission to cry or to be angry, it may not necessarily make them feel good. What it will do is 'take away or alleviate "feeling bad about feeling bad"' (p .4).

As a general principle, paying attention to a patient's grief in relation to the voice problem is best undertaken by the SLP who has the in-depth knowledge of the different voice disorders and how specific aspects of loss may become more pronounced during different stages of the therapeutic process. This grief counselling should not be seen as being separate from the direct voice work. However, in rare cases the sense of loss may be so profound that the person shows signs of anxiety or depressed mood that prevents him/her from moving forward with voice therapy or in other domains of life. Here, it may be appropriate to refer on to a SLP with specialised training in counselling, singing, theatre voice, traumatic brain injury, or progressive neurological disorders as befits the particular difficulty. Alternatively, referral to a psychologist or psychiatrist with a sound knowledge of problems associated with voice disorders would be appropriate. In an ideal situation this would be in a multi-disciplinary setting where a collaborative approach is fostered and where the mental health professionals work closely alongside the SLP as the traditional voice work continues (Baker, 1998, 2002; Butcher *et al.*, 2007; J. Miller, 2003; Nichol *et al.*, 1993; Rammage *et al.*, 2001; Rosen & Sataloff, 1997).

To recognise indications for mentoring collaboration, supervision or referring on

The issues related to more severe levels of grieving that signal the need for seeking help highlight the importance of identifying other possible restraints to change. These can impede a patient's level of motivation and commitment, block their progress in gaining insights, or prevent the person from generalising and sustaining the changes they have made beyond the clinical setting. They may even put the patient at risk of relapse.

As outlined in some of the case examples throughout this chapter, when we fail to achieve the desired outcomes, therapists hypothesise about possible *internal restraints to change* such as *unconscious resistance* on the part of the patient, or a number of *external restraints to change* that have been contributing to the person being stuck. Some of these may be contextual factors, such as the patient's family situation or their occupational setting, where larger systemic issues mitigate against a person obtaining full resolution.

Some examples where I have found it essential to seek supervision are mentioned below:

1. Direct voice work was totally unsuccessful with an 8 year-old boy presenting with vocal nodules, where his exhausted and frustrated parents openly declared that they had completely lost control over the discipline of their children, and had no success in gaining their son's co-operation with respect to his vocal behaviour. By going with the family to an experienced family therapist who helped the parents to reassert their rights to be 'boss of the house', and then the boy to assert himself and his rights to become 'boss of his own voice', this facilitated the changes that were needed to enable voice therapy to continue.

2. No progress had been made with a 28 year-old woman presenting with severe MTVD and Reinke's oedema. She was married with two young children and her marital situation was dire. She revealed that much of her vocal strain was occurring during vehement arguments and screaming matches with her husband, and she feared for her emotional and physical safety. I met with the husband on one occasion and after this session I recognised that the degree of nastiness and marital conflict was outside my experience at the time. I was scared too. We booked a conjoint session with an experienced male family therapist (also known for his reputation in dealing with domestic violence) for an assessment and advice on how best to proceed. The couple argued, yelled and screamed at each other in front of both us, and it was of some relief to me to hear the family therapist confront the couple quite directly about their behaviour, to state that no progress could ever be made while this level of animosity and verbal violence continued, and only to consider coming back when they decided that they wanted to make some changes in their relationship. He reassured me there was no way I would get anywhere with my patient with her vocal nodules and in effect gave me permission to end therapy which I did.

In other cases, the most influential restraints to change will be those emerging from the *dynamics of the therapeutic alliance* and in particular, issues related to the *therapist's way of being*. In reflecting upon these crucial aspects, it is the therapist's responsibility to be alert to *transference* and *countertransference* issues, and how these may influence the way therapy proceeds or falters (Crago & Gardner, 2012). It is not so difficult to recognise when the behaviour of a patient suggests transference issues related to aspects of their relationship with parental figures, close siblings, or other highly influential people in their lives, such as teachers. It is more difficult to acknowledge a therapist's *countertransference issues* that may stall or damage a collaborative working relationship. In these instances the patient may no longer feel that the therapeutic environment is the right place for them to change, triggering their emotional withdrawal, or their decision to leave therapy without any warning. SLPs often report that this is a common trend amongst voice patients, but rarely raise questions about why this may be so. Maybe the answer lies with therapists becoming more aware of the impact that the dynamics of transference and countertransference will have on the therapeutic process, and engaging in more stringent self-reflection about a therapist's role in determining outcomes. 'The analysis of treatment failure is an important way of developing therapeutic skill' (Carr, 2012) (p. 254).

Seeking collaboration, supervision, or referring on does not signify ineptitude

Given our respective codes of ethics, it is an absolute given that we should always review our practice and seek help when we are not achieving positive outcomes. Recognising the patient's unconscious resistance and some of the other external restraints to change is a good start, and deciding to seek help in some form or other is desirable. Realising that we may be one of the key players in blocking progress may be less palatable, and our own resistance may hold us back from pursuing this aspect for some time.

Furthermore, it is not always easy to know exactly *when* to do this or *to whom* we should turn. In some settings, mentoring, working collaboratively, or having regular supervision is fostered and enjoyed. In other settings, possibly more so in private practice, clinicians will describe the process of deciding to seek help as being fraught. They often report mixed feelings of frustration towards the patient and with themselves, and in many cases, a sense of shame (Cavicchia, 2010). A therapist's ambivalence about whether or not to seek help reflects similar processes to those that many patients go through before they too decide to come to therapy. Learning to recognise the phenomena of *parallel processes* that may operate between therapy and supervision can be a revelation to a therapist when attending supervision for the first time. It may even inspire the clinician to shift from deep-seated emotions of shame or ineptitude to feelings of excitement and exuberance as he or she embarks on new ways of exploring the therapeutic process.

Some of the constructs in the discussion above are captured most effectively in the inspiring work of the Executive Coaching supervisor Alison Hodge (2013, 2014, 2016) and as depicted in her *The Three Pillars of Supervision* model (Fig. 12.7.)

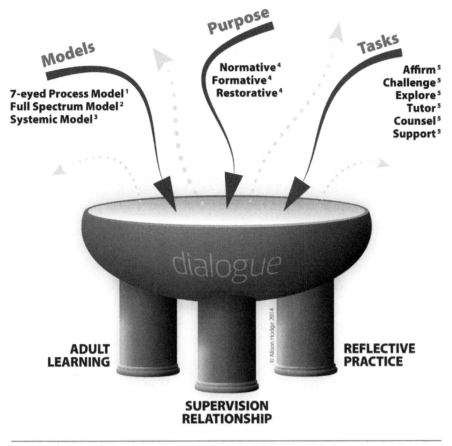

Fig. 12.7 The Three Pillars of Supervision model © Alison Hodge (2014, 2016)

Reproduced with kind permission Alison Hodge

This model is best understood by referring to the full explanation of the formative processes and action research project that led to its development in the publications cited above. For the purposes of this text, I have chosen to highlight some of the key constructs underpinning the model, and suggest that it has much to offer voice practitioners or other mental health professionals working with therapists and their patients with vocal disorders.

As proposed by Hodge (2016), the overall purpose of supervision is to learn new skills, maintain standards, and promote the overall well-being of those seeking supervision. The three pillars that underpin the coaching supervision model are:

- *Pillar 1: The Supervision relationship* where emphasis is given to creating an environment of trust and safety so that coaches can both share their practice while also disclosing their concerns and vulnerability. Here, the author highlights how issues related to *parallel processes* between the supervision relationship and the coach/client system may emerge, and how *observation, modelling* and *feedback about relational phenomena* in the supervision relationship may create new ways of dealing with these issues in their relationship with clients.

- *Pillar 2: Creating the core conditions of adult learning* where emphasis is given to supervision being a process that is sought voluntarily, that is collaborative, and that fosters reflective practice. The learning space gives permission 'not to know' and to be open, curious and to explore.

- *Pillar 3: Promoting the value of reflective practice* where emphasis is given to preparing for the supervision session and writing up reflections on the process. This process fosters new insights for work with clients and also enables a deeper appreciation of the personal and professional development gained from being in supervision.

Together, these pillars support the container that holds the background knowledge and principles of the different models of supervision, the specific purposes and focus of supervision that might be appropriate at the time, and the tasks that may be undertaken in this complex process. It is within this context of 'the container' with the interactions between these specific ingredients that the important generative dialogue can take place, enabling 'new knowledge', 'insights', 'self-awareness', and 'learning' to emerge.

Hodge (2016) also reports most interesting findings on other processes involved in supervisors and executive coaches '*keeping fit for purpose*'. Her data show that while ongoing one-to-one supervision is a crucial ingredient, it is not enough on its own. 'Keeping fit for purpose' also requires the support of a team that may include a number of professional advisors on the one hand, and a network of critical friends, peers, and family members with an appreciation of the work that is being undertaken on the other.

The *Three Pillars of Supervision* model, and the principles that underpin keeping fit for purpose, support the training and practice of SLPs where clinicians are required to reflect carefully on their clinical practice, to be up-to-date when engaging with patients, and to be alert to signs of professional burnout. The emphasis given by Hodge to ongoing supervision fostering 'generative dialogue', and these processes being 'formative', 'normative', and 'restorative', is both energising and refreshing. It most effectively reinforces a number of constructs introduced throughout this current text where it has been noted that master clinicians from both *vocology* and mental health disciplines are generally open and transparent about their practice, willing to persevere in the face of ambiguity and not knowing, undertake their own personal therapy, and reach out to learn from others (Baker, 2008, 2010b; Butcher & Cavalli, 1998; Butcher *et al.*, 2007; Crago & Gardner, 2012; DiLollo, 2014; Fourie, 2011b; Gibney, 2010). A summary of the counselling components involved in this action phase of intervention is shown in Box 12.6.

Box 12.6 Stage 3: The action phase, seeking solutions and gaining insights

Main purposes

- To enhance conventional therapies by generating changes in behaviours, thoughts and feelings that enable patients to find their physiological and metaphorical voice again
- To integrate counselling with creative and traditional approaches to restore phonation
- To prepare the person for strategies designed to facilitate improved phonation
- To identify and deal with any restraints to change that may include the therapist
- To gain further insights into precipitating or perpetuating psychosocial factors
- To recognise impact of vocal problems and grieve different forms of loss
- To recognise indications for mentoring, collaboration, supervision or referring on

Levels of counselling

- Supportive counselling with empathetic listening, seeking to understand throughout
- Psycho-educational counselling with information and advice where appropriate
- Motivational counselling that inspires the person to draw upon their strengths
- Further grief counselling to help resolve sense of loss or altered sense of identity
- Relational counselling to deal with interpersonal conflicts and coping with stress

Different intensities of therapeutic engagement

- Creates a holding environment that enables implicit emotions to become explicit
- Enables deepening of the therapeutic alliance in dealing with restraints to change
- Develops a therapeutic relationship that becomes the nexus of change

Therapist skills, strategies, qualities and 'ways of being' to facilitate change

- Responds to clues that patients have different ways of learning
- Integrates *bottom-up* and *top-down* approaches to counselling with direct voice work
- Reframes and externalises the problem; collapses time; amplifies change; raises dilemmas; restrains change; predicts collapse; confronts; highlights inner strengths
- Inspires, encourages, motivates, persists, remains present, realistic and humble

Stage 4: Closing phase that entails consolidating changes and ending therapy

The primary purpose of integrating counselling during this final phase of intervention is to facilitate a satisfactory ending for the person with the vocal problem and for the therapist too. As emphasised earlier in this chapter, the rather arbitrary allocation of neat and sequential stages does not always reflect the reality of the therapeutic process. For instance, issues related to ending therapy may well have been pre-empted even in the very first session, and attention to generalising beyond the clinical setting or activities to consolidate aspects of vocal change will often be interwoven throughout the action phase. In addition, learning to cope with the possibility of residual dysphonia, and some interpersonal or psychosocial issues being too difficult to resolve, may also have become evident much earlier than this final phase. The consolidation of vocal and personal changes is a collaborative process that is generally a most positive experience for both concerned. However, many patients, especially those with PVD, may require more sophisticated psychological support from the SLP in stabilising their voice in different social or emotional contexts. Likewise, ending therapy is an active and mutually negotiated process that can proceed with a logical and inevitable finality, but in other situations it may be neither negotiated, nor logical. When this occurs it will require deeper levels of counselling in order to appreciate the impact that ending therapy has upon the patient, and in some cases, on the therapist too. Some of these different issues are highlighted below.

To consolidate changes and generalisation with psychosocial support

One of the key purposes of integrating counselling with traditional voice work in this closing phase is to help patients to consolidate the changes they have made outside the clinical setting. This is often a most enjoyable process for both parties, and as the person becomes increasingly confident in maintaining improvements in their vocal technique they often return to follow-up appointments with a spring in their step.

With others, such as those with PVD, using their newly recovered voice can be extremely threatening, especially if they have been dysphonic for weeks, months or even years (as in case examples 12.2 and 12.4). These people may find the path to consolidation very slow, with variable success in maintaining their normal phonation. Sometimes it may be markedly inconsistent and at other times, it may disintegrate or completely relapse into the former dysphonia. This can be disappointing for the patient and equally troubling for the therapist.

In situations like this the counselling work will involve coming to understand the context in which it is most threatening for the person. Is it related to being with and talking to particular people? Is it to do with the social context where they are put on the spot and required to perform to a certain level where they feel inept and out of control? Is it related to a specific topic of conversation that becomes too difficult to put into words and to voice out aloud? Or is it due to the sheer embarrassment of hearing their 'normal' voice that has not as yet become embodied into 'the self' they previously knew themselves to be?

Once some of these possible issues have been explored, the therapist and patient may decide together on how to introduce different levels of challenge. This will draw upon the therapist's sensitivity to the concerns of the patient but in generating different challenges, it can be a creative and enjoyable process for both.

As in case example 12.2, some of these activities included inviting 'safe' family members or friends into the therapy sessions, small tasks to use his voice in a 'safe setting' such as on the telephone, and then in a Skype conversation. This was then extended beyond the clinical setting where the therapist encouraged him to use his voice where he was not known, such as in a café to order a coffee or from a stranger to ask for directions. Later, he was invited to walk vigorously outside in a large open park with the therapist, where no one else would be likely to hear him, but where the pace of the walking and animation in the conversation acted to distract him from listening too carefully to his voice as it began to stabilise with more confidence.

As in the case example 12.4, the therapist contacted the lecturers in the drama school and conservatorium to prepare the other students for the changes that they were going to hear in the speaking and singing voice of their colleague, and to invite their support when he used his 'new voice' for the first time rather than resorting to cajoling or jeering, which young people of that age might normally do with no malice intended.

In themselves, these day-to-day activities are not new to SLPs who are always helping patients to generalise improvements in their communication skills in more functional ways. What matters here is the rationale for introducing the different levels of challenge and threat, keeping in mind the constructs outlined earlier in this chapter in relation to the involuntary closing down of the laryngeal valve in the face of threat as the person freezes, or prepares for flight or fight.

To evaluate the vocal and personal changes which have been achieved

Another key purpose of counselling work during this final phase is to reflect upon and evaluate the changes that have been made. At a more superficial level these will involve changes or improvements to the person's voice. At a deeper level the changes may be related to the ways in which the person is now coping differently with a range of psychosocial factors such as attending to their overall general health and well-being, dealing with stressful situations in a less anxious and more proactive manner, or finding new ways to deal with interpersonal conflicts at home or at work that had previously felt insurmountable.

When patients experience dramatic or substantial changes to their voice and/or their personal situation, there is often a sense of celebration that can be enjoyed by both parties and the likelihood of ending therapy becomes a matter of fact decision. At other times, achieving improvements in vocal function is very slow, whether due to organic and other neurophysiological considerations, psychological issues where a patient's family or work setting continues to be problematic, or as previously mentioned, due to some degree of failure within the therapeutic relationship itself. Reaching a level of acceptance that these restraints to change may be too difficult to overcome may generate sensitive counselling conversations to help the patient achieve a balance between realistic expectations, hope, and despair, and to prepare themselves for ending therapy (Bergin & Walsh, 2005; O'Hara, 2011; Wiles, Cott, & Gibson, 2008). These very issues will be of equal significance for the therapist, and may well be somewhat confronting too.

To consider the implications of ending therapy for both patient & therapist

'The end of therapy is a crucial time for speech–language pathologists and can impact upon their sense of achievement and satisfaction' (Hersh, 2010b) (p. 283).

In a most interesting lead article for a Scientific Forum, Deborah Hersh raises a number of important issues in relation to ending therapy across the spectrum of SLP interventions, and then invites commentary from clinicians from the different areas of specialty (Hersh, 2010a, 2010b). She acknowledges that *discharge from therapy*, *termination of therapy*, or *ending of therapy* can be a significant time for patients, especially those who may have been in therapy for a very long time. She places particular emphasis on the impact of therapeutic endings *on the therapist* and suggests that while under ideal circumstances ending of therapy is negotiated in a collaborative way with a natural sense of closure, it is not always this neat. On the contrary, sometimes a patient terminates therapy suddenly without any warning. At other times it is difficult to reach an agreed time to end therapy where progress has been very slow, where there is a residual disability, when prognosis for further change is poor, or where expectations may be unrealistic. Hersh suggests that the discharge process or ending of therapy is often 'a complex negotiation for clinicians which involves a great deal of emotional energy' (p. 283), and proposes that three main areas of tension underpin this process. These are:

1. Real versus ideal endings
2. Balancing their personal and professional selves in making and breaking of therapeutic relationship
3. Respecting client autonomy while retaining control over caseloads and fair allocation of resources (Hersh, 2010b) (p. 290)

Terminologies related to therapeutic endings

Hersh highlights the conundrum over terminology that refers to this very final phase of therapy where clinicians from SLPs and other areas of mental health may use terms such as *'discharge'*, *'treatment termination'* or *'closure*, all of which imply therapist control or the finality of ending therapy. Other practitioners refer to *'leaving therapy' 'celebration'*, *'finishing well'*, *'rite of passage'* or *'reintegration'*. These rather euphemistic terms suggest that the final phase of therapy is something experienced primarily by the patient, and that ending therapy need not necessarily mean being totally cut off from further contact. Rather, it may be construed as a developmental or transitional phase.

In my commentary on Hersh's excellent lead paper, I have proposed that a term such as *discharge* is best used in an administrative sense. In my clinical practice I prefer to discuss the *ending of therapy* with a patient in a transparent manner, both at the outset of our therapeutic encounter and then, 'whatever the outcome, whether it is positive or negative, it is a process that is negotiated and determined by both, with the door left open for the client to return' (Baker, 2010a) (p. 310). This position seems to resonate with recent discussions in the psychoanalytic literature where it has been suggested by Medenhall (2009) that the notions of *discharge* or *termination* no longer reflect current analytic perspectives. These therapists now give stronger emphasis to the clinical principle that the client should be able to initiate and sustain more complex modes of connection and relatedness both during and after therapy. Medenhall suggests that the therapeutic relationship should be like a dyad that is constantly evolving, and that termination is incongruent with this more modern approach to analysis.

> *'The analysand [client undergoing analysis] may cease contact for some time, but the sustaining emotional bond remains, and resumption of contact may now be viewed as a reflection of this positive state of affairs'* (Medenhall, 2009) (p. 128).

Other analysts have also suggested that the final phase of therapy should be construed as a healthy developmental process, with the main task for both client and therapist as one of *letting go* or simply *ending therapy*.

> *'The term "termination" has seemed oddly cold and sterile for describing the moment when two individuals, upon reaching the end of a profound and caring shared human experience, and with one, at least, likely facing a richer beginning than was possible before, go their (sometimes) separate ways'* (Frank, 2009) (p.150).

Real versus ideal endings

Hersh (2010b) also discusses the tensions that exist between those endings that may be ideal, where there is 'an experience of successfully achieving agreed goals, a sense of closure and a job well done' (p. 283), or others that are less than satisfactory. She describes these as being more real, and it is a helpful concept to keep in mind.

In the field of voice disorders and in other areas of mental health, there is always the juggling of values around *ideal criteria* versus *working realities* (Shane, 2009). For example, we all recognise those situations when enforced endings may occur if the patient leaves due to further illness or job-related reasons, if they request a second opinion, if they drift away with no explanation, or leave suddenly feeling belligerent or dissatisfied. While rationalisation or even attending supervision may soften the blow after clients drop out or leave unhappily, the reflective therapist is left with uncomfortable questions about his or her level of competence and possibly too a lingering sense of shame or humiliation (Baker, 2010a).

The impact of ending therapy on the therapist

In researching the fascinating question about the impact of therapeutic endings on the therapist, it has been surprising to find that there is virtually no published literature that addresses this topic in relation to voice disorders. It could be argued that in comparison with aphasia therapy, many voice problems are more discrete, the time spent in therapy is shorter, and the thrust of therapy is focused on education, improvements in vocal techniques and moderate behavioural changes. While the quality of the therapeutic relationships is no less important in forming the foundation for such work to take place, the ending of therapy for both patient and therapist does not seem to be so fraught .

In others areas of voice however, where dysphonias may arise from TBI, progressive neurological disorders, psychogenic factors, or work-related issues where third party insurers become enmeshed in the process of rehabilitation, therapy is likely to be longer-term. Likewise, where a severe and intractable dysphonia has implications for further neurological deterioration, loss of career, or difficulties in interpersonal relationships, such work draws upon every facet of knowledge, skill, and creativity, and requires a willingness to persevere in the face of considerable uncertainty. Here, the strength of the therapeutic relationship is crucial and in these more complex disorders, it requires deeper and more sustained levels of involvement from the clinicians in holding the patient as he or she struggles to resolve the problem.

As exemplified in some of the case examples throughout this text, the impact upon the therapist in doing this work can be very demanding and while many authors have described the struggles and very real frustrations associated with the work, we rarely acknowledge or write about how rewarding it can be when resolution of the voice disorder is finally achieved (Aronson, 1990; Baker, 1998, 2002, 2003; Butcher *et al.*, 2007; Elias *et al.*, 1989; Kollbrunner, Menet, & Seifert, 2010; Neemuchwala, 1998).

However, the demands, rewards and sense of fulfillment are not just associated with the successful resolution of the vocal problem. With this longer-term work, the therapist comes to know the patient very well, and no doubt the patient comes to know the therapist quite well too, perhaps better than we imagine. It seems strange then that the published literature does not pay due attention to the positive and intense intellectual and emotional gains that can come from such special relationships, or the possibility that this whole process is also nurturing to the therapist. Similarly, voice therapists rarely write about feelings related to their own separation anxiety or sense of loss that they may experience as these longer-term therapeutic relationships come to a natural end. Ironically, it is often our speech pathology students who express such feelings so passionately when they face handing over their clients to the next student, and when they admit how much they have come to treasure a therapeutic relationship.

Perhaps too there is much to learn from our psychiatric colleagues who more readily acknowledge the therapist's reactions in anticipating termination of therapy, the therapist's love for the patient, and the emotional challenge that they also face with the loss of a special and valued relationship when analysis comes to an end. Analysts and psychotherapists reflect honestly about the struggles, regrets, and recriminations with respect to the ending of therapy, but they also acknowledge the positive rewards that they have derived from the intense intellectual and emotional investment in the therapeutic relationship.

> *"Through our involvement with our patients' struggles and growth, we come to know them, and they us deeply; we are often experienced by analysands as knowing them more profoundly than anyone else. (Have no illusions. They often come to know us deeply too, sometimes, despite themselves.) It is often difficult for us to lose patients with whom we have worked deeply* (Frank, 2009).

I support the view put forward by Deborah Hersh (2010b) that if SLPs are to deal with therapeutic endings more effectively, the implicit processes and emotions associated with the final phase of therapy need to be made more explicit. I suggest that this will be achieved more easily when therapists acknowledge that they too experience rewards and losses in the therapeutic relationship. While for some clinicians the end of therapy is finite, my own belief is that the door is always open and that the therapeutic relationship, once established, need never be broken (Baker, 2010a). A summary of the components involved in this final stage of our therapeutic work is summarised in Box 12. 7.

Box 12.7 Stage 4: Consolidating changes and ending therapy

Main Purposes
- To consolidate changes and generalisation with psychosocial support
- To evaluate the vocal and personal changes which have been achieved
- To consider the implications of ending therapy for both patient and therapist
- To end therapy leaving the door open for the person to return

Levels of counselling
- Supportive counselling in acknowledgement of all that the patient has achieved
- Grief counselling with respect to residual problems still unresolved
- Psychoeducational counselling related to terminating therapy or referring on
- Counselling focused upon weaning from therapy and ending therapy

Different intensities of therapeutic engagement
- Encourages healthy separation
- Deals with invitations to continue the relationship outside bounds of therapy
- Acknowledges the therapeutic relationship and what it means for the person

Therapist skills, strategies, qualities and 'ways of being'
- Offers creative approaches to consolidation of changes and generalising
- Enables collaborative appraisal of what has been achieved
- Negotiates appropriate follow up
- Reflects upon situations where patients terminate therapy with no warning
- Celebrates mutually agreed upon timing and manner for ending of therapy
- Recognises that the therapeutic relationship once established is never broken

Conclusion

'You don't put your life into books you find it there' (Bennett, 2007) (p.104).

Vocology is a burgeoning field and one to which many disciples contribute so generously, making it such a vibrant professional community. The advances in medicine, surgery, technology, and assessment, along with the more stringent attention to principles of perceptual-motor learning in facilitating phonatory behavioural change, are most exciting. More sophisticated functional imaging studies of the brain are now throwing new light on many cognitive and emotional processes that were hypothesised so many years ago, with new evidence confirming the postulated interactions between the different levels of the brain under various conditions of thinking, feeling, and doing. Sigmund Freud and Pierre Janet were not so wrong after all.

Running parallel to this process is an equally welcome emphasis on new ways of integrating both quantitative and qualitative approaches in our research. This is helping us to be much more accountable in evaluating outcomes, and it is refreshing to witness inspiring efforts to tease out the essential components of the therapeutic process. Some of these clinical processes are related to the role of counselling in the management of voice disorders. Recent evidence shows that counselling and psychotherapy bring about measurable changes in the brain, with concomitant improvements in the physical and mental well-being of individuals regardless of the theoretical models being used. It is the quality of the therapeutic relationship that has been shown to be the key ingredient in assuring successful therapeutic outcomes.

When I think of the great master practitioners I have observed, or the writings of some of our finest scholars in the fields of medicine, speech pathology, vocology, vocal pedagogy, otolaryngology, neurology, psychology and psychiatry, family therapy, and executive coaching, the essence of what they have always conveyed is twofold.

One is the emphasis on the capacity of practitioners in the respective disciplines to integrate left and right brain approaches, with close attention to scientific and objective detail on the one hand and longer-shot perspectives that draw upon intuition, sensitivity to emotions, and the context of the individual on the other. The other key emphasis is on the importance of understanding what it is about the *quality of the relationship* and the *practitioner's way of being* that enables each person to flourish and for change to take place. Whether it is in the context of clinical or vocal teacher-student relationships, the supervisory relationship, or the therapeutic relationship, this is what matters the most.

For me, there is nothing more important than the relationship. It is reflected in our different worlds of art and sculpture, music and song, opera and theatre, and in the wonderful world of poetry and literature. It is the foundation of our lives, at home with family and friends, and with our colleagues at work. The relationship is the basis of all our work with our patients, and with our students and colleagues in nurturing their development to fully realise who they are and in supporting them to become all that they want to be.

The question remains, can the special skills and ways of being that engender a therapeutic relationship be taught, or can this be learned? Of course they can. We may need to move outside our personal comfort zone to do so, and we may well have to reach out beyond the confines of our own profession to learn from the wisdom and brilliance of others. Or if we look closely, it might be right there in front of us.

References

American Psychiatric Association. (2013). *Diagnostic and statistical manual of mental disorders DSM-5* (5th ed.). Arlington: American Psychiatric Association.

Aronson, A. E. (1990). Psychogenic voice disorders. In *Clinical voice disorders: An interdisciplinary approach.* (3rd ed., pp. 116–159). New York: Thieme.

Aronson, A. E., & Bless, D. M. (2009). *Clinical voice disorders* (4th ed.). New York: Thieme.

Baker, J. (1998). Psychogenic dysphonia: Peeling back the layers. *Journal of Voice, 12*(4), 527–535.

Baker, J. (1999). Changes to women's voices following hormonal therapy. A report on alterations to the speaking and singing voices of four women. *Journal of Voice, 13*(4), 496–507.

Baker, J. (2002). Persistent dysphonia in two performers affecting the singing and projected speaking voice: A report on a collaborative approach to management. *Logopedics, Phoniatrics, Vocology, 27,* 179–187.

Baker, J. (2003). Psychogenic voice disorders and traumatic stress experience: A discussion paper with two case reports. *Journal of Voice, 17*(3), 308–318.

Baker, J. (2008). The role of psychogenic and psychosocial factors in the development of functional voice disorders. *International Journal of Speech-Language Pathology, 10*(4), 210–230.

Baker, J. (2010a). The therapeutic relationship once established need never be broken. *International Journal of Speech-Language Pathology, 12*(4), 309–312.

Baker, J. (2010b). Women's voices: Lost or mislaid, stolen or strayed? *International Journal of Speech-Language Pathology, 12*(2), 94–106.

Baker, J. (2016). Functional voice disorders: Clinical presentations and differential diagnosis. In M. Hallet, J. Stone & A. Carson (Eds.), *Functional neurologic disorders.* Amsterdam: Elsevier.

Baker, J., Ben-Tovim, D. I., Butcher, A., Esterman, A., & McLaughlin, K. (2013). Psychosocial risk factors which may differentiate between women with Functional Voice Disorder, Organic Voice Disorder, and Control group. *International Journal of Speech-Language Pathology, 15*(6), 547–563.

Baker, J., & Lane, R. D. (2009). Emotion processing deficits in functional voice disorders. In K. Izdebski (Ed.), *Emotions in the human voice* (Vol. 3, pp. 105–136). San Diego: Plural Publishing.

Behrman, A., Dahl, L. D., Abramson, A. L., & Schutte, H. K. (2003). Anterior-posterior and medial compression of the supraglottis: Signs of nonorganic dysphonia or normal postures? *Journal of Voice, 17*(3), 403–410.

Bennett, A. (2007). *The uncommon reader*. London: Faber & Faber and Profile Books.

Bergin, L., & Walsh, S. (2005). The role of hope in psychotherapy with older adults. *Aging and Mental Health, 9*(1), 7–15.

Bickford, J., Coveney, J., Baker, J., & Hersh, D. (2013). Living with the altered self. *International Journal of Speech-Language Pathology, 15*(3), 324–333.

Boss, P., & Carnes, P. (2012). The myth of closure. *Family Process, 51*(4), 456–469.

Brown, G. W., Bifulco, A., & Harris, T. O. (1987). Life events, vulnerability and onset of depression: Some refinements. *British Journal of Psychiatry, 150*, 30–42.

Brown, G. W., & Harris, T. O. (1978). *Social origins of depression*. London: Tavistock Publications.

Butcher, P., & Cavalli, L. (1998). Fran: Understanding and treating psychogenic dysphonia from a cognitive-behavioural perspective. In D. Syder (Ed.), *Wanting to talk*. London: Whurr.

Butcher, P., Elias, A., & Cavalli, L. (2007). *Understanding and treating psychogenic voice disorder: A CBT framework*. Chichester: Wiley.

Butcher, P., Elias, A., Raven, R., Yeatman, J., & Littlejohns, D. (1987). Psychogenic voice disorder unresponsive to speech therapy: Psychological characteristics and cognitive-behaviour therapy. *British Journal of Disorders of Communication, 22*, 81–92.

Carr, A. (2012). *Family therapy: Concepts, process and practice*. Chichester: Wiley-Blackwell.

Cavicchia, S. (2010). Shame in the coaching relationship: Reflections on organisational vulnerability *Journal of Management Development, 29*(10), 877–890.

Couture, S., & Sutherland, O. (2006). Giving advice on advice-giving: A conversation analysis of Karl Tomm's practice. *Journal of Marital and Family Therapy, 32*(3), 329–344.

Crago, H., & Gardner, P. (2012). *A safe place for change. Skills and capacities for counselling and therapy*. Melbourne: IP Communications.

D'Angelo, J. (2000). *Healing with the voice*. London: Thorsons.

Damasio, A. R. (2000). A second chance for emotion. In R. D. Lane & L. Nadel (Eds.), *Cognitive neuroscience of emotion* (pp. 12–23). New York: Oxford University Press.

Damasio, A. R. (2003). *Looking for Spinoza: Joy, sorrow, and the feeling brain*. New York: Harcourt, Inc.

de Jong, F. I. C. R. S., Cornelius, B. E., Wuyts, F. L., Kooijman, P. G. C., Schutte, H. K., Oudes, M. J., & Graamans, K. (2003). A psychological cascade model for persisting voice problems in teachers. *Folia Phoniatrica et Logopaedia, 55*(2).

Dietrich, M., Andreatta, R. D., Jiang, Y., Joshi, A., & Stemple, J. C. (2012). Preliminary findings on the relation between the personality trait of stress reaction and the central neural control of vocalization. *International Journal of Speech-Language Pathology, 14*(4), 377–389.

Dietrich, M., & Verdolini Abbott, K. (2014). Psychobiological stress reactivity and personality with high and low stressor-induced extralaryngeal reactivity. *Journal of Speech, Language and Hearing Research, 57*, 2076–2089.

DiLollo, A. (2014). Constructivism and adaptive leadership: Framing an approach for clinicians to overcome barriers to counseling. In R. J. Fourie (Ed.), *Therapeutic processes for communcation disorders* (pp. 139–152). New York: Psychology Press.

DiLollo, A., & Neimeyer, R. A. (2014). *Counseling in Speech-Language Pathology and Audiology*. San Diego: Plural Publishing.

Eastwood, C., Madill, C., & McCabe, P. (2015). The behavioural treatment of muscle tension voice disorders: A systematic review. *International Journal of Speech-Language Pathology, 17*(3), 287–303.

Egan, G. (2009). *The skilled helper* (9th ed.). Belmont: Brooks Cole.

Elias, A., Raven, R., Butcher, P., & Littlejohns, D. (1989). Speech therapy for psychogenic voice disorder: A survey of current practice and training. *British Journal of Disorders of Communication, 24*, 61–76.

Elkan, E. D. (1995). *The effects of upper respiratory dysfunction on the laryngeal condition*, Masters Thesis, Northeast Missouri State University.

Epstein, R., Hirani, S. P., Stygall, J., & Newman, S. P. (2009). How do individuals cope with voice disorders? Introducing the Voice Disability Coping Questionnaire. *Journal of Voice, 23*(2), 209–217.

Flasher, L. V., & Fogle, P. T. (2012). *Counseling skills for speech-language pathologists and audiologists* (2nd ed.). New York: Delmar, Cengage Learning.

Flaskas, C. (2011). The therapeutic relationship and use of the self. In P. Rhodes & A. Wallis (Eds.), *A practical guide to family therapy* (pp. 1–15). Melbourne: IP Communications.

Fourie, R. J. (2011a). From alienation to therapeutic dialogue. In R. J. Fourie (Ed.), *Therapeutic processes for communication disorders*. New York: Psycholgoy Press.

Fourie, R. J. (Ed.). (2011b). *Therapeutic processes for communication disorders*. New York: Psychology Press.

Frank, K. A. (2009). Ending with options. *Psychoanalytic Inquiry, 29*(2), 136–156.

Gelech, J. M., & Desjardins, M. (2011). I am many: The reconstruction of self following acquired brain injury. *Qualitative Health Research, 21*(1), 62–74.

Geller, E. (2011). Using oneself as a vehicle for change in relational and reflective practice. In R. J. Fourie (Ed.), *Therapeutic processes for communcication diosrders* (pp. 195–212). New York: Psychology Press.

Geller, E., & Foley, G. M. (2009). Expanding the "ports of entry" for speech-language pathologists: A relational and reflective model for clinical practice. *American Journal of Speech Language Pathology, 18*(1), 4–21.

Gelso, C. J. (2009). The real relationship in a postmodern world: Theoretical and empirical explorations. *Psychotherapy Research, 19*(3), 253–264.

Gibney, P. (2010). *The pragmatics of therapeutic practice.* Melbourne: Psychoz Publications

Hatcher, S., & House, A. (2003). Life events, difficulties and dilemmas in the onset of chronic fatigue syndrome: A case-control study. *Psychological Medicine, 33,* 1185–1192.

Helou, L. B. (2014). *Intrinsic laryngeal muscle response to a speech preparation stressor: Personality and autonomic predictors.* (Ph.D. Doctoral Dissertation), University of Pittsburgh.

Helou, L. B., Wang, W., Ashmore, R. C., Rosen, C. A., & Verdolini Abbott, K. (2013). Intrinsic laryngeal muscle activity in response to autonomic nervous system activation. *The Laryngoscope, 123,* 2756–2765.

Hersh, D. (2010a). Finishing well: The personal impact of ending therapy on speech-language pathologists. *International Journal of Speech-Language Pathology, 12*(4), 329–332.

Hersh, D. (2010b). I can't sleep at night with discharging this lady: The personal impact of ending therapy on speech-language pathologists. *International Journal of Speech-Language Pathology, 12*(4), 283–291.

Hodge, A. (2013). Coaching supervision – an ethical angle. In E. Murdoch & J. Arnold (Eds.), *Full spectrum supervision: "Who you are, is how you supervise"* (pp. 1–32). St Albans: Panoma Press.

Hodge, A. (2014). *An action research inquiry into what goes on in coaching supervision to the end of enhancing the coaching profession.* (DProf. thesis), Middlesex University. Available at: http://eprints.mdx.ac.uk/13707/ [Accessed October 2016]

Hodge, A. (2016). The value of coaching supervision as a development process and its contribution to continued professional and personal wellbeing for executive coaches. *International Journal of Evidence Based Coaching and Mentoring, 14*(2).

Holland, A. L. (2007). *Counselling in communication disorders.* San Diego: Plural Publishing.

House, A., & Andrews, H. B. (1988). Life events and difficulties preceding the onset of functional dysphonia. *Journal of Psychosomatic Research, 32*(3), 311–319.

Jacobs, M., & van Biene, L. (2015). Psychogenic voice disorder: A view through the lens of self. *European Journal for Person Centered Healthcare, 3*(2).

Kleinman, A. (2012). The art of medicine: Culture, bereavement, and psychiatry. *The Lancet, 379,* 608–609.

Kollbrunner, J., Menet, A., & Seifert, E. (2010). Psychogenic aphonia: No fixation even after a lengthy period of aphonia. *Swiss Medical Weekly, 140,* 12–17.

Kollbrunner, J., & Seifert, E. (2015). Encouragement to increase the use of psychosocial skills in the diagnosis and therapy of patients with functional dysphonia. *Journal of Voice.* doi: doi:10.1016/l.jvoice.2015.11.021

Lane, R. D. (2000). Neural correlates of conscious emotional experience. In R. D. Lane & L. Nadel (Eds.), *Cognitive neuroscience of emotion.* (pp. 345–370). Oxford: Oxford University Press.

Linklater, K. (2006). *Freeing the natural voice* (2nd ed.). London: Nick Hern Books.

Lombard, E. (1911). Le signe do l'elevation do al voix. *Annals Maladiers Oreille, Larynx, Nez, Pharynx, 37,* 101–119.

Luterman, D. (2011). Ruminations of an old man: A 50-year perspective on clinical practice. In R. J. Fourie (Ed.), *Therapeutic processes for communication disorders* (pp. 3–8). New York: Psychology Press.

MacLean, P. D. (1990). *The triune brain in evolution: Role in paleocerebral functions.* New York: Plenum Press.

Mathieson, L. (2001). *Greene and Mathieson's: The voice and its disorders.* (6th ed.). London: Whurr.

McDonald Klimek, M., Obert, K., & Steinhauer, K. (2005a). *Estill voice training workbook: Level one – Figures for voice control*: Estill Voice Training Systems International, LLC

McDonald Klimek, M., Obert, K., & Steinhauer, K. (2005b). *Estill voice training workbook: Level two – Figure combinations for six voice qualtities*: Estill Voice Training Systems International, LLC.

McLeod, J. E., & Clarke, D. M. (2007). A review of psychosocial aspects of motor neurone disease. *Journal of Neurological Sciences, 258,* 4–10.

Medenhall, S. (2009). From termination to the evolution of a relationship: A new understanding. *Psychoanalytic Inquiry, 29*(2), 117–135.

Miller, J. (2003). The crashed voice – a potential for change: A psychotherapeutic view. *Logopedics Phoniatrics Vocology, 28,* 41–45.

Miller, T., Deary, V., & Patterson, J. (2014). Improving asscess to psychological therapies in voice disorders: A cognitive behavioural therapy model. *Current Opinion in Otolaryngology and Head and Neck Surgery, 22*(3), 201–205.

Miller, W. R., & Rollnick, S. (2013). *Motivational interviewing* (3rd ed.). NY: Guilford Publications.

Moyns, C. L. (2015). *Speech pathologists use of behaviour change techniques in voice therapy.* (B. Health Science (Honours)), La Trobe University, Bundoora, Victoria Australia.

Neemuchwala, P. (1998). Psychogenic factors in dysphonia. In T. Harris, S. Harris, Rubin, J.S. & D. M. Howard (Eds.), *The Voice Clinic Handbook* (pp. 246–265). London: Whurr.

Nichol, H., Morrison, M. D., & Rammage, L. (1993). Interdisciplinary approach to functional voice disorders: The psychiatrist's role., *108,* 643–647.

O'Hara, D. (2011). Counselling & psychotherapy in action: Psychotherapy and the dialects of hope and despair. *Counselling Psychology Quarterly, 24*(4), 323–329.

Oliveira, G., Hirani, S. P., Epstein, R., Yazigi, L., & Belhau, M. (2012). Coping strategies in voice disorders of a Brazilian population. *Journal of Voice, 26,* 205–213.

Pemberton, C., Oates, J., & Russell, A. (2009). *Cost effective provision of vocal hygiene information: Preliminary evaluation of the Voice Care for Teachers Package as a prevention tool.* Paper presented at the The Occupational Voice Symposium: Protecting your voice in the workplace, University College, London.

Ramig, L. O., & Verdolini, K. (1998). Treatment efficacy: Voice disorders. *Journal of Speech, Language, and Hearing Research, 41*, s101.

Rammage, L., Morrison, M., & Nichol, H. (2001). *Management of the voice and its disorders.* San Diego: Singular Publishing Group.

Riley, J. (2002). Counseling: An approach for speech-language pathologists. *Contemporary Issues in Communication Science and Disorders, 29*, 6–16.

Rosen, D. C., & Sataloff, R. T. (1997). *Psychology of voice disorders.* San Diego: Singular Publishing Group.

Roy, N. (2008). Assessment and treatment of musculoskeletal tension in hyperfunctional voice disorders. *International Journal of Speech-Language Pathology, 10*(4), 195–209.

Roy, N., & Bless, D. M. (2000b). Personality traits and psychological factors in voice pathology: A foundation for future research. *Journal of Speech, Language, and Hearing Research, 43*, 737–748.

Sama, A., Carding, P. N., Price, S., Kelly, P., & Wilson, J. A. (2001). The clinical features of functional dysphonia. *The Laryngoscope, 111*(3), 458–463.

Sanders, C. (2012). *What lies beneath – The hidden foundations of family therapy.* Paper presented at the Australian Association of Family Therapy Conference, Perth.

Sasaki, C. T. (2006). Anatomy and development and physiology of the larynx. *GI Motility Online.* doi: 10.1038/gim07

Sataloff, R. T. (1991). *Professional voice. The science and art of clinical care.* New York: Raven Press.

Shane, E. (2009). Approaching termination: Ideal criteria versus working realities. *Psychoanalytic Inquiry, 29*(2), 167–173.

Shewell, C. (2009). *Voice work: Art and science in changing voices.* Chichester: Wiley-Blackwell.

Stemple, J. C., Roy, N., & Klaben, B. K. (2014). *Clinical voice pathology* (Fifth ed.). San Diego: Plural Publishing Inc..

Stone, J. (2016). Functional neurological disorders: The neurological assessment as treatment. *Practical Neurology, 16*, 7–17. doi: 10.1136/practneurol-2015-001241

Sullivan, B. (2008). *Counsellors and counselling: A new conversation.* Sydney: Pearson Education Australia.

Sutherland, O., Dienhart, A., & Turner, J. (2013). Responsive persistence Part II. Practices of postmodern therapists. *Journal of Marital and Family Therapy, 39*(4), 488–501.

Sutherland, O., Turner, J., & Dienhart, A. (2013). Responsive persistence Part I: Therapist influence on postmodern practice. *Journal of Marital and Family Therapy, 39*(4), 470–487.

Titze, I. R., & Verdolini Abbott, K. (2012). *Vocology. The science and practice of voice habilitation.* Salt Lake City: National Center for Voice and Speech.

Tomm, K. (1988). Interventive interviewing Part III. Intending to ask lineal, circular, strategic, or reflexive questions? *Family Process, 27*(1), 1–15.

van Mersbergen, M. (2011). Voice disorders and personality: Understanding their interactions. In T. L. Eadie (Ed.), *Perspectives on voice and voice disorders* (Vol. 21, pp. 31–38). Rockville: ASHA Publications.

Ward, P. R., Muller, R., Tsouros, G., Hersh, D., Lawn, S., Winefield, A. H., & Coveney, J. (2011). Additive and subtractive resilience strategies as enablers of biographical reinvention: A qualitative study of ex-smokers and never-smokers. *Social Science and Medicine, 72,* 1140–1148.

Wendler, J. (2015). Voice therapy: From past to the present from a phoniatrician's perspective. *Logopedics Phoniatrics Vocology, 40*(2), 56–63.

Wiles, R., Cott, C., & Gibson, B. E. (2008). Hope, expectations and recovery from illness: A narrative synthesis of qualitative research. *Journal of Advanced Nursing,* 564–573.

Zollinger, S. A., & Brumm, H. (2011). The lombard effect. *Current Biology, 21*(16), R614–R615.

About the author

Janet Baker L.A.C.S.T., M.Sc., Ph.D.
Speech Pathologist and Family Therapist; Consultant in Voice and Supervision of Professional Practice; Adjunct Associate Professor, Flinders University, South Australia

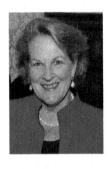

Adjunct Associate Professor Jan Baker is a speech pathologist and family therapist with post-graduate qualifications in psychotherapy. She studied classical singing through the Elder Conservatorium for over 10 years and has enjoyed performing as soloist in the mezzo soprano repertoire of recital and oratorio. Jan has specialized in the area of voice and counselling for over 40 years and is a Fellow of Speech Pathology Australia (SPA).

Jan was one of a small group involved in establishing the Australian Voice Association (1991) and she has been the president on two occasions. She has served as a member of the Scientific Committee – Voice for the International Association of Logopedics and Phoniatrics; a member of the Fellowships Committee for SPA; a member of Trust Fund and selection committee for scholarship offered by the International Federation of University Women in SA; and has been appointed as a Medical Expert for the Expert Review Panel of the Lifetime Support Authority by the Minister of Health.

Jan was the inaugural lecturer for Bachelor of Applied Science in Speech Pathology at Sturt College, now Flinders University, and she has taught at undergraduate and post-graduate levels in Australia and overseas. After completing her Ph.D. in 2006, Jan was appointed as Associate Professor and Co-ordinator for the Graduate Entry Master of Speech Pathology at Flinders University from 2007–2011.

She has presented at many national and international conferences seeking to integrate and share her knowledge in the practices of speech pathology, psychotherapy, family therapy and professional voice. Jan's clinical work, research interests and publications have been focused on the etiology and management of functional and psychogenic voice disorders, on working with the professional singers and understanding the psychological processes involved in the therapeutic relationship. Jan continues to teach nationally and internationally, and to supervise research in the areas of voice and counselling. She now offers services as Consultant in Voice and Supervision of Professional Practice to speech pathologists and mental health professionals throughout Australia and from overseas.

Lightning Source UK Ltd.
Milton Keynes UK
UKOW07f1538241016

286026UK00001B/1/P